Genes, Brain, and Development
The Neurocognition of Genetic Disorders

Genes, Brain, and Development

The Neurocognition of Genetic Disorders

Edited by

Marcia A. Barnes

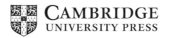

CAMBRIDGE
UNIVERSITY PRESS

CAMBRIDGE UNIVERSITY PRESS
Cambridge, New York, Melbourne, Madrid, Cape Town, Singapore,
São Paulo, Delhi, Dubai, Tokyo

Cambridge University Press
The Edinburgh Building, Cambridge CB2 8RU, UK

Published in the United States of America by Cambridge University Press, New York

www.cambridge.org
Information on this title: www.cambridge.org/9780521685368

First published 2010

Printed in the United Kingdom at the University Press, Cambridge

A catalogue record for this publication is available from the British Library

Library of Congress Cataloguing in Publication data
Genes, brain, and development : the neurocognition of genetic disorders / [edited by] Marcia A. Barnes.
p. cm.
Includes bibliographical references.
Summary: "Genetic disorders that affect neurodevelopment are informative for understanding the relations
between genes, brain, and behavior and for testing cognitive models. The chapters in the first section of this volume
deal with three major neurogenetic disorders, fragile X diagnosed through its genotype often as a consequence of
developmental delays, spina bifida identified in utero or at birth based on its physical phenotype – the spinal lesion,
and autism, diagnosed through its behavioral phenotype in childhood, increasingly in the early preschool years" –
Provided by publisher.
ISBN 978-0-521-68536-8 (pbk.)
1. Developmental disabilities – Genetic aspects.   2. Neurologic manifestations of general diseases.
3. Genetic disorders.   4. Psychophysiology – Genetic aspects.   I. Barnes, Marcia A., 1958–.   II. Title.
[DNLM: 1. Developmental Disabilities – genetics.   2. Brain – growth & development.   3. Genetic Diseases,
Inborn.   4. Human Development.   5. Models, Neurological.
WM 140 G32695 2010]
RJ506.D47G45   2010
616.85'88042–dc22
                                                                                              2009039345

ISBN 978-0-521-68536-8 Paperback

Additional resources for this publication at www.cambridge.org/9780521685368

For Stephanie Lane (1971–2006)

Contents

List of Contributors	*page* ix
Preface	xi
Acknowledgments	xvi

Section 1 Connecting genes, brain, and behavior in neurodevelopmental disorders — 1

1 Intergenerational effects of mutations in the fragile X mental retardation 1 gene. Fragile X: A model of X-linked mental retardation and neurodegeneration — 3
Mariya Borodyanskaya, Sarah Coffey, Michele Y. Ono, and Randi J. Hagerman

2 Autism: Genes, anatomy, and behavioral outcome — 19
Emma Esser, Saasha Sutera, and Deborah Fein

3 Development in spina bifida: Neurobiological and environmental factors — 53
Marcia A. Barnes, Heather B. Taylor, Susan B. Landry, and Lianne H. English

Section 2 Genetic disorders and models of neurocognitive development — 83

4 Language and communication in autism spectrum disorders — 85
Susan Ellis Weismer

5 Language development in children with Williams syndrome: New insights from cross-linguistic research — 105
Stavroula Stavrakaki

6 Language in Down syndrome: A life-span perspective — 122
Jean A. Rondal

7   Genetic disorders as models of mathematics learning disability:
      Fragile X and Turner syndromes   143
      Melissa M. Murphy, Michèle M. M. Mazzocco, and Michael McCloskey

8   A developmental approach to genetic disorders   175
      Sarah J. Paterson

9   The use of strategies in embedded figures: Tasks by boys with and without
      organic mild mental retardation: A review and some experimental
      evidence   199
      Anastasia Alevriadou and Helen Tsakiridou

      Index   216

Contributors

Anastasia Alevriadou
Department of Early Childhood Education,
University of Western Macedonia, Greece

Marcia A. Barnes
Department of Pediatrics,
Children's Learning Institute,
University of Texas Health Science Center at
Houston, Houston, Texas, USA

Mariya Borodyanskaya
MIND (*Medical Investigation of
Neurodevelopmental Disorders*) Institute,
University of California at Davis Medical
Center, Sacramento, California, USA

Sarah Coffey
MIND (*Medical Investigation of
Neurodevelopmental Disorders*) Institute,
University of California at Davis Medical
Center, Sacramento, California, USA

Susan Ellis Weismer
Department of Communicative
Disorders/Waisman Center,
University of Wisconsin-Madison,
Madison, Wisconsin, USA

Lianne H. English
Department of Psychology, University of
Guelph, Guelph, Ontario, Canada

Emma Esser
Department of Psychology,
University of Connecticut, Storrs,
Connecticut, USA

Deborah Fein
Department of Psychology,
University of Connecticut, Storrs,
Connecticut, USA

Randi J. Hagerman
MIND (*Medical Investigation of
Neurodevelopmental Disorders*) Institute,
Department of Pediatrics,
University of California at Davis Medical
Center Sacramento, California, USA

Susan B. Landry
Department of Pediatrics,
Children's Learning Institute,
University of Texas Health Science Center at
Houston, Houston, Texas, USA

Michèle M. M. Mazzocco
Department of Psychiatry and Behavioral
Sciences, Johns Hopkins University School of
Medicine, Director, Math Skills Development
Project, Kennedy Krieger Institute, Baltimore,
Maryland, USA

Michael McCloskey
Department of Cognitive Science,
Johns Hopkins University, Baltimore,
Maryland, USA

Melissa M. Murphy
Department of Education,
College of Notre Dame of Maryland,
Baltimore, Maryland, USA

Michele Y. Ono
MIND (*Medical Investigation of
Neurodevelopmental Disorders*) Institute,
University of California at Davis Medical
Center, Sacramento, California, USA

Sarah J. Paterson
Center for Autism Research,
Children's Hospital of Philadelphia and
University of Pennsylvania School of
Medicine, Philadelphia,
Pennsylvania, USA

Jean A. Rondal
Psycholinguistic Unit, Department of
Cognitive Sciences, University of Liege,
Liege, Belgium

Stavroula Stavrakaki
Department of Italian Linguistics and
Literature, Aristotle University of
Thessaloniki, Greece

Saasha Sutera
Department of Psychology, University of
Connecticut, Storrs, Connecticut, USA

Heather B. Taylor
Department of Pediatrics,
Children's Learning Institute,
University of Texas Health Science Center at
Houston, Houston, Texas, USA

Helen Tsakiridou
Department of Primary Education,
University of Western Macedonia, Greece

Preface

The study of genetic disorders that affect neurodevelopment has led to a rich body of interdisciplinary research in genetics, neuroscience, and psychology. These collaborations have not only promoted a better understanding of genetic disorders themselves, but have also resulted in new discoveries about the connections between genes, brain, and cognition. When people consider genetic disorders that affect cognitive development they often think about single gene disorders such as fragile X syndrome or chromosome disorders such as Down syndrome. However, there is a growing recognition that many neurodevelopmental disorders have strong genetic components even though their genetic underpinnings may be less well understood than those diagnosed through genetic testing. And, increasingly, cross-disorder comparisons with overlapping phenotypic variability are proving to be useful models for understanding the interplay of genes, brain, and behavior across development. Given the increasing recognition of the role that genes play in developmental disorders, an exhaustive survey of disorders that affect cognitive development is beyond the scope of any one book. The purpose of this book is to represent some of the ways in which a number of disorders, both those diagnosed through genetic testing, and those identified through their physical and behavioral phenotypes, are being used to test models of neurobehavioral development and to understand relations between genes, brain, and behavior.

Introduction

Organization of the book

Genetic disorders that affect neurodevelopment are informative for understanding the relations between genes, brain, and behavior and for testing cognitive models. The chapters in Section 1 of this volume deal with three major neurogenetic disorders: fragile X diagnosed through its genotype often as a consequence of developmental delays; spina bifida identified in utero or at birth based on its physical phenotype – the spinal lesion; and autism, diagnosed through its behavioral phenotype in childhood, increasingly in the early preschool years. The evidence connecting genes, neural phenotypes, and cognitive/behavioral phenotypes are reviewed for each disorder. Section 2 of the book is devoted to studies and reviews of research that use neurogenetic disorders to test cognitive and developmental models. These chapters consider language and mathematical cognition in Down syndrome, autism, Williams syndrome, fragile X syndrome, and Turner syndrome.

In Chapter 1, Borodyanskaya, Coffey, Ono, and Hagerman review what is known about the relation of genotype, the neural phenotype, and cognitive and social–emotional phenotypes in fragile X syndrome (FXS). FXS represents one neurogenetic disorder in which these relations have been extensively studied such that much is also known about the molecular basis of FXS as well as other disorders related to the fragile X premutation. The authors show how FXS as a neurogenetic disorder of childhood has led to discoveries about the genetic underpinnings of two quite different disorders of adulthood: both a reproductive disorder called primary ovarian insufficiency and a neurodegenerative disorder called fragile X associated tremor/ataxia syndrome related to the fragile X premutation. The chapter also covers current issues in treatment and screening.

Esser, Sutera, and Fein present a review of autism in Chapter 2 that covers what is known about the genetics, neural and cognitive/behavioral phenotypes, and interventions in this disorder. In addition to discussing what is understood about the factors that lead to variability in outcomes in autism, the authors address new areas of research in autism, including functional imaging studies of the mirror neuron system, providing a balanced interpretation of what recent findings might mean. Interventions for autism are explained in some detail, highlighting the available evidence for their effectiveness. The authors end by suggesting some mechanisms by which interventions could be affecting neurodevelopment and pose the interesting question: If autism is a neurogenetic disorder how can children be said to "recover" from their autism?

In Chapter 3, Barnes, Taylor, Landry, and English show how an understanding of spina bifida myelomeningocele (SBM), best known in the past as a birth defect affecting the spine, has benefited from a research enterprise that links variability in genotype to variability in the physical, neural, and behavioral/cognitive phenotypes. They review studies that have used SBM to test neurocognitive models in domains such as attention and reading comprehension. This chapter also provides examples of how longitudinal studies of a neurogenetic disorder that is identified before or at birth can be used to understand developmental precursors of learning disabilities and the separate and interactive effects of neurobiological and environmental factors on development. Issues related to clinical care and interventions across the life span are discussed.

The first three chapters in Section 2 of the book provide reviews or investigations of language functioning in autism, Down syndrome, and Williams syndrome. Ellis Weismer's review of studies of language development in autism in Chapter 4 tackles issues similar to those raised in the preceding chapter on autism; that is, how best to capture phenotypic variability in autism to predict and understand developmental trajectories and language outcomes. Ellis Weismer discusses various models for how these questions can be answered, including studies of language using the common diagnostic categories in autism, longitudinal studies that follow children with autism categorized according to language phenotypes in early childhood, and comparisons of children with autism to disorders that share phenotypic overlap such as Specific Language Impairment. In Chapter 5, Stavrakaki presents a detailed analysis of syntactic comprehension in Greek-speaking children with Williams syndrome. In order to test models of delay, impairment, or normal development of syntactic comprehension consistent with mental age, Stavrakaki compares the comprehension of a number of syntactic structures in children with Williams syndrome to typically developing children both at and below the mental ages of the group with Williams syndrome. In Chapter 6, Rondal provides a review of language in Down syndrome across the life span. He covers what is known about the development of components of language from prelinguistic skills, phonology, and lexical development to grammar, pragmatics, and discourse. Rondal also uses Down syndrome to address theoretical questions about a critical period for language development, and he reviews the evidence for and against premature language aging in this disorder.

In Chapter 7, Murphy, Mazzocco, and McCloskey compare math performance in two neurogenetic disorders associated with mathematical learning disability – fragile X and Turner syndromes – to each other and also to mathematical performance in typically developing children. Murphy and her colleagues test models of mathematical disability by looking at the relation of mathematical outcomes to the differing cognitive phenotypes associated with each disorder. Their chapter shows that, although models of mathematical learning disabilities are informative for understanding mathematical functioning in neurogenetic conditions, the study of mathematical processing in these neurogenetic conditions can also inform the broader field of research on mathematical learning disabilities.

In Chapter 8, Paterson shows the benefits of taking a developmental approach to the study of neurogenetic disorders, particularly one that starts very early in development, in her comparisons of Williams and Down syndromes for language and number and in comparisons of these disorders and autism for face processing. Paterson uses this research to argue that an understanding of the cognitive phenotype is only possible through knowing the starting point of development, the developmental trajectory of cognitive skills, and their end states. In effect, Paterson expands the behavioral phenotypes of these conditions, which are often viewed as being somewhat static, into developmental behavioral phenotypes that are marked by principled changes over early and later developmental time windows.

In Chapter 9, Alevriadou and Tsakiridou make the point that the investigation of *strengths* in the profiles of children with intellectual disability is informative not only for understanding the cognitive phenotype in those children but also for understanding those cognitive abilities more generally. Although the focus of the book is on neurogenetic disorders of childhood, there is also much to be learned from looking at constructs, such as strategy use, that are not typically studied in children with disorders causing intellectual disability[1], whether arising from neurogenetic or other neurobiological causes.

Common themes

Heterogeneity in genes, brain, and behavior

Several common themes emerge across these chapters. One of these is what can be learned from exploiting the considerable heterogeneity in genes, brains, and behavior *within* neurogenetic disorders as illustrated in the chapters in Section 1 of the book. The chapters on fragile X and autism show that it is not only the full syndrome that is associated with the behavioral phenotype. For example, the premutation of fragile X is associated with some overlapping, but also some quite different physical and behavioral phenotypes that emerge later in life. Some aspects of the autism phenotype are more common in parents and siblings of children with autism than they are in families without a child with autism. In spina bifida, the environment moderates the effects of lesion level that is connected to the genetics of the disorder, leading to considerable phenotypic heterogeneity. Although heterogeneity is seen as providing important information for scientific study, the heterogeneity that comes along with disorders that are defined according to the behavioral phenotype, as is the case for autism, may not always be so tractable. Esser, Sutera, and Fein note that *almost too much is known* about the neural and behavioral phenotypes associated with autism, leading to many contrasting findings and interpretations. Both they and Ellis Weismer in her chapter on language in autism suggest that working from well-defined behavioral phenotypes in addition to diagnostic categories may be one way to organize and promote understanding of the connections between the genotype, neural and behavioral phenotypes, and responses to interventions.

---

[1] The terms mental retardation and intellectual disability are used interchangeably in this volume. The reader is referred to Schalock, Luckasson, Shogren *et al.* (2007) for discussion.

Comparisons of behavioral phenotypes across disorders

Another commonality across several chapters is related to what can be gleaned by comparing neural and behavioral phenotypes *across* neurogenetic disorders and to the behavioral phenotypes of general developmental disorders such as learning disabilities. The success of this approach depends on careful attention to the behavioral phenotype and to the use of cognitive models to guide these investigations. This approach is explicit in the chapter by Murphy and her colleagues, who delineate similarities and differences in the mathematical phenotype itself across neurogenetic disorders. Other examples of this general approach are contained in the chapters by Paterson, Stavrakaki, Barnes and colleagues, and Ellis Weismer. These chapters demonstrate the importance of *dissecting* the behavioral phenotype using experimental measures derived from cognitive, developmental, and neuro-cognitive models.

Paying attention to development in neurogenetic disorders

The importance of developmental and life span perspectives for understanding neurogenetic disorders is the main topic of the chapter by Paterson. Chapters by Rondal, Borodyanskaya and colleagues, Ellis Weismer, and Barnes and colleagues provide examples of how longitudinal studies and life-span studies in neurogenetic disorders are useful for generating disorder-specific knowledge on behavioral and neural phentotypes, and for providing information relevant for general developmental theories of ability and disability. Importantly, studies that show that the behavioral phenotype can change over the course of development suggest that developmental trajectories and timing of biological and environmental influences on behavioral phenotypes ought to be important foci in studies mapping genes, brain, and behavior in neurogenetic disorders.

References

Schalock, R. L., Luckasson, R. A., Shogren, K. A. *et al.* (2007). The renaming of mental retardation: Understanding the change to the term intellectual disability. *Intellectual and Developmental Disabilities*, **45**, 116–124.

Acknowledgments

I would like to acknowledge the role that Dr. Andrew Papanicolaou and the Vivian Smith Advanced Studies Institute of the International Neuropsychological Society played in the development of this book. The bringing together of faculty and graduate students and trainees in neuropsychology and neurology led to many vibrant discussions that are reflected in its contents. I thank Kimberly Raghubar and Landa Marks for editorial assistance and Richard Marley at Cambridge University Press for his patience and persistence. Finally, this book could not have been done without the dedication of Margaret Wilkinson and Stephanie Lane to our spina bifida research program. The preparation of this book was supported by grants from the Canadian Institutes of Health Research and from NIH (P01 HD35946) and NINDS (R01HD046609–04).

Connecting genes, brain, and behavior in neurodevelopmental disorders

Intergenerational effects of mutations in the fragile X mental retardation 1 gene. Fragile X: A model of X-linked mental retardation and neurodegeneration

Mariya Borodyanskaya, Sarah Coffey, Michele Y. Ono, and Randi J. Hagerman

Introduction

There have been remarkable advances in genetics over the past decade including the sequencing of the human genome which was completed in 2003, 50 years after the discovery of the double-helix structure of DNA by Watson and Crick (Valle, 2004). These advances have furthered our understanding of many forms of mental retardation, including X-linked mental retardation of which fragile X syndrome (FXS) is the most common type.

There are approximately 30,000 genes in the human genome, and approximately 1000 genes on the X chromosome. Over 200 of these genes on the X chromosome have been associated with mental retardation. The X chromosome has more genes associated with mental retardation than any other chromosome. Approximately 20–25% of all cases of mental retardation are X-linked. Because males only have one X chromosome, they are much more vulnerable to the effects of an abnormal gene on the chromosome. There are approximately 20% more males with mental retardation than females in the general population. In this chapter we will review the most common inherited cause of mental retardation and neurodegeneration; fragile X associated tremor/ataxia syndrome (FXTAS), the most common cause of ataxia in those over 50 years of age; and the fragile X mental retardation 1 gene (*FMR1*), the most common gene associated with X-linked mental retardation.

This work was supported by NICHD (grants HD36071, HD02274), NINDS (grant NS044299), NIDCR DE019583, NIA AG032115, NCRR CTSC RR024146, and the MIND Institute at the University of California, Davis.

There have been significant advances in our knowledge of the molecular basis of both FXS, caused by a full mutation of the *FMR1* gene, and newly identified disorders related to the fragile X premutation. The disorders related to the fragile X premutation include FXTAS and primary ovarian insufficiency (POI). The disorders associated with the *FMR1* gene provide an important model for gene, brain, and behavior relationships that are further described here.

Molecular biology of fragile X syndrome

Normally, individuals have 5 to 44 CGG repeats in the 5'-untranslated region of the *FMR1* gene on the X chromosome. A full mutation CGG-repeat expansion, exceeding 200 repeats, causes FXS. For full mutation alleles, there is usually complete methylation of the CGG repeat and promoter region, leading to a dramatic decrease or elimination in transcription, with little or no *FMR1* mRNA and little or no *FMR1* protein (FMRP) produced (Tassone *et al.*, 1999, 2000a, 2000b). It is the lack or deficiency of FMRP that leads to the physical and behavioral phenotype of FXS.

It is also possible that upregulation of the metabotropic glutamate receptor (mGluR5) system may explain features of FXS. When there is a deficit or an absence of FMRP, as in FXS, there is a molecular response that ultimately weakens synaptic connections (Huber *et al.*, 2002). The processes involved in this response can cause growth of long, thin, and immature dendritic spine structures. There is also a lack of pruning or an overgrowth of synaptic connections. This leads to dendritic overgrowth in inappropriate areas of the brain, particularly the hippocampus and the limbic system (Bear *et al.*, 2004; Huber *et al.*, 2002).

Spectrum of involvement

Fragile X syndrome

The physical phenotype of FXS includes prominent ears, long face, and hyperextensible finger joints. Retrospective studies have found that many males with FXS have various medical conditions, e.g., approximately 85% have otitis media, 36% have strabismus, 31% have emesis, 23% have a history of sinusitis, and 15% have failure to thrive in infancy. Loose connective tissue is thought to lead to some of these features (e.g., otitis media), in addition to other common characteristics (e.g., hyperextensible finger joints, soft or velvet-like skin, and flat feet). The most common neurologic abnormality in FXS is seizures, which affect approximately 15–22% of children with FXS (Hagerman, 2002a). Epilepsy in individuals with FXS may be related to the dysregulation of the gamma-aminobutyric acid$_a$ (GABA$_a$) receptor whose message binds to FMRP.

Because some of the above features of FXS are not present until childhood and the cognitive and behavioral characteristics are often not obvious until late in the first or second year of life, most children are not diagnosed until 3 years of age or older (Bailey, 2004). From 80% to 90% of male children with FXS have IQs in the borderline to mildly mentally retarded range (Hagerman, 2002a). Language impairment has also been recognized as a characteristic hallmark associated with FXS. In addition, children with FXS have difficulty with auditory processing, e.g., the ability to filter out irrelevant noises (Hagerman, 2002a).

Young males with FXS often present with hypotonia (low muscle tone), which can affect joint stability, fine and gross motor coordination, and sensory integration. This can lead to a delay in developmental milestones, e.g., crawling and walking. Approximately 60–90% of boys with FXS are tactile defensive, meaning they do not like people to touch them, the feeling of their clothing, and/or the texture of food (Hatton *et al.*, 2002).

The full mutation is also frequently accompanied by severe emotional problems, including anxiety and mood instability. Anxiety may be manifested by gaze aversion in new social situations, withdrawn behavior and social isolation, distress with changes in routine and desire for sameness, obsessive–compulsive behavior, and repetitive and tangential speech. Hyperarousal and anxiety in children with FXS can often lead to aggression and tantrums. Studies have shown as many as 42% of young males and 28% of young females with FXS have aggression (Hagerman, 2002a).

During periods of increased anxiety, stress, or excitement, some stereotypic behaviors associated with autism, e.g., hand-flapping and hand-biting, are displayed. Studies have shown that 25–60% of males (Abbeduto *et al.*, 2007; Bailey *et al.*, 2000; Cohen, 1995; Denmark *et al.*, 2003; Kaufmann *et al.*, 2004; Rogers *et al.*, 2001; Turk & Graham, 1997) and 3–17% of females (Hatton *et al.*, 2006; Mazzocco *et al.*, 1997) with FXS have autistic behavior or a diagnosis of autism or autism spectrum disorder (ASD). These individuals with both FXS and autism have poorer cognitive abilities and lower adaptive functioning than individuals with FXS alone (Hatton *et al.*, 2003; Kau *et al.*, 2004; Kaufmann *et al.*, 2004; Rogers *et al.*, 2001). For example, it has been found that children with FXS with autism have more impairment in nonverbal cognition and expressive language compared to children with FXS alone or autism alone (Abbeduto *et al.*, 2007, 2008; Philofsky *et al.*, 2004). The amount of problem behavior is also higher in individuals with FXS with autism than in individuals with FXS alone (Hatton *et al.*, 2006). See Chapter 2 on autism and Chapter 7 on math in FXS.

The premutation

Individuals with premutation alleles express 55 to 200 CGG repeats, and exhibit translational inhibition, consequently producing *increased* levels of *FMR1* mRNA

(Tassone *et al.*, 2000a). These mRNA levels increase from 2 to 10 times the normal levels with increasing CGG repeat size over the premutation range (Tassone *et al.*, 2000a). Moderate deficits in FMRP levels in individuals with the larger premutation alleles appear in both peripheral blood leucocytes (Allen *et al.*, 2004; Tassone *et al.*, 2000a) and in lymphoblastoid cells (Kenneson *et al.*, 2001). However, the majority of individuals with the premutation have FMRP levels within normal limits (Tassone *et al.*, 2000a). Individuals with the premutation exhibit a continuum of neurological, neuropsychiatric, and magnetic resonance imaging phenotypes (Hagerman, 2006; Roberts *et al.*, 2009).

The premutation may be unstable, expanding from one generation to the next. Expansion can lead to a full mutation, causing FXS when passed on by a female. Since this is an X-linked disorder, males are more severely affected by the *FMR1* mutations than females. The premutation is more common in the general population (1 per 130 females and 1 per 250 males) (Dombrowski *et al.*, 2002; Hagerman, 2008; Rousseau *et al.*, 1995) than the full mutation (FXS; 1 per 2500) (Hagerman, 2008); thus, the impact of the problems associated with the premutation may be greater than the problems associated with the full mutation.

In the past, carriers of the premutation were considered to be unaffected by cognitive deficits (Bennetto *et al.*, 1996; Franke *et al.*, 1999; Reiss *et al.*, 1993). However, current research indicates that fragile X premutation carriers may present with attention deficit hyperactivity disorder (ADHD), learning disabilities, mental retardation, or ASD (Farzin *et al.*, 2006; Hagerman, 2002a). Furthermore, premutation carriers with subtle deficits in FMRP (Hagerman & Hagerman, 2002a; Loesch *et al.*, 2004) can exhibit some characteristics of FXS, including poor eye contact, hand-flapping, hand-biting, perseverative speech, sensory hyperarousal, and anxiety (Hull & Hagerman, 1993; Riddle *et al.*, 1998).

Past case studies showed children with the premutation were occasionally diagnosed with autism, mental retardation, ADHD, or severe learning disabilities (Hagerman *et al.*, 1996; Tassone *et al.*, 2000d). With advancements in the technique for diagnosing autism, researchers now discover more individuals with autism or ASD and the premutation (Goodlin-Jones *et al.*, 2004). One study found that the rate of ASD, in both the proband (73%) and nonproband premutation carriers (8%), is significantly higher compared to siblings without the premutation (0%) (Farzin *et al.*, 2006). Additionally, ADHD diagnosis in proband individuals (93%) is significantly more common compared to controls (0%) (Farzin *et al.*, 2006).

Elevated *FMR1* mRNA, not CGG repeat size or reduced FMRP, is significantly associated with increased psychological symptoms, predominantly obsessive–compulsive symptoms and psychoticism, in adult males with the premutation (Hessl *et al.*, 2005). Interestingly, this effect is more prominent in younger men without FXTAS, suggesting that psychological symptoms may precede the neuro-degenerative disease (Hessl *et al.*, 2005).

There are strong positive associations between both CGG repeat size and *FMR1* mRNA, and psychological symptoms. The *FMR1* mRNA level is predominantly associated with obsessive–compulsive symptoms, anxiety, and interpersonal sensitivity. In summary, we find evidence of a toxic gain-of-function effect leading to psychological symptoms in premutation males with and without FXTAS, as well as females with the premutation with skewed activation, especially women with symptoms of FXTAS (Hessl *et al.*, 2005).

Female premutation carriers

Females with the premutation may display emotional problems such as anxiety, social phobia, depression, and subtle neurological difficulties, including sensory deficits/neuropathy, and hormonal changes (Roberts *et al.*, 2009). Additionally, approximately 15–20% of female carriers develop POI (Cronister *et al.*, 1991; Sherman, 2000; Sullivan *et al.*, 2005; Welt *et al.*, 2004). POI is not seen in individuals with the full mutation, and may thus be related to the toxic effects of the elevated *FMR1* mRNA, which occurs almost exclusively in the premutation range (Allen *et al.*, 2004; Hagerman & Hagerman, 2004a). Because *FMR1* is more highly expressed in ovarian follicles compared to other organs (Hinds *et al.*, 1993), the ovary is more vulnerable to *FMR1* mRNA toxicity.

While 15–20% of carriers have POI, the remaining carriers that are cycling normally may have endocrine dysfunction or subclinical ovarian dysfunction (Allingham-Hawkins *et al.*, 1999; Murray *et al.*, 2000; Schwartz *et al.*, 1994; Sherman, 2000; Vianna-Morgante & Costa, 2000; Welt *et al.*, 2004), which includes a significantly shortened cycle, elevated follicle-stimulating hormone (FSH) throughout the cycle, elevated inhibin B in the follicular phase, and elevated inhibin A and progesterone in the luteal phase. This may be the result of a decreased number of follicles and granulosa cell dysfunction, or decreased cell number in the corpus luteum. Additionally, nearly half of female carriers report a history of infertility, as defined by 1 year of unprotected intercourse without pregnancy (Sherman, 2000).

There is an association between CGG repeat number and prevalence of POI (Sullivan *et al.*, 2005). Those with 100 or more repeats exhibited a decrease in prevalence of POI. This discrepancy may be because some cells have early methylation at a lower CGG repeat number, which may protect those cells from the toxicity of the premutation. Additionally, CGG repeat size has effects on the age of menopause, with low-end CGG repeats demonstrating menopause 2.5 years earlier than the average woman, and medium- to high-end premutation carriers demonstrating menopause 4 years earlier than low-end carriers (Sullivan *et al.*, 2005). For cycling women, there is a CGG repeat effect on the FSH level. The activation ratio (the percentage of cells that have the normal X as the active X) also correlates with FSH levels.

The issue of psychological and emotional problems in premutation carriers has been controversial for years because the stress of raising a child with FXS can cause significant emotional problems that are difficult to separate from the effects of the premutation itself. Approximately one fourth of female premutation carriers report problems of shyness, social anxiety, and depression (Roberts *et al.*, 2009; Sobesky *et al.*, 1994, 1996). The rates of depression are similar in women with or without the premutation who had children with developmental disabilities. Females with greater than 100 CGG repeats with correspondingly lower levels of FMRP had higher rates of depression and interpersonal sensitivity than women with less than 100 CGG repeats (Derogatis, 1994; Johnston *et al.*, 2001).

Approximately 8% of females with the premutation are also found to have FXTAS. Those females with FXTAS also have a high rate of hypothyroidism (50%) and fibromyalgia (43%) (Coffey *et al.*, 2008).

Male premutation carriers
Males with the premutation but without FXTAS show significant memory deficits and problems in executive function compared to age-matched controls (Moore *et al.*, 2004a). Also, in premutation males, increased CGG repeat size and decreased FMRP are significantly associated with decreased gray matter density in brain areas such as the cerebellum, brainstem, amygdalo–hippocampal complex, caudate and insula bilaterally, left thalamus and inferior temporal cortex, right pre- and post-central gyri, and inferior parietal cortex extending to the precuneus; however, *FMR1* mRNA is not significantly associated with gray matter density (Jakala *et al.*, 1997; Moore *et al.*, 2004b). A recent study (Murphy *et al.*, 1999) supports the hypothesis that the premutation causes structural changes in the brain in both young and old male and female carriers.

Males with the premutation display a pattern of deficit similar in profile, however milder in presentation, to that of individuals with the full mutation (FXS). Problems include impairment on a social cognition task, obsessive–compulsive traits, and executive function problems including inhibitory control (Cornish *et al.*, 2005). In the past, the theme of lowered FMRP causing problems in a limited number of premutation carriers was supported by the finding of an occasional child with the premutation who presented with mental retardation or autism/ASD and lowered FMRP levels (Aziz *et al.*, 2003; Goodlin-Jones *et al.*, 2004; Tassone *et al.*, 2000b). However, these individuals often had only mild deficits of FMRP and all had significant elevations of *FMR1* mRNA when measured (Goodlin-Jones *et al.*, 2004; Tassone *et al.*, 2000d). Currently, research shows a high rate of both ASD and ADHD in male premutation carriers (Farzin *et al.*, 2006).

FXTAS

Discovery of FXTAS

Studies of adult males with the premutation have dramatically improved our understanding of the effects of elevated *FMR1* mRNA in carriers. Originally, only females with the premutation were studied because they were the ones who presented to clinic with their children affected by FXS, and were therefore the easiest to evaluate. Grandfathers who are carriers rarely came to clinic. Therefore, it was initially a retrospective study of the histories that daughters gave about their fathers, including those with and without the premutation, which first suggested psychiatric difficulty in the carriers (Dorn *et al.*, 1994). Alcoholism, depression, reclusive behavior, ADHD, and social deficits were more prevalent in grandfathers with the premutation compared to grandfathers without the premutation (Dorn *et al.*, 1994).

The discovery of FXTAS has had a remarkable effect on the fragile X field from many perspectives, including genetic counseling, clinical care, and research endeavors. The RNA toxicity mechanism leading to FXTAS (Hagerman & Hagerman, 2004a) is now supported by animal research in both premutation mouse and *Drosophila* models.

Investigations of neurological and cognitive involvement in premutation carriers led to the discovery of FXTAS (Jacquemont *et al.*, 2003a). While arising from the same gene, the pathogenesis and clinical presentation of FXTAS is entirely distinct from FXS. Although the *FMR1* gene is involved in both disorders, the mRNA level is increased in all premutation carriers, whereas mRNA levels are reduced or absent in FXS (Hagerman & Hagerman, 2004b; Tassone *et al.*, 2000c). The risk of developing FXTAS increases with age (Jacquemont *et al.*, 2004). Significant correlations exist between CGG repeat number and the age at which neurological symptoms arise, the age of ataxia onset, and the age of tremor onset (Tassone *et al.*, 2005). Tremor and ataxia are found in 17% of the male carriers in their 50s, 38% in their 60s, 47% in their 70s, and 75% in their 80s (Jacquemont *et al.*, 2004).

Diagnostic criteria

We have developed diagnostic criteria for definite, probable, and possible FXTAS (Jacquemont *et al.*, 2003b), based on the presence of major and minor criteria. Tremor and ataxia are major clinical criteria and the characteristic symmetric white matter disease in the middle cerebral peduncles (the MCP sign) are major radiological criteria (Brunberg *et al.*, 2002). The minor radiological diagnostic criterion is global brain atrophy, and the minor clinical diagnostic criteria include memory and executive function deficits, and parkinsonism (Jacquemont *et al.*, 2003b). The

FXTAS inclusions seen on neuropathologic study have also been added as major criteria (Hageman and Hagerman, 2004a).

Radiological features

Magnetic resonance imaging in eight males with FXTAS demonstrated a significant reduction in the volumes of cerebrum, cerebellum, and cerebral cortex in premutation carriers (Loesch *et al.*, 2005). There was a significant relationship between cerebral volumes and the number of CGG repeats as seen in the autopsy studies by Greco *et al.* (2006). This provides further evidence that the size of the premutation in the *FMR1* gene is a major determinant of the neurodegeneration associated with FXTAS. There is an increased hippocampal volume in one study of carriers, suggesting the coexistence of both neurodevelopmental and neurodegenerative processes (Loesch *et al.*, 2005). Recent functional magnetic resonance imaging studies of memory and hippocampal function show decreased activation of the hippocampus in male carriers compared to controls (Koldewyn *et al.*, 2008).

Pathological features

FXTAS is an inclusion disorder (Greco *et al.*, 2002). Inclusion-bearing neural cell loads correlate positively with the CGG repeat number. The greatest number of inclusions is in the hippocampus, specifically the pyramidal cell layer and the hilus (Greco *et al.*, 2006). Inclusions are also seen in cranial nerve nuclei XII and in the autonomic neurons of the spinal cord. White matter disease is associated with spongiosis, particularly in the subcortical regions and in the MCP. There is also evidence of astrocyte pathology with significant activation of the astrocytes in areas of white matter disease (Greco *et al.*, 2006). Current research suggests age of death correlates inversely with CGG repeat number. One recent case study patient died at age 87 with only mild ataxia in the last year of his life and no tremor. He had only an occasional inclusion, without spongiosis, and he also had the lowest number of CGG repeats, 65. His case is instructive and provides further evidence that there is a CGG repeat dependence of disease and that mild disease can be subclinical (Greco *et al.*, 2006).

FXTAS has been studied occasionally in females with the premutation. Five cases were reported in 2004 (Hagerman *et al.*, 2004), and subsequently 8% of female premutation carriers from a cohort of 146 females were found to have FXTAS (Coffey *et al.*, 2008). Females displayed symptoms of intention tremor, ataxia, parkinsonism, and peripheral neuropathy. One female died at age 85, and a study of her brain demonstrated inclusions that were identical to the inclusions in the males.

Molecular studies have identified a variety of proteins within the inclusions, including αB crystallin and myelin basic protein (MBP) (Iwahashi *et al.*, 2006). Inclusions contain *FMR1* mRNA (Tassone *et al.*, 2004), which is consistent with the hypothesis of RNA gain-of-function toxicity leading to FXTAS. The inclusions contain a number of neurofilament proteins, including lamin A/C, MBP, and at least two RNA binding proteins, heterogeneous nuclear ribonucleoprotein A2 (hnRNPA2), and muscleblind-like protein l (Iwahashi *et al.*, 2006). One or more of these proteins may mediate the RNA gain-of-function mechanism of disease in FXTAS. Elevated *FMR1* mRNA levels found in premutation carriers may lead to sequestration and/or dysregulation of a number of proteins that are important for neuronal function (Arocena *et al.*, 2005; Hagerman & Hagerman, 2004b). This dysregulation would in turn lead to white matter disease, potentially from the involvement of MBP and hnRNPA2, and neuronal cell death leading to the brain atrophy in FXTAS.

There is cellular evidence that lamin A/C is dysregulated in neurons with the premutation, and this dysregulation disturbs the nuclear architecture of the cell, making the cell more sensitive to oxidative stress and subsequent cell death (Arocena *et al.*, 2005). Interestingly, neurons with the premutation initially grow faster than normal neurons, possibly due to the effect of dysregulation of lamin A/C. The enhanced growth in premutation neurons could have an important effect on brain function in development, particularly the social deficits seen in young males with the premutation (Farzin *et al.*, 2006).

Treatment

The advances within the past 5 years related to the neurobiological changes associated with fragile X are also leading to new treatment endeavors that represent specific interventions for FXS (Hagerman *et al.*, 2009; Hagerman *et al.*, 2005). Clinical monitoring and a number of interventions should be considered standard once an individual is identified as having FXTAS or FXS. These include treatment for specific neurological and psychiatric symptoms; referral to psychiatry, gerontology, and occupational therapy; and genetic counseling for the patient and family (Hagerman, 2002b).

For the school-aged child with FXS, a thorough assessment of speech/language, occupational therapy, and academic needs is necessary to develop optimal interventions. An exploration of peer tutoring, social skills training, and assistive technology resources is helpful in developing a comprehensive and integrated program for these children (Hagerman & Hagerman, 2002b).

Many psychopharmacological agents are currently being used to treat individuals with the full mutation and premutation, including stimulants, selective serotonin-reuptake inhibitors (SSRIs), and atypical antipsychotics. For FXTAS, there is not one medication that is effective for all of the neurological symptoms, but medications used for other movement disorders are used to provide symptomatic control (Hagerman & Hagerman, 2002b; Hagerman *et al.*, 2008).

Parents, patients, and clinicians hold hope for a specific treatment that could reverse the neurobiological abnormalities in FXS. However, until such hope is fulfilled, advances in neurobiology have fueled the search for specific treatments. Agents that may be able to regulate the mGluR5 pathway are currently being evaluated for human trials (Hagerman, 2006; Hagerman *et al.*, 2005, 2009). These agents include fenobam and lithium. Recent studies of lithium have demonstrated cognitive and neurological benefits in the fragile X animal models (Hagerman, 2006; Hagerman *et al.*, 2005). An open trial of lithium in patients demonstrated it was helpful for behavior and improved cognitive measures in patients with FXS (Berry-Kravis *et al.*, 2008). A recent single-dose clinical trial of fenobam in 12 adults with FXS did not find any safety problems and supports implementation of controlled trials of fenobam in adults with FXS (Berry-Kravis *et al.*, 2009).

Cascade testing and screening

A defined treatment for FXS would stimulate newborn screening for FXS. However, such screening efforts are currently being evaluated on a research pilot-basis domestically and internationally (Hagerman *et al.*, 2005).

Our understanding of disorders associated with the premutation has led to recommendations regarding high-risk screening. Recommendations that have been in the literature for a number of years include screening all individuals with mental retardation or autism of unknown etiology (McConkie-Rosell *et al.*, 2005). It is now being recommended that males and females over the age of 50 with tremor or ataxia be screened for the *FMR1* premutation (Jacquemont *et al.*, 2006; Sherman *et al.*, 2005). We are also recommending testing of all women with POI (Wittenberger *et al.*, 2007). Because of the frequency of anxiety disorders and phobias in individuals with the premutation and the full mutation, we propose high-risk screening of these psychiatric populations.

Genetic counseling remains a critical component for fragile X testing and screening because of the disorder's complex multigenerational inheritance pattern, variable phenotype, and implications for the family. A detailed family pedigree must be obtained by a genetic counselor in order to provide genetic risk assessment for carrier status and risk of having affected offspring (McConkie-Rosell *et al.*, 2005).

Discussion

As research continues, we will have a better understanding of the modifying genes and protective factors involved in the variable phenotypes seen in FXS and FXTAS. Advances in the area of molecular biology in FXS are leading to new and better treatments. Advances in screening of high-risk populations and newborn screening will further our knowledge of the prevalence of this disorder and lead to intensive interventions that can take place right after diagnosis, at the time of birth.

REFERENCES

Abbeduto, L., Brady, N., & Kover, S. T. (2007). Language development and fragile X syndrome: Profiles, syndrome-specificity, and within-syndrome differences. *Mental Retardation and Developmental Disabilities Research Reviews*, **13**, 36–46.

Abbeduto, L., Murphy, M. M., Kover, S. T., *et al.* (2008). Signaling noncomprehension of language: A comparison of fragile X syndrome and Down syndrome. *American Journal on Mental Retardation*, **113**, 214–30.

Allen, E. G., He, W., Yadav-Shah, M., & Sherman, S. L. (2004). A study of the distributional characteristics of FMR1 transcript levels in 238 individuals. *Human Genetics*, **114**, 439–47.

Allingham-Hawkins, D. J., Babul-Hirji, R., Chitayat, D., *et al.* (1999). Fragile X premutation is a significant risk factor for premature ovarian failure: The international collaborative POF in fragile X study- preliminary data. *American Journal of Medical Genetics*, **83**, 322–5.

Arocena, D. G., Iwahashi, C. K., Won, N., *et al.* (2005). Induction of inclusion formation and disruption of lamin A/C structure by premutation CGG-repeat RNA in human cultured neural cells. *Human Molecular Genetics*, **14**, 1–11.

Aziz, M., Stathopulu, E., Callias, M., *et al.* (2003). Clinical features of boys with fragile X premutations and intermediate alleles. *American Journal of Medical Genetics*, **121B**, 119–27.

Bailey, D. B., Jr. (2004). Newborn screening for fragile X syndrome. *Mental Retardation and Developmental Disabilities Research Reviews*, **10**, 3–10.

Bailey, D. B., Jr., Hatton, D. D., Mesibov, G., Ament, N., & Skinner, M. (2000). Early development, temperament and functional impairment in autism and fragile X syndrome. *Journal of Autism and Developmental Disorders*, **30**, 49–59.

Bear, M. F., Huber, K. M., & Warren, S. T. (2004). The mGluR theory of fragile X mental retardation. *Trends in Neuroscience*, **27**, 370–7.

Bennetto, L., Pennington, B. F., & Rogers, S. J. (1996). Intact and impaired memory functions in autism. *Child Development*, **67**, 1816–35.

Berry-Kravis, E., Hessl, D., Coffey, S., *et al.* (2009). A pilot open label, single dose trial of fenobam in adults with fragile X syndrome. *Journal of Medical Genetics*, **46**, 266–71.

Berry-Kravis, E., Sumis, A., Hervey, C., *et al.* (2008). Open-label treatment trial of lithium to target the underlying defect in fragile X syndrome. *Journal of Developmental and Behavioral Pediatrics*, **29**, 293–302.

Brunberg, J. A., Jacquemont, S., Hagerman, R. J., *et al.* (2002). Fragile X premutation carriers: Characteristic MR imaging findings in adult males with progressive cerebellar and cognitive dysfunction. *American Journal of Neuroradiology*, **23**, 1757–66.

Coffey, S. M., Cook, K., Tartaglia, N., *et al.* (2008). Expanded clinical phenotype of women with the FMR1 premutation. *American Journal of Medical Genetics*, **146A**, 1009–16.

Cohen, I. L. (1995). Behavioral profiles of autistic and non autistic fragile X males. *Developmental Brain Dysfunction*, **8**, 252–69.

Cornish, K. M., Kogan, C., Turk, J., *et al.* (2005). The emerging fragile X premutation phenotype: Evidence from the domain of social cognition. *Brain and Cognition*, **57**, 53–60.

Cronister, A., Schreiner, R., Wittenberger, M., Amiri, K., Harris, K., & Hagerman, R. J. (1991). Heterozygous fragile X female: Historical, physical, cognitive, and cytogenetic features. *American Journal of Medical Genetics*, **38**, 269–74.

Demark, J. L., Feldman, M. A., & Holden, J. J. (2003). Behavioral relationship between autism and fragile X syndrome. *American Journal on Mental Retardation*, **108**, 314–26.

Derogatis, L. R. (1994). *Symptom Checklist-90-R (SCL-90-R): Administration, Scoring, and Procedures Manual*. Minneapolis: National Computer Systems.

Dombrowski, C., Levesque, S., Morel, M. L., Rouillard, P., Morgan, K., & Rousseau, F. (2002). Premutation and intermediate-size FMR1 alleles in 10 572 males from the general population: Loss of an AGG interruption is a late event in the generation of fragile X syndrome alleles. *Human Molecular Genetics*, **11**, 371–8.

Dorn, M. B., Mazzocco, M. M., & Hagerman, R. J. (1994). Behavioral and psychiatric disorders in adult male carriers of fragile X. *Journal of American Academy of Child and Adolescent Psychiatry*, **33**, 256–64.

Farzin, F., Perry, H., Hessl, D., *et al.* (2006). Autism spectrum disorders and attention-deficit/ hyperactivity disorder in boys with the fragile X premutation. *Journal of Developmental and Behavioral Pediatrics*, **27**, S137–44.

Franke, P., Leboyer, M., Hardt, J., *et al.* (1999). Neuropsychological profiles of FMR-1 premutation and full-mutation carrier females. *Psychiatry Research*, **87**, 223–31.

Goodlin-Jones, B., Tassone, F., Gane, L. W., & Hagerman, R. J. (2004). Autistic spectrum disorder and the fragile X premutation. *Journal of Developmental Behavioral Pediatrics*, **25**, 392–8.

Greco, C. M., Berman, R. F., Martin, R. M., *et al.* (2006). Neuropathology of fragile X-associated tremor/ataxia syndrome (FXTAS). *Brain*, **129**(Pt. 1), 243–55.

Greco, C. M., Hagerman, R. J., Tassone, F., *et al.* (2002). Neuronal intranuclear inclusions in a new cerebellar tremor/ataxia syndrome among fragile X carriers. *Brain*, **125**, 1760–71.

Hagerman, P. J. (2008). The fragile X prevalence paradox. *Journal of Medical Genetics*, **45**, 498–9.

Hagerman, R. J. (2002a). Physical and behavioral phenotype. In R. J. Hagerman & P. J. Hagerman (Eds.), *Fragile X Syndrome: Diagnosis, Treatment and Research*, 3rd edn. (pp. 3–109). Baltimore: The Johns Hopkins University Press.

Hagerman, R. J. (2002b). Medical follow-up and pharmacotherapy. In R. J. Hagerman & P. J. Hagerman (Eds.), *Fragile X Syndrome: Diagnosis, Treatment and Research*, 3rd edn. (pp. 287–338). Baltimore: The Johns Hopkins University Press.

Hagerman, R. J. (2006). Lessons from fragile X regarding neurobiology, autism, and neurodegeneration. *Journal of Developmental and Behavioral Pediatrics*, **27**, 63–74.

Hagerman, R. J. & Hagerman, P. J. (2002a). The fragile X premutation: Into the phenotypic fold. *Current Opinion in Genetics and Development*, **12**, 278–83.

Hagerman, R. J. & Hagerman, P. J. (2002b). *Fragile X Syndrome: Diagnosis, Treatment, and Research*, 3rd edn. Baltimore: The Johns Hopkins University Press.

Hagerman, P. J. & Hagerman, R. J. (2004a). The fragile-X premutation: A maturing perspective. *American Journal of Human Genetics*, **74**, 805–16.

Hagerman, P. J. & Hagerman, R. J. (2004b). Fragile X-associated tremor/ataxia syndrome (FXTAS). *Mental Retardation and Developmental Disabilities Research Reviews*, **10**, 25–30.

Hagerman, R. J., Berry-Kravis, E., Kaufmann, W. E., *et al.* (2009). Advances in the treatment of fragile X syndrome. *Pediatrics*, **123**, 378–90.

Hagerman, R. J., Hall, D. A., Coffey, S., *et al.* (2008). Treatment of fragile X-associated tremor ataxia syndrome (FXTAS) and related neurological problems. *Clinical Interventions in Aging*, **3**, 251–62.

Hagerman, R. J., Leavitt, B. R., Farzin, F., *et al.* (2004). Fragile-X-associated tremor/ataxia syndrome (FXTAS) in females with the FMR1 premutation. *American Journal of Human Genetics*, **74**, 1051–6.

Hagerman, R. J., Ono, M. Y., & Hagerman, P. J. (2005). Recent advances in fragile X: A model for autism and neurodegeneration. *Current Opinion in Psychiatry*, **18**, 490–6.

Hagerman, R. J., Staley, L. W., O'Conner, R., *et al.* (1996). Learning-disabled males with a fragile X CGG expansion in the upper premutation size range. *Pediatrics*, **97**, 122–6.

Hatton, D., Hooper, S. R., Bailey, D. B., Skinner, M. L., Sullivan, K. M., & Wheeler, A. (2002). Problem behavior in boys with fragile X syndrome. *American Journal of Medical Genetics*, **108**, 105–16.

Hatton, D. D., Sideris, J., Skinner, M., *et al.* (2006). Autistic behavior in children with fragile X syndrome: Prevalence, stability, and the impact of FMRP. *American Journal of Medical Genetics A*, **140**, 1804–13.

Hatton, D. D., Wheeler, A. C., Skinner, M. L., *et al.* (2003). Adaptive behavior in children with fragile X syndrome. *American Journal on Mental Retardation*, **108**, 373–90.

Hessl, D., Tassone, F., Loesch, D. Z., *et al.* (2005). Abnormal elevation of FMR1 mRNA is associated with psychological symptoms in individuals with the fragile X premutation. *American Journal of Medical Genetics B Neuropsychiatric Genetics*, **139**, 115–21.

Hinds, H. L., Ashley, C. T., Sutcliffe, J. S., *et al.* (1993). Tissue specific expression of FMR-1 provides evidence for a functional role in fragile X syndrome. *Nature Genetics*, **3**, 36–43 [published erratum appears in Nature Genetics, 5, 312].

Huber, K. M., Gallagher, S. M., Warren, S. T., & Bear, M. F. (2002). Altered synaptic plasticity in a mouse model of fragile X mental retardation. *Proceedings of the National Academy of Sciences of the United States of America*, **99**, 7746–50.

Hull, C. & Hagerman, R. J. (1993). A study of the physical, behavioral, and medical phenotype, including anthropometric measures, of females with fragile X syndrome. *American Journal of Diseases of Children*, **147**, 1236–41.

Iwahashi, C. K., Yasui, D. H., An, H. J., *et al.* (2006). Protein composition of the intranuclear inclusions of FXTAS. *Brain*. **129**, 256–71.

Jacquemont, S., Hagerman, R. J., Leehey, M. A., *et al.* (2003a). Penetrance of the fragile X-associated tremor/ataxia syndrome (FXTAS) in a premutation carrier population: Initial results from a California family-based study. *American Journal of Human Genetics, 53rd Annual Meeting, Los Angeles, CA.*, **73**(Suppl), A10:163.

Jacquemont, S., Hagerman, R. J., Leehey, M., *et al.* (2003b). Fragile X premutation tremor/ataxia syndrome: Molecular, clinical, and neuroimaging correlates. *American Journal of Human Genetics*, **72**, 869–78.

Jacquemont, S., Hagerman, R. J., Leehey, M. A., *et al.* (2004). Penetrance of the fragile X-associated tremor/ataxia syndrome in a premutation carrier population. *Journal of the American Medical Association*, **291**, 460–9.

Jacquemont, S., Leehey, M. A., Hagerman, R. J., Beckett, L. A., & Hagerman, P. J. (2006). Size bias of fragile X premutation alleles in late-onset movement disorders. *Journal of Medical Genetics*, **43**, 804–9.

Jakala, P., Hanninen, T., Ryynanen, M., *et al.* (1997). Fragile-X: Neuropsychological test perform-ance, CGG triplet repeat lengths, and hippocampal volumes. *Journal of Clinical Investigation*, **100**, 331–8.

Johnston, C., Eliez, S., Dyer-Friedman, J., *et al.* (2001). Neurobehavioral phenotype in carriers of the fragile X premutation. *American Journal of Medical Genetics*, **103**, 314–9.

Kau, A. S., Tierney, E., Bukelis, I., *et al.* (2004). Social behavior profile in young males with fragile X syndrome: Characteristics and specificity. *American Journal of Medical Genetics*, **126A**, 9–17.

Kaufmann, W. E., Cortell, R., Kau, A. S., *et al.* (2004). Autism spectrum disorder in fragile X syndrome: Communication, social interaction, and specific behaviors. *American Journal of Medical Genetics*, **129A**, 225–34.

Kenneson, A., Zhang, F., Hagedorn, C. H., & Warren, S. T. (2001). Reduced FMRP and increased FMR1 transcription is proportionally associated with CGG repeat number in intermediate-length and premutation carriers. *Human Molecular Genetics*, **10**, 1449–54.

Koldewyn, K., Hessl, D., Adams, J., *et al.* (2008). Reduced hippocampal activation during recall is associated with elevated FMR1 mRNA and psychiatric symptoms in men with the fragile X premutation. *Brain Imaging and Behavior*, **2**, 105–16.

Loesch, D. Z., Huggins, R. M., & Hagerman, R. J. (2004). Phenotypic variation and FMRP levels in fragile X. *Mental Retardation and Developmental Disabilities Research Reviews*, **10**, 31–41.

Loesch, D. Z., Litewka, L., Brotchie, P., Huggins, R. M., Tassone, F., & Cook, M. (2005). Magnetic resonance imaging study in older fragile X premutation male carriers. *Annals of Neurology*, **58**, 326–30.

Mazzocco, M. M., Kates, W. R., Baumgardner, T. L., Freund, L. S., & Reiss, A. L. (1997). Autistic behaviors among girls with fragile X syndrome. *Journal of Autism and Developmental Disorders*, **27**, 415–35.

McConkie-Rosell, A., Finucane, B., Cronister, A., Abrams, L., Bennett, R. L., & Pettersen, B. J. (2005). Genetic counseling for fragile X syndrome: Updated recommendations of the National Society of Genetic Counselors. *Journal of Genetic Counseling*, **14**, 249–70.

Moore, C. J., Daly, E. M., Schmitz, N., *et al.* (2004a). A neuropsychological investigation of male premutation carriers of fragile X syndrome. *Neuropsychologia*, **42**, 1934–47.

Moore, C. J., Daly, E. M., Tassone, F., *et al.* (2004b). The effect of pre-mutation of X chromosome CGG trinucleotide repeats on brain anatomy. *Brain*, **127**, 2672–81.

Murphy, D. G., Mentis, M. J., Pietrini, P., *et al.* (1999). Premutation female carriers of fragile X syndrome: A pilot study on brain anatomy and metabolism. *Journal of American Academy of Child and Adolescent Psychiatry*, **38**, 1294–301.

Murray, A., Ennis, S., MacSwiney, F., Webb, J., & Morton, N. E. (2000). Reproductive and menstrual history of females with fragile X expansions. *European Journal of Human Genetics*, **8**, 247–52.

Philofsky, A., Hepburn, S. L., Hayes, A., Hagerman, R., & Rogers, S. J. (2004). Linguistic and cognitive functioning and autism symptoms in young children with fragile X syndrome. *American Journal of Mental Retardation*, **109**, 208–18.

Reiss, A. L., Freund, L., Abrams, M. T., Boehm, C., & Kazazian, H. (1993). Neurobehavioral effects of the fragile X premutation in adult women: A controlled study. *American Journal of Human Genetics*, **52**, 884–94.

Riddle, J. E., Cheema, A., Sobesky, W. E., *et al.* (1998). Phenotypic involvement in females with the FMR1 gene mutation. *American Journal on Mental Retardation*, **102**, 590–601.

Roberts, J. E., Bailey, D. B., Jr., Mankowski, J., *et al.* (2009). Mood and anxiety disorders in females with the FMR1 premutation. *American Journal of Medical Genetics Neuropsychiatric Genetics*, **150B**, 130–9.

Rogers, S. J., Wehner, E. A., & Hagerman, R. J. (2001). The behavioral phenotype in fragile X: Symptoms of autism in very young children with fragile X syndrome, idiopathic autism, and other developmental disorders. *Journal of Developmental Behavioral Pediatrics*, **22**, 409–17.

Rousseau, F., Rouillard, P., Morel, M. L., Khandjian, E. W., & Morgan, K. (1995). Prevalence of carriers of premutation-size alleles of the FMRI gene–and implications for the population genetics of the fragile X syndrome. *American Journal of Human Genetics*, **57**, 1006–18.

Schwartz, C. E., Dean, J., Howard-Peebles, P. N., *et al.* (1994). Obstetrical and gynecological complications in fragile X carriers: A multicenter study. *American Journal of Medical Genetics*, **51**, 400–2.

Sherman, S. L. (2000). Premature ovarian failure in the fragile X syndrome. *American Journal of Medical Genetics*, **97**, 189–94.

Sherman, S., Pletcher, B. A., & Driscoll, D. A. (2005). Fragile X syndrome: Diagnostic and carrier testing. *Genetics in Medicine*, **7**, 584–7.

Sobesky, W. E., Pennington, B. F., Porter, D., Hull, C. E., & Hagerman, R. J. (1994). Emotional and neurocognitive deficits in fragile X. *American Journal of Medical Genetics*, **51**, 378–85.

Sobesky, W. E., Taylor, A. K., Pennington, B. F., Bennetto, L., Porter, D., & Hagerman, R. J. (1996). Molecular-clinical correlations in females with fragile X. *American Journal of Medical Genetics*, **64**, 340–5.

Sullivan, A. K., Marcus, M., Epstein, M. P., *et al.* (2005). Association of FMR1 repeat size with ovarian dysfunction. *Human Reproduction*, **20**, 402–12.

Tassone, F., Greco, C., Berman, R. F., *et al.* (2005). *Clinical and Molecular Correlations in FXTAS*. Paper presented at 55th Annual Meeting of the American Society of Human Genetics, October 25–29. Salt Lake City, UT.

Tassone, F., Hagerman, R. J., Chamberlain, W. D., & Hagerman, P. J. (2000a). Transcription of the FMR1 gene in individuals with fragile X syndrome. *American Journal of Medical Genetics*, **97**, 195–203.

Tassone, F., Hagerman, R. J., Loesch, D. Z., Lachiewicz, A., Taylor, A. K., & Hagerman, P. J. (2000b). Fragile X males with unmethylated, full mutation trinucleotide repeat expansions have elevated levels of FMR1 messenger RNA. *American Journal of Medical Genetics*, **94**, 232–6.

Tassone, F., Hagerman, R. J., Taylor, A. K., Gane, L. W., Godfrey, T. E., & Hagerman, P. J. (2000c). Elevated levels of FMR1 mRNA in carrier males: A new mechanism of involvement in fragile X syndrome. *American Journal of Human Genetics*, **66**, 6–15.

Tassone, F., Hagerman, R. J., Taylor, A. K., *et al.* (2000d). Clinical involvement and protein expression in individuals with the FMR1 premutation. *American Journal of Medical Genetics*, **91**, 144–52.

Tassone, F., Iwahashi, C., & Hagerman, P. J. (2004). FMR1 RNA within the intranuclear inclusions of fragile X-associated tremor/ataxia syndrome (FXTAS). *RNA Biology*, **1**, 103–5.

Tassone, F., Longshore, J., Zunich, J., Steinbach, P., Salat, U., & Taylor, A. K. (1999). Tissue-specific methylation differences in a fragile X premutation carrier. *Clinical Genetics*, **55**, 346–51.

Turk, J. & Graham, P. (1997). Fragile X syndrome, autism, and autistic features. *Autism*, **1**, 175–97.

Valle, D. (2004). Genetics, individuality, and medicine in the 21st century. *American Journal of Human Genetics*, **74**, 374–81.

Vianna-Morgante, A. M. & Costa, S. S. (2000). Premature ovarian failure is associated with maternally and paternally inherited premutation in Brazilian families with fragile X [see comments] [letter]. *American Journal of Human Genetics*, **67**, 254–5; discussion 256–8.

Welt, C. K., Smith, P. C., & Taylor, A. E. (2004). Evidence of early ovarian aging in fragile X premutation carriers. *Journal of Clinical Endocrinology Metabolism*, **89**, 4569–74.

Wittenberger, M. D., Hagerman, R. J., Sherman, S. L., *et al.* (2007). The FMR1 premutation and reproduction. *Fertility and Sterility*, **87**, 456–65.

2

Autism: Genes, anatomy, and behavioral outcome

Emma Esser, Saasha Sutera, and Deborah Fein

Introduction

Autism is a highly heritable disorder with variable physiological, behavioral, and cognitive expression, and a widely variable set of outcomes. In some ways, not enough is known about each of these levels of expression of the disorder; in some ways, however, too much is known – many findings at the genetic, anatomical, and neurochemical levels have been reported, but are often not replicated or are directly opposite to each other (low vs. high chemical levels, increased vs. decreased volume of particular brain structures), and no successful synthesis of findings across or within levels has yet been made. Given this complex and disjointed set of studies, we have not attempted a comprehensive or synthetic review.

We will not address studies on neurochemistry or other physiological factors that have been raised as possibilities in autism, such as inflammatory processes (Vargas *et al.*, 2005), but will focus on genetics, anatomy, and behavioral/cognitive outcome. We will first describe the basic phenomenology and epidemiology of the autistic syndromes. Second, we will review what is known about the genetic basis of autism. Third, we will describe the current state of knowledge about the neuro-anatomy of autism. Finally, we will address outcome: what is known about the outcome of affected children; and most intriguingly, if autism has a genetic basis, which seems to affect basic neuroanatomy, how is it possible that some children "recover" from their autism? (Discussion of autism associated with fragile X syndrome can be found in Chapter 1.)

In 1943, Kanner described 11 children with "extreme autistic aloneness" (p. 242), failure to use language in a communicative fashion, and an obsessive desire for the maintenance of sameness. These three features (social isolation, failure to communicate, and perseverative behavior) still form the basis for diagnosis of ASD in DSM-IV-TR (American Psychiatric Association, 2000). Social isolation is a key and

This work was done with support from the NIMH to Dr. Fein ("Language Functioning in Optimal Outcome Children with a History of Autism")

necessary feature for diagnosis of any ASD. It includes impairment in nonverbal communication, such as failure to make appropriate eye contact or to use gestural communication to compensate for verbal impairments. It also includes poor peer relationships and insensitivity to the displayed emotions of others. Perhaps most pathognomonically, children with autism seldom point, either to share their interest in something with another person (joint attention) or to request, with pointing for joint attention most impaired. In the realm of communication impairment, language is marked by delays (or total absence of language); a repetitive and stereotyped quality; a failure to hold reciprocal conversations (even when sufficient language is present); and impoverished, absent, or delayed pretend play. In the domain of repetitive behaviors, the child may show unreasonable insistence on meaningless routines, resistance to change in the environment, preoccupations with certain topics or collections, stereotyped motor movements (hand-flapping, rocking, spinning), and visual preoccupations (staring at lights, spinning wheels, lining up toys). A child can meet criteria for autistic disorder by having two social symptoms and at least one in each of the other domains, with a minimum of six symptoms in total (American Psychiatric Association, 2000). Such children can range from severely retarded, nonverbal, and unrelated to others, to having a high IQ, excellent language, and attempts to interact (albeit strangely) with others.

The autism spectrum is called pervasive developmental disorder (PDD) in DSM-IV-TR (2000), although ASD is coming to replace PDD in the literature. In addition to autistic disorder, a commonly used diagnosis is Asperger disorder; in this syndrome, normal intellect is present, with no language delay, along with marked perseverative and obsessive interests. Rett syndrome is a disorder almost exclusively found in girls, with at least a large minority showing a mutation in the MECP2 gene on the X chromosome. After a few months of normal development, regression of skills and characteristic hand-wringing behavior and loss of purposeful hand use appear, with a generally poor outcome (Amir *et al.*, 1999). A remaining category, pervasive developmental disorder–not otherwise specified (PDD-NOS) is applied to children who have some autistic features (including at least one symptom in the social domain) but do not meet criteria for another ASD disorder.

In addition to the diagnostic criteria, many children with ASD show abnormalities in their responses to sensory input: they may be underresponsive, ignoring sounds and painful stimuli; overresponsive, responding strongly to what others perceive as mild (usually auditory) stimuli; and engaging in behavior that seems to provide sensory input such as staring at shadows or lights, or piling weighted objects (e.g., heavy blankets) on top of themselves (Liss *et al.*, 2006).

Children with ASD often show disturbed sleep patterns (Elia *et al.*, 2000; Williams *et al.*, 2004) and abnormally strong food preferences and restricted diets. Some children with ASD have significant mood problems, with irritability and inconsolable crying, especially when young. When older, they may be at increased risk for anxiety and depression (Kim *et al.*, 2000), as well as other psychiatric disorders, such as obsessive–compulsive disorder and Tourette syndrome (Comings & Comings, 1991; Lainhart, 1999). Although figures are changing as early intervention improves, at least half of children with ASD have IQs in the mentally retarded range (Muhle *et al.*, 2004). Although the idea that ASD is fundamentally a disorder of language is no longer accepted as widely as it once was, it does appear that many children with ASD resemble those with developmental language disorder in their marked deficits in phonology and syntax (Kjelgaard & Tager-Flusberg, 2001; see Chapter 4). Finally, attentional impairments, such as poor ability to shift attention from one topic or stimulus to another and poor ability to sustain attention to uninteresting tasks, are extremely prevalent in ASD (Landry & Bryson, 2004; Zwaigenbaum *et al.*, 2005); a recent paper (Fein *et al.*, 2005) describes a clinical phenomenon in 11 children, where the clinical picture evolved from ASD to ADHD.

As many as 29% of children with ASD will have seizures (Volkmar & Nelson, 1990), with most having their onset in either early childhood or in adolescence. Although there is still some debate about the possibility of autistic behaviors in Landau-Kleffner syndrome, where children show pronounced regression in language accompanied by characteristic EEG abnormalities, most neurologists will assess children with autistic behaviors and marked language regression for this syndrome (Trevathan, 2004).

The gender ratio of ASD is consistently found to be about 4:1 boys to girls, but the incidence remains an area of debate and disagreement. Significant increases in the incidence of ASD have been reported (Newschaffer *et al.*, 2005), but others (Chakrabarti & Fombonne, 2005) argue that changes in how diagnostic criteria are applied, the pressures for an ASD diagnosis to obtain educational services, and variations in the ascertainment methods account for most or all of this apparent increase. Current estimates of the prevalence of ASD are as high as 0.6% (Chakrabarti & Fombonne, 2005).

Genetics

A significant minority, approximately 10%, of the cases of autism are accounted for by rare medical conditions, both genetic and nongenetic, that are single gene disorders or caused by disruptions at known chromosomal sites that affect the development of the brain. These include tuberous sclerosis, Angelman syndrome, fragile X, Rett syndrome, and neurofibromatosis (Barton & Volkmar, 1998; Folstein & Rutter, 1988; Konstantereas & Homatidis, 1999; Lauritsen *et al.*, 1999;

Smalley, 1998; Weidmer-Mikhail *et al.*, 1998; Wing & Gould, 1979). With these disorders, the autistic clinical picture occurs more often than expected by chance. Although the exact etiology is not known, there is compelling evidence that the majority of the remaining 90% of cases also have a genetic etiology, although a significantly more complex one than the single gene disorders listed above.

In finding that monozygotic (MZ) twins have a higher concordance rate than dizygotic (DZ) twins, the study by Folstein and Rutter (1977) of same-sex twins provided initial evidence suggesting that autism's etiology is both complex and genetic. Subsequent twin studies have replicated their findings (Bailey *et al.*, 1995; Ritvo *et al.*, 1985; Steffenburg *et al.*, 1989), and estimates of heritability are now 60% or higher in MZ twins, when ASDs rather than strictly defined autistic disorder are included, and 0% in DZ twins, although Folstein (1999) posits that "only about 65 pairs of twins have been studied in total, so the 0% concordance is probably a type-II error"; the expected DZ rate is 3–6%, the same as the recurrence risk to siblings (Bailey *et al.*, 1995; Folstein & Rutter, 1977; Steffenburg *et al.*, 1989). These differing concordance rates suggest the involvement of multiple genes.

Given that not all MZ twins are concordant, it has been suggested that environmental factors may also play a role. Initial studies suggested that obstetric complications may contribute to differential risk (Gillberg & Gillberg, 1983; Lord *et al.*, 1991; Piven *et al.*, 1993). In a few early twin studies, there was a history of perinatal injury in the affected twin (Folstein & Rutter, 1977; Steffenberg *et al.*, 1989). Those with autism were more likely to have suffered perinatal injury (Deykin & MacMahon, 1980; Finnegan & Quarrington, 1979). However, it now appears that such mild complications do not result in damage to the developing brain (Bailey *et al.*, 1995; Bolton *et al.*, 1994, 1997; Rutter *et al.*, 1999). Therefore, some researchers have concluded that such complications do not play a causative role in the development of autism.

The increased risk extends to non-twin siblings as well but decreases significantly moving from siblings to more distant relatives (Szatmari *et al.*, 1998). Rates of sibling concordance are in the range of about 2–10%, many times higher than the rate of autism in the general population, with risk of related but less severe effects, such as language delay, found in up to 35% of siblings (see below) (Jones & Szatmari, 1988; Ritvo *et al.*, 1985, 1989; see Rutter *et al.*, 1999, for review).

The pattern of heritability as observed in twin and family studies suggests the involvement of multiple genes. Pickles and colleagues (2000) combined data from twin and family studies, concluding that it is most likely that 3–5 susceptibility genes must act in combination. Similarly, Santangelo and Folstein (1999) estimate that 2–4 genes are involved. However, estimates range from 3 to 15 involved genes to more than 100 (Risch *et al.*, 1999).

Twin and family studies also revealed the presence of the broader autism phenotype (BAP). That is, many relatives, especially siblings and parents, of autistic probands do not meet criteria for a diagnosis of an ASD but currently exhibit and have a history of social and communicative impairments, especially pragmatics, and, to a lesser degree, repetitive behaviors and interests (Bolton *et al.*, 1994; Landa *et al.*, 1991, 1992; Piven & Palmer, 1997; Piven *et al.*, 1990, 1991, 1994, 1997a,b; Szatmari *et al.*, 1998). These subthreshold traits often occur in the absence of mental retardation (Fombonne *et al.*, 1997; Szatmari *et al.*, 1993). When MZ twins are discordant, the unaffected twin often has subthreshold traits, including deficits in communication and social skills, providing evidence that the genetic liability extends well beyond the strict initial diagnostic criteria for autistic disorder (Bailey *et al.*, 1995; Folstein & Rutter, 1977). There has been some question as to what specific impairments or traits are a part of BAP (see Rutter *et al.*, 1999). Dawson and colleagues (2002) suggest that six traits be considered components of the BAP, including deficits in face processing and social affiliation. The existence of the BAP also suggests the involvement of multiple genes (Fombonne *et al.*, 1997). As Folstein (1999) observed, "It is unlikely that all the genes will be inherited again in another child in the same sibship. However, it is equally unlikely for another child to inherit NONE of the contributing genes." Therefore, parents and siblings may exhibit some traits of autism (Folstein, 1999).

As of 2004, ten independent genome-wide linkage screens of autism had been completed, with reports of an association between autism and anomalies on most chromosomes, which is further evidence of the heterogeneity of autism (see Wassink *et al.*, 2004, for review, and Dawson, 2008, for an update). Nicolson and Szatmari (2003) and Polleux and Lauder (2004) also review results of genome scans and association studies. Regions from 7q and 2q are the most frequently cited across studies, while others suggest there is evidence for the involvement of chromosomes 13q and 15q (Tager-Flusberg *et al.*, 2001). There is evidence that chromosome 7q is a locus related to the development of language in individuals with autism (Alarcon *et al.*, 2002; Bradford *et al.*, 2001). Furthermore, there is some evidence that suggests a locus at 7q31 for autism and developmental language disorder, also known as specific language impairment (SLI; see Folstein & Mankoski, 2000, for review). Folstein and Mankoski (2000) posit that "autism and SLI appear to be genetically related; both disorders occur much more often than expected by chance within the same family, and some cases exist that have phenotypes that cannot be distinctly differentiated."

Genetic results, in general, are difficult to replicate, in part due to the probability of multiple genes contributing to susceptibility and because of the relative weakness of results. On the other hand, reducing phenotypic hetero-geneity in participant samples may increase the replicability of genetic findings.

In an attempt to decrease heterogeneity, Molloy *et al.* (2005) studied a sample of individuals with autism characterized by regression, finding evidence of linkage on chromosomes 21q and 7q.

Candidate gene studies assess the potential contribution of specific genes to autism susceptibility and are examined because, based on the gene's function, there is evidence of their involvement. Strong candidate genes have included Neurologin 3 and 4, chromosome 15 q11-q13 (gamma-aminobutyric acid receptor subunits), and a gene in the serotonin system (Wassink *et al.*, 2004). However, results have been mixed, with some studies yielding positive linkage results while others fail to replicate these findings. Morrow *et al.* (2008) studied a sample of autistic individuals whose parents tended to share ancestors, magnifying the power to detect inherited factors. They found several chromosome regions implicated in these cases, and argue that a common link among these sites, and others identified by other groups, is that the genes play a role in synapse function and nervous system response to experience.

One important recent study (Sebat *et al.*, 2007) reported de novo copy number variants in multiple genes, higher in autistic individuals from families with only one affected individual than in families with multiple, or no, affected individuals, suggesting a possibly different mechanism in some simplex families, that would be hard to detect with linkage studies.

In sum, twin and family studies established that autism is a highly heritable disorder with the BAP present in siblings and parents. Linkage and candidate gene studies have implicated numerous chromosomes, but results have often not been replicated (see Cook, 2001; Maestrini *et al.*, 2000; Muhle *et al.*, 2004, for recent reviews).

Neuroanatomical findings

There is considerable evidence to suggest structural and functional differences in the brains of children with autism vs. children without autism; however, inconsistency is the hallmark of this literature as well (Palmen *et al.*, 2004). This inconsistency may be due to several factors. Past studies examining magnetic resonance imaging use different methodologies and lack power due to small sample sizes and the inherent heterogeneity of the disorder. In addition, several studies include subjects with neurological disease, and fail to match subjects based on characteristics such as age, sex, and cognitive ability. Instead, selection of comparison groups is often driven by feasibility.

Although there are extremely heterogeneous findings across brains, the most consistent finding has been macrocephaly in children with ASD. Between 19% and 53% of individuals with ASD have a head circumference above the 97th percentile at some point in development (Courchesne *et al.*, 2003; Dementieva *et al.*, 2005). At birth, children later diagnosed with an ASD tend to have a smaller than normal head circumference (Courchesne *et al.*, 2001, 2003). By the age of 14 months, these same children have a larger than normal head circumference, which some hypothesize suggests a failure of pruning of neuronal connections (Courchesne *et al.*, 2003). The macrocephaly seems to be due to a large volume of gray, and especially white, matter (Herbert, 2005), rather than enlarged ventricles, as is often the case with macrocephaly.

Findings regarding the implications of macrocephaly on the functioning of children with ASD vary. Dementieva *et al.* (2005) found that 35% of autistic individuals displayed an accelerated head growth, which was defined by more than a 25 percentile increase between two consecutive measurements, and 19% were macrocephalic. The children with accelerated head growth were a higher functioning group. Similarly, children on the autism spectrum who have a larger head circumference also tend to have higher nonverbal than verbal scores on a measure of cognitive ability (Deutsch & Joseph, 2003). Courchesne *et al.* (2003), in contrast, found the children with steeper head circumference growth curves to be more impaired on a few of the developmental variables measured.

When compared to typically developing and developmentally delayed children, children with autism show increased cerebellar and cerebral volume (Sparks *et al.*, 2002). In addition, they also show enlarged amygdalae and hippocampi (Sparks *et al.*, 2002). Akshoomoff *et al.* (2004) examined similar anatomical differences in young children as predictors of outcome at the age of 5 years. Whole brain volume was largest in children with low-functioning autism, compared to typically developing children. In terms of cerebral volume, children with high-functioning autism had the greatest cerebral white matter volume, although this difference did not reach significance. Cerebral gray matter volume, however, was larger for the children with low-functioning autism, compared to the control group. In terms of cerebellar volume, children on the autism spectrum and typically developing children did not differ in cerebellar gray matter volume. However, the children within the autism spectrum had enlarged cerebellar white matter volume. In addition, children on the autism spectrum displayed a larger than normal area of the anterior vermis, and children with low-functioning autism displayed a smaller area of the posterior vermis, compared to those with high-functioning autism. In this instance, variability in brain structure was correlated with diagnostic outcome in young children with autism. Cerebellar white matter volume was important in separating the low-functioning autism group from the control group, while size of the anterior and posterior cerebellar vermis and cerebral white matter volume were important predictors in separating high-functioning autism group from the control group and the low-functioning autism group.

In both children and adults, findings include small, densely packed cells in the limbic system, specifically the hippocampus, amygdala, subiculum, entorhinal cortex, septal nuclei, anterior cingulate gyrus, septum, and mamillary body (see Bauman & Kemper, 2005, for review). Another finding is a decreased number of Purkinje cells in the cerebellum and brainstem across age, sex, and cognitive ability (Bauman & Kemper, 2005).

Some anatomical findings have differed between children and adults. Depending upon the area of the brain, young children display increased brain volume in white and gray matter (Aylward *et al.*, 2002; Courchesne *et al.*, 2001; Herbert *et al.*, 2003). Total brain volume normalizes in older children and adults, but their head circumference remains large, suggesting earlier brain overgrowth (Aylward *et al.*, 2002).

Decreased gray matter in the right paracingulate gyrus, left occipito-temporal cortex, and left inferior frontal sulcus, and increased gray matter in the left amygdala, right inferior temporal gyrus, left middle temporal gyrus, and cerebellum may be another correlate of autism (Abell *et al.*, 1999). With the exception of the cerebellum, these brain structures project to or from the amygdala, which may impact regulation of emotional states (Abell *et al.*, 1999). A shortening of the brainstem and an absence of facial nuclei have also been found to be associated with autism (Rodier, 2002). However, after correcting for brain volume, Herbert *et al.* (2003) found the thalamus, cerebellum GD-putamen, and brainstem to be of normal size. In addition, the cerebral white matter was larger, while the cerebral cortex and amygdala–hippocampal complex were smaller. In high-functioning children with autism between the ages of 7 and 15 years, Palmen *et al.* (2005) found enlarged gray matter, cerebellum, and ventricles, but not enlarged white matter.

White matter abnormalities appear to be found across studies. Casanova *et al.* (2002) examined the number and packing density of minicolumns in the frontal and temporal cortex and found an increased number of columns, which were smaller and less compact with reduced neuropil space, possibly leading to excessive white matter. Gustafsson (1997, 2004) theorizes that the abnormality of minicolumns might result from irregular excitatory and inhibitory processes in the cortex, an early low capacity of producing serotonin, or insufficient production of nitric oxide. In addition, white matter abnormalities might result from irregular development or maintenance of unnecessary connections (Just *et al.*, 2004).

Underconnectivity (Just *et al.*, 2004) between or within cognitive, perceptual, and motor circuits could be the result of disruptions in gray matter circuitry or white matter communications systems. Koshino *et al.* (2005) found normal amounts of connectivity on functional magnetic resonance images on a working memory task, but prefrontal activation was connected to right posterior activity in people with autism and left posterior activity in normal controls.

In sum, the structural neuroanatomical studies show that specific areas of the brain are consistently implicated in autism; however, specific abnormalities vary. While the amygdala and hippocampus have been implicated, increased, decreased, and normal size of the amygdala and hippocampus have all been reported. Other anatomical findings include structural and functional abnormalities in the cerebellum and parietal cortex (Courchesne *et al.*, 2001). Some find increased cerebellar size (Sparks *et al.*, 2002), and others find decreased cerebellar size (Hashimoto *et al.*, 1995; Murakami *et al.*, 1989). Also implicated is increased size of the basal ganglia, although different areas are implicated in different studies (Herbert *et al.*, 2003; Sears *et al.*, 1999) and decreased size of the corpus callosum, both anterior and posterior (Egaas *et al.*, 1995; Harden *et al.*, 2000; Manes *et al.*, 1999; Piven *et al.*, 1997c). The most consistent finding thus far appears to be increased brain size in children with autism, which suggests a more global abnormality in brain development (Courchesne *et al.*, 2001, 2003; Dementieva *et al.*, 2005).

Functional imaging studies of autism are in their infancy (see Rumsey & Ernst, 2000; Schultz & Robins, 2005, for reviews). There have been some provocative findings of reduced activity in frontal areas (Horwitz *et al.*, 1988), as well as findings of activation in adjacent areas to those normally activated by specific tasks, such as face processing (Schultz *et al.*, 2000) and theory of mind tasks, using positron emission tomography scanning (Happe *et al.*, 1996). Williams *et al.* (2006) found different patterns of activation in adolescent boys with ASD vs. controls, in an imitation paradigm, including differences in an area associated with mirror neuron function in the right temporo-parietal junction, as well as in the left amygdala. Mundy (2003) reviews much of this literature, especially with relation to activation of medial (also thought to be associated with mirror neuron activity and related to social cognition) and lateral frontal cortex, with a focus on joint attention. Ramachandran and Oberman (2006) review some of this work and describe some of their recent findings of abnormal activation of "mirror neuron" regions in children with autism who are watching others' actions. This work is fascinating and will eventually contribute to our understanding of how the brain functions differently in autism. However, the interpretation of these findings seems usually to be that, if the "mirror neuron" system or "theory of mind module" are not functioning normally, this means that autism results from fundamental abnormalities in these systems. However, we also need to consider the alternative possibility that, if motivational abnormalities drive attention to an unusual set of idiosyncratic stimuli and away from social stimuli, then the "mirror neuron" system will be deprived of its normal input during development. This would be consistent with the possibility that the cells in the mirror neuron system are not physiologically or morphologically abnormal in and of themselves, but respond to an abnormal set of inputs, namely that they respond to the child's own intentions and goals but not to the intentions and goals of others. This would suggest that the mirror neuron system dysfunction, and perhaps dysfunction in other social cognition systems as well, is a downstream consequence of a problem at an earlier stage of processing.

Given the marked heterogeneity of the apparent genetic contributions to autism, as well as the heterogeneity of the brain structure of affected children, one would expect a resulting heterogeneity in functional outcome, and this is indeed the case.

Initial outcome studies

Initial outcome studies established the somewhat varied, but generally poor outcome of children with autism. In the first studies of this kind, Rutter *et al.* (1967) and Lockyer and Rutter (1969, 1970) examined the social, behavioral, cognitive, psychological, and educational/work outcome of 63 children diagnosed with "infantile psychosis," generally accepted as autism spectrum disorders, at a 5- to 15-year follow-up (mean age 15 years, 7 months). At follow-up, 14% had achieved a "good" adjustment, 25% had a "fair" adjustment, 13% "poor," and almost half (48%) were "very poorly" adjusted according to the following criteria: a "good" outcome was described as leading a normal or near-normal social life and functioning satisfactorily at school or work; a "fair" outcome was described by the researchers as "making social and educational progress in spite of significant, even marked, abnormalities in behavior or interpersonal relationships"; a "poor" outcome was described as "severely handicapped and unable to lead an independent life, but where there was still some measure of social adjustment and it was felt that some potential for social progress remains"; and a "very poor" outcome was described as "unable to lead any kind of independent existence."

Educationally, adjustment was equally poor for most children; IQ and schooling were not correlated, in part because of comorbid behavioral problems as well as the lack of adequate educational options at the time the study was conducted. For these reasons, the educational achievement of most children was below what would be expected today. Socially, all children with "infantile psychosis" were initially described as "autistic." At follow-up, 14% of children had sufficient social skills that this description was no longer appropriate. Another 38% improved. However, approximately 10% became socially more "autistic." Speech impairments were more stable, with approximately half showing neither improvement nor deterioration. At follow-up, approximately half the children had not developed functional speech and onset of seizures was sometimes accompanied by regression in speech. Although usually improved, most children still exhibited some level of ritualistic and compulsive behaviors. Cognitively, those children diagnosed with infantile psychosis performed better on measures of performance ability than on those of verbal ability.

In an epidemiological study, Lotter (1974a,b) followed 32 children with autism from initial diagnosis at 8 to 10 years of age to follow-up approximately 8 years later, comparing three groups: a group with definite autism (n=15), a less well-defined group with autism (n=17), and a comparison group (n=22). They examined outcomes as described by Rutter *et al.* (1967). For the combined group (i.e., the definite plus less well-defined groups) with autism, outcome was similar to that of Rutter *et al.* (1967): 14% had a "good" outcome, 24% had a "fair" outcome, and 62% had a "poor" or "very poor" outcome. They noted that no females demonstrated a "good" or "fair" outcome. Again, IQ and speech were related to outcome. A number of individuals experienced later adolescent onset of seizures, often during adolescence, a finding also reported by Rutter *et al.* (1967). By follow-up, one-third exhibited strong symptoms of neurological abnormalities (Rutter *et al.*, 1967).

In a similar study, DeMyer and colleagues (1973) followed 126 children initially evaluated at a mean of 5 years of age and re-examined at a mean of 12 years of age. Consistent with other studies, the majority of participants (60–75%) had a poor outcome and a very small minority (1–2%) had a "normal" recovery. The higher functioning the children were initially, the more likely they were to improve in speech and social skills. The best predictor of functioning in work and educational settings was initial functioning in this area, and many did not show improvement. Gillberg and Steffenberg (1987), in a follow-up study of children between the ages of 16 and 23 years originally diagnosed with infantile autism or other childhood psychoses, also found that early speech and IQ were closely associated with outcome. Similar to previous results, of the children diagnosed with infantile autism, 44% had a "poor" or "very poor" outcome and 17% had a "fair" or "good" outcome. The remaining 35% had a "restricted but acceptable outcome."

These initial follow-up studies established several important and currently accepted facts regarding the outcome of individuals who would, for the most part, meet criteria for autistic disorder. The likelihood of a positive outcome, in general, is low for children with autism. Those who function higher initially demonstrate more improvement with age. Early cognitive functioning and early development of functional speech are important predictors of outcome, while family situation is not a significant predictor. Finally, while the majority of children exhibit mental retardation (approximately 75%), performance IQ is generally better than verbal IQ (Filipek *et al.*, 1999). In fact, a substantial minority of individuals with autism will never be able to communicate verbally.

Changes in autistic symptoms

Research is generally consistent in demonstrating continuity over time of an ASD diagnosis, but there is also evidence of change in symptom severity, especially during adolescence (McGovern & Sigman, 2005). While most children diagnosed with an ASD in childhood continue to meet criteria during adolescence, parent report indicates improvements in several areas related to social functioning, adaptive functioning, and repetitive/stereotyped interests, with the most change noted in higher-functioning adolescents. In contrast, Gillberg and Steffenberg (1987) found that some individuals experienced an aggravation of symptoms (35%) or deterioration continuing through puberty (22%). This pattern was more prevalent in females. Waterhouse and Fein (1984) also documented loss of cognitive skills in some children with autism around puberty, which generally recovered by later adolescence. Furthermore, in the Gillberg and Steffenberg (1987) study, of those who deteriorated, 60% developed epilepsy during puberty. In total, 26% of their sample with autism had epilepsy. This is somewhat higher than more recent estimates that are around 15% (Howlin *et al.*, 2004). However, some parents and clinicians have reported increases in sociability at puberty (Park, 1967). The changes occurring at puberty may be the result of brain maturation and/or hormonal changes that occur during puberty. These may reflect the onset of affective disorder at that time, resulting in exacerbation of symptoms and deterioration of skills (Lainhart & Folstein, 1994), or the expression of the normal emotional turbulence of puberty in children with pre-existing social isolation, aggression, and inability to communicate verbally.

Fecteau and colleagues (2003) found significant improvements in social, communication, and restricted interest/repetitive interests with improvement varying across domains and among items using the Autism Diagnostic Interview-Revised (ADI-R: Lord *et al.*, 1994). Similarly, Piven and colleagues (1996b) examined autistic symptoms in high-IQ adolescents and young adults with autism and retrospectively at age 5 using the ADI-R and found that behaviors generally improved over time. In both studies, more participants exhibited improvement in communication and social behaviors than in ritualistic/repetitive behaviors. This is consistent with the pattern noted by Rutter *et al.* (1967).

As children with an ASD grow older, many, particularly those who are high-functioning, begin to perceive that they are different from their typically developing peers. This can have implications for their socio-emotional health. For example, Bauminger and Kasari (2000) investigated loneliness and friendship in 22 high-functioning children with autism (ages 8–14) compared to controls and found that the children with autism reported greater feelings of loneliness. While all children with autism reported having at least one friend, their friendships were of poor quality. Likewise, adolescents with ASD are generally at higher risk for depression and anxiety (Kim *et al.*, 2000).

Stability of early diagnosis

Some of the studies mentioned previously (DeMyer *et al.*, 1973; Piven *et al.*, 1996a) address whether individuals no longer meet criteria for ASD as they enter later childhood, adolescence, and adulthood. Following this, studies have examined the stability of the early diagnosis of autistic disorder and have found that the diagnosis is generally stable in children ages 3 and 4 years (Charman *et al.*, 2005; Cox *et al.*, 1999; Gillberg, 1990; Lord, 1995; Moore & Goodson, 2003; Sigman & Ruskin, 1999; Stone *et al.*, 1999). However, the diagnosis of ASD is less stable, presumably because it includes less-affected children. A diagnosis of an ASD includes children who meet criteria for autistic disorder as well as those children who evidence significant impairment in social skills and either an impairment in communication or stereo-typed behaviors but do not meet criteria for autistic disorder (American Psychiatric Association, 2000).

Recently, Eaves and Ho (2004) evaluated the reliability of early diagnoses. Two-year-olds with symptoms of autism were given an evaluation and were then re-evaluated at age 4½ years. Eighty-eight percent were initially diagnosed with an ASD. Between the two evaluations, 79% remained in the same diagnostic category, while about 10% moved in either direction. Five children became more autistic (PDD-NOS to autistic disorder), and five children became less autistic (autism to PDD-NOS and ASD to non-ASD). Notably, no children moved onto the spectrum between initial and follow-up assessments. Reliability was higher for autistic disorder than for PDD-NOS. In agreement with other studies, higher-functioning children improved the most, but improvement was unrelated to intervention. IQ was not stable, with two-thirds changing in both directions by over 20 points, providing evidence that measures of cognitive ability may not be very reliable at age 2 in children with autism. However, performance IQ at 4 years has been found to be highly correlated with performance IQ at age 10 in children with autistic disorder (Lord & Schopler, 1989).

Moore and Goodson (2003) also found that a diagnosis of an ASD at age 2 is reliable. Like Eaves and Ho (2004), they found that, although some children moved in both directions in terms of diagnoses, diagnosis was relatively stable. All children with an ASD at age 2 continued to meet criteria for an ASD at follow-up. Furthermore, social and communication skills were fairly stable. This study, as well as others, supports the idea that symptom presentation may change with age; repetitive behaviors are apparent by age 4 to 5, but at age 2 are rarely observed (Cox *et al.*, 1999). Generally, it is understood that children with an ASD at 2 years may have less prominent repetitive and stereotyped behaviors, but are characterized by greater impairments in social communicative behaviors, especially joint attention (e.g., Charman *et al.*, 1997, 1998; Charman & Baird, 2002; Mundy *et al.*, 1994;

Swettenham *et al.*, 1998). In fact, because repetitive behaviors are rare in 2-year-olds, different diagnostic criteria may be needed for very young children (Stone *et al.*, 1999).

Although there is the possibility of change in either direction, in general, the early diagnosis of autism has been found to be reliable and is crucial for the implementation of early intervention (Charman *et al.*, 2005; Cox *et al.*, 1999; Eaves & Ho, 2004; Gillberg, 1990; Lord, 1995; Moore & Goodson, 2003; Sigman & Ruskin, 1999; Stone *et al.*, 1999). In addition, research has also demonstrated that the symptoms exhibited by young children vary to some degree from the clinical picture exhibited by older children with an ASD.

Adult outcomes

Research has also attempted to extend outcome findings into adulthood. In a recent study examining adult outcomes for individuals with autism, it was found that 22% had "very good" or "good" outcome, while 58% had "poor" or "very poor" outcome (Howlin *et al.*, 2004). Again, IQ was found to be an important predictor of outcome. Even for those adults with improved outcome, impairments remain (Howlin *et al.*, 2000, 2004). Most individuals with autism are unable to live independently (Howlin *et al.*, 2000; Wolf & Goldberg, 1986). For example, Wolf and Goldberg (1986) found that 69% of their sample (mean age, 17 years) was living in an institutional or group home, while the rest were living at home. Ruble and Dalrymple (1996) found that approximately half of their sample (17 years or older) was living at home. When compared to those with developmental receptive language disorder in adulthood, those with autism continue to demonstrate greater impairments in many domains, with a majority having severe social impairments (Howlin *et al.*, 2000).

According to the traditional definition of a "good outcome," generally defined as the "achievement of independence and a normal social life" (DeMyer *et al.*, 1973; Gillberg & Steffenburg, 1987; Kobayashi *et al.*, 1992; Rutter, 1970), all 46 of the participants in the study by Ruble and Dalrymple (1996) had a poor outcome, although many were participating in community and family activities and reported being generally happy. While the authors acknowledge the ongoing impairments and difficulties these individuals continue to experience through adulthood, they suggest, like Lord and Venter (1992), that a definition of outcome should also include other criteria, such as self-report of happiness.

Subgroups of children with ASDs

Lotter (1974b) was one of the first to explore the possibility of subgroups of children with autism. Since this time, researchers have often suggested that high- and low-functioning autism be considered separately (Cohen *et al.*, 1987; Tsai,

1992). Indeed, Fein and colleagues found that these two subtypes are divided based on cognitive functioning and have different developmental trajectories (Fein *et al.*, 1999; Stevens *et al.*, 2000). Greater improvements were found in the higher functioning group, especially in the social and communication domains (similar to the findings of McGovern & Sigman, 2005). Furthermore, this group was more likely to no longer meet criteria for an ASD by school age. The trajectory for the lower functioning group was more stable in terms of symptom severity and declined somewhat in cognitive functioning. Similarly, a hierarchical cluster analysis resulted in two subgroups of school-age children, a low- and high-functioning group, differing in social, language, and nonverbal ability (Stevens *et al.*, 2000). The higher functioning group had near normal cognitive scores and behavior. This group did not differ from the worse outcome group on the severity of their autism at preschool, but were higher functioning cognitively at preschool.

Other researchers have examined the differing trajectories that may be expected for children with different ASDs, namely autism or Asperger syndrome. High-functioning children diagnosed with autism or Asperger syndrome at age 4–6 years were assessed 2 years later and again at age 10–13 years (Starr *et al.*, 2003; Szatmari *et al.*, 2000, 2003). Between initial assessment and first follow-up, they found that the groups follow developmental trajectories that are, in general, parallel, with both groups improving but the Asperger group functioning better (Starr *et al.*, 2003; Szatmari *et al.*, 2000). Furthermore, they found that the degree to which early language and nonverbal skills predicts outcome differs between the two diagnoses in that it was stronger for those with autism (Szatmari *et al.*, 2003).

Optimal outcome

Is "recovery" or a truly optimal outcome possible for children diagnosed with ASD in early childhood? In many of the studies described above, there is a small group described as having "good," "excellent," or "optimal" outcome, or a small group who are no longer diagnosable with ASD. Sometimes this is taken as evidence of some unreliability in the early diagnosis, but it is equally possible that the early diagnosis was correct and that the individual did indeed move off the autism spectrum. Definitions of good outcome vary widely by study, and in many cases, good outcome means holding a job, living independently, and having some meaningful relationships, but still being diagnosable with an ASD. However, excluding this group, there appear to be many studies documenting children who move off the ASD spectrum some time during childhood. In addition to the studies described above, there are several carefully done treatment studies (described below) that document these outcomes.

Ongoing work by our group has documented "optimal outcome" in several studies. Optimal outcome is considered to be moving off the ASD spectrum and functioning in the normal range on standardized measures of cognitive, language, and adaptive functioning. It does not exclude residual or comorbid deficits, for example, residual language problems, obsessionality, social awkwardness, or psychiatric conditions such as anxiety or depression. Kelley *et al.* (2006) studied 14 children with well-described autism spectrum conditions in early childhood who had optimal outcomes by age 6–9. All were mainstreamed with no one-on-one assistance, and scored in the normal range on all standardized tests of language, cognition, and adaptive (including social) functioning. A detailed examination of their language, however, revealed residual language deficits in many of the children, including problems with understanding mental state verbs ("guess", "estimate"), inductive reasoning about animate objects, second-order theory of mind, and narrative production. An ongoing study is following these children in early adolescence and generally showing that they are continuing to close the gap with normal controls, showing even fewer and milder residual language problems. Fein *et al.* (2005), described 11 children (2 overlapping with Kelley *et al.*, 2006) with clear ASD who evolved into an ADHD clinical picture, but no longer met criteria for ASD. One of our ongoing studies (Sutera *et al.*, 2007) using an early detection sample is finding that about 20% of children diagnosed with ASD at age 2 move off the spectrum by age 4. So far, we have not been able to identify any developmental or symptomatic variables that can predict this movement (including head circumference), except for better motor functioning at age 2. It is difficult to believe that little in their clinical presentation would differ from the children with less optimal outcomes, but at least it does confirm the validity of their diagnoses, since they did not differ from the children with continued ASD diagnoses. All of the children did receive significant amounts of early intervention, but of different types and intensity, and probably differing in quality, so perhaps some answers to their variable outcomes will lie in analysis of intervention. Helt *et al.* (2008) discuss mechanisms that might underlie the behavioral recovery of such children.

Intervention

Individuals with an ASD present a diverse array of symptoms; therefore, a single effective intervention method for individuals with an ASD may not be found. Despite the social deficits inherent in a diagnosis of an ASD, effective interventions have historically focused on building cognitive and academic skills. Recently, however, treatment methods have begun to emphasize social relatedness and relationship building, which are the key deficits in ASD. The most effective interventions probably need to address both cognitive and social deficits.

Behavioral interventions

Applied behavior analysis (ABA), and related methods, use a stimulus–response learning technique and break down complex tasks into basic, achievable steps. Positive reinforcers are used to shape, achieve, maintain, and generalize behavioral goals. Maladaptive behaviors are decreased or eliminated by replacing unwanted behaviors with prompted appropriate behaviors, which are then positively re-inforced. ABA is structured by adults who are working with the child, and the child's progress is monitored by objective measurement. The goal of ABA is to teach cognitive and social skills, as well as providing pleasurable social experiences, and to decrease maladaptive behaviors, with the assumption that social relatedness and positive feelings toward other people will follow. ABA as a treatment for individuals with ASD is the most evidence-supported method for improving outcomes.

An early and important empirical study that identified an effective treatment for individuals with autism used ABA (Lovaas, 1987). In this study, principles of behavioral analysis were applied to 38 children with autism. The treatment team consisted of all individuals in the child's environment, including the child's thera-pist, parents, and teachers. Intensive intervention consisted of 40 hours per week, lasting for more than 2 years. In the intensive treatment group, Lovaas (1987) reported that 47% of the children achieved normal intellectual and educational functioning, whereas, only 2% of the control group showed similar improvement. Lovaas' results were unique at the time due to his use of a control group and close-to random assignment of participants. (Participants were assigned to the experimental group unless there were an insufficient number of staff members available to provide treatment.) Lovaas' outcome measures, however, did not assess play skills and communicative language.

Sallows and Graupner (2005) have replicated Lovaas' findings by using the method developed by Lovaas and comparing a clinic-directed group to a parent-directed group of children receiving intervention. Both groups were similar in hours of treatment per week, with children receiving 39 hours per week in the clinic-directed group and 32 hours per week in the parent-directed group during year 1. During year 2, hours of intervention per week decreased 1 to 2 hours, and each year thereafter, intervention hours gradually decreased as children were integrated into a school setting.

Across groups, 48% of the children attained an IQ above 85 after 4 years of treatment. All of these children displayed rapid acquisition of new material early in treatment. Pretreatment characteristics, rather than clinic- vs. parent-directed intervention and hours per week of intervention, were most likely to predict outcome. Higher levels of pretreatment imitative skills, receptive language, IQ, social interaction, and adaptive skills predicted posttreatment IQ, adaptive skills, and language scores. Additionally, the authors reported that many of these children had their diagnosis of an ASD removed by their referring psychiatrist post-treatment.

Smith *et al.* (2000) also attempted to replicate Lovaas' impressive findings and compared a group of children who received an average of 24.5 hours per week of ABA to a group of children who received parent training consisting of ABA techniques as their sole intervention. All children were between the ages of 18 and 42 months at the time of referral. Although not as impressive as Lovaas' results, they found that children who received ABA intervention made more gains in cognitive and academic skills than the group of children who received only parent-training intervention. Additionally, children diagnosed with PDD-NOS made more gains than children diagnosed with autistic disorder. However, neither treatment group made gains in adaptive skills.

Further attempts have been made to examine the effects of ABA in older children. Eikeseth *et al.* (2002) assigned children with ASD to receive either behavioral intervention or eclectic intervention, both of which occurred at the child's elementary school. Children in both groups received a minimum of 20 hours per week of treatment. In addition to 20 weekly hours of treatment, children in both groups were mainstreamed with his/her typical classmates, while being shadowed by a therapist in order to promote generalization of acquired skills. The ABA group's treatment was based on Lovaas' method, with the additional emphasis on play and social skills. The eclectic treatment group incorporated elements from TEACCH (please see description of TEACCH later in this chapter), sensory–motor integration, and ABA. Findings revealed that children in the ABA treatment group made greater gains in IQ, language, and adaptive behavior than children in the eclectic treatment group. An additional recent study (Howard *et al.*, 2005) also compared intense ABA-type treatment with eclectic intensive and less intensive treatments. Although there were some limitations in the study's methodology (parent-selected rather than random assignment, and children in the ABA group starting on average 6 months younger), the results were quite dramatic: children in the ABA group showed much steeper learning rates over the year and a half of the study, and showed average scores in the normal range for most skills (with language skills lagging behind in the mildly delayed range). The study does not report how many children in any of the groups showed normal-range skills in all areas, or how many had lost their autistic symptomatology, but examination of the individual scores presented for receptive and expressive language reveals that there was a small group of children in each group who did especially well and a small group in the ABA group who made little improvement, but that, for the majority of children, the ABA treatment was clearly more effective for all skills.

Recent variations on Lovaas' discrete trial method have focused on the generalization, motivation, and functions of language. The Assessment of Basic Language and Learning (ABLLS) (developed by Sundberg and Partington, 1998) is based on B. F. Skinner's analysis of verbal behavior. The ABLLS program provides guidance in assessing a child's current level of functioning and designing an effective intervention plan in the areas of language, imitation, play, social, academic, and adaptive skills (focusing on achieving fluency and automaticity) and learning in natural environments. This program has not yet been evaluated to see if language outcomes can be enhanced by this specialized form of ABA.

Developmental interventions

Whereas behavioral interventions are driven by adult-directed activities, developmental interventions are child-driven and more naturalistic. The goal of developmental interventions is to encourage social relatedness, with the assumption that cognitive and other skills will follow. One popular developmental intervention, Floor Time (Greenspan & Wieder, 2000), focuses on the therapist engaging in shared experiences with the child. The therapist follows the child's lead in an attempt to create a meaningful relationship. The gains that a child makes using this type of therapy are less objectively measurable than with ABA.

The SCERTS model (Prizant *et al.*, 2000) also involves allowing the child to direct the activities in a naturalistic manner. However, the therapist takes advantage of the child's intrinsic motivation to communicate with the therapist, structuring the environment in such a way that the child is required to communicate in order to meet his/her needs. The therapist relies on naturally occurring events to elicit communication, while also incorporating behavioral strategies. The therapist models appropriate behavior, and often incorporates social stories or scripts to teach the child necessary skills.

Relationship development intervention (RDI) assumes that "individuals with autism spectrum disorders can participate in authentic emotional relationships if they are exposed to them in a gradual, systematic way." There are several books and a website devoted to RDI (Gutstein, 2001; Gutstein & Sheely, 2002a,b) describing this program, which is increasing in popularity. However, there are no controlled studies demonstrating its comparative effectiveness.

The Denver model (developed by Sally Rogers and colleagues) emphasizes the development of play, positive affect, interpersonal relationships, and language. The child is engaged in constant, coordinated social relatedness so that symbolic and interpersonal communication can be established. Language development is targeted by the adult being sensitive to the child's self-directed activities in a natural environment, and using these activities to create a need for the child to communicate. Additionally, nonverbal communication is stressed. Rogers and DiLalla (1991) report accelerating developmental gains, such as symbolic play and affective, reciprocal exchanges, for children enrolled in the program.

Social stories

Social stories (see Sansosti *et al.*, 2004, for a review of the literature), are commonly used to present appropriate social behaviors to children with autism in the form of a story. They are useful for teaching children routines, conversational exchanges, idioms, others' intentions and perspectives, how to do an activity, how to ask for help, and how to handle emotions such as anger and frustration. Descriptive sentences are used to describe what people do in particular social scenarios, and directive sentences state, in positive terms, what the desired behavior is. Perspective sentences present others' reactions to a situation. After the social story is reviewed with the child, control sentences identify strategies to facilitate memory and comprehension. For every directive or control sentence, there are typically two to five descriptive or perspective sentences. Stories are then faded by reviewing them less frequently with the child and replacing control and directive sentences with descriptive and perspective sentences. Social stories is easily combined with other intervention programs and can be a useful adjunct to behavioral or developmental approaches.

TEACCH

The Treatment and Education of Autistic and Related Communication Handicapped Children (TEACCH) was developed at the University of North Carolina by Eric Schopler (Mesibov, Shea, & Schopler, 2004). TEACCH recognizes the heterogeneity of individuals with autism and is individually tailored to each child's unique strengths (such as visuo-spatial processing and interest in routine and repetitive activities) rather than focusing on deficits. The TEACCH method involves using structured teaching to teach functional skills that the individual shows a readiness to learn. In addition, part of the TEACCH philosophy is to accommodate the environment to the individual's autism-related deficits and allow them to use his/her strengths to compensate for such deficits. When combined with an intensive behavioral program, skills such as imitation, perception, cognition, and motor skills improve (Ozonoff & Cathcart, 1998).

Peer training

Peer training has also been used to enhance the treatment of preschool and early elementary age children with an ASD (Kohler *et al.*, 1997; Strain & Hoyson, 2000). Educating peers on developmental disabilities and differences, as well as the strengths that children with disabilities often have, can aid in a child's success in an inclusion setting. Prior to mainstreaming, peers are often brought into a small setting to work on social skills training, with an emphasis on the peers modeling appropriate behavior. Children with an ASD are then mainstreamed into a typical classroom where adults coach and prompt, when necessary, appropriate behavior.

Several rigorous research programs are currently evaluating the effectiveness of several different peer interventions and social skills groups in improving social skills in autism.

In sum, there are many factors that contribute to treatment outcome, and intervention does not independently lead to a positive outcome. While intervention is highly important, prognosis depends upon as-yet unknown relations between child characteristics, such as initial language and joint attention skills, and amount and type of intervention (Bono *et al.*, 2004). Koegel *et al.* (2001) hypothesize that there are pivotal areas that influence outcome. Such pivotal skills, such as spontaneous self-initiations, are related to a positive response to treatment (Mundy *et al.*, 1994). Furthermore, children can be taught these pivotal skills, thereby leading to more favorable treatment outcomes (Koegel *et al.*, 1999).

Behaviorally based programs have the most empirical support for treating children with an ASD. Crucial elements seem to include intensive, behaviorally based, structured interventions with specific goals, plans for promoting maintenance and generalization of skills, involvement of parents, reducing interfering behaviors, and the development of positive relationships with therapists, and later, with other children (Dawson & Osterling, 1997; Rogers, 1998). Last, beginning intervention as early as possible for children diagnosed with an ASD seems critical to a positive outcome (e.g., Harris & Handleman [2000] found better outcomes in children starting behavioral programs at a mean age of 3.5 years vs. those starting at 4.5 years), although controlled studies of age at start of treatment are few.

Although full normalization of behavior and cognition are the exception rather than the rule, longitudinal studies of diagnostic stability, while reporting generally stable diagnosis, also report children moving off the spectrum, as do studies reporting successful treatment outcome. As described above, our group has also described two groups of children who moved off the ASD spectrum (Fein *et al.*, 2005; Kelley *et al.*, 2006), and our ongoing studies are finding that approximately 20% of young children are moving off the spectrum during early childhood. Given the anatomic and genetic abnormalities outlined above, how is such movement possible?

Mechanisms of improvement

The answer, of course, is that no one knows, and even speculation on this question is in its infancy. Few papers have addressed this issue, and the few that have are speculative; no neurobiological mechanisms have directly been tested in this group of individuals with optimal outcome.

Mundy and Crosson (1997) were among the first to consider the theoretical implications of the "recovery hypothesis," namely that children with autism could essentially recover. They argue that, since impaired joint attention is perhaps the most pathognomonic sign of autism, improvement to normal levels in joint attention and other social communication skills should be essential in considering a child "recovered." They also suggest that infrequent initiation of joint attention acts in young children with autism may reflect a gap in their inherent social motivation system. They speculate that there is a "transient disturbance" in neurological functioning at a time when social interaction and social cognition are rapidly developing and that, consequently, the child is severely deprived of the necessary complex social input. In addition to severely impacting the development of social behavior, this deflects the child further and further from the path of normal development in many other ways. The initial, primary disturbance produces a cascading downstream series of effects in other behavioral systems. The effectiveness of early intervention, they suggest, lies in its ability to provide social input, preventing the secondary neurological disturbances. Behavioral treatment, they suggest, acts as a scaffolding for the development of other skills, such as cognitive and linguistic skills, during the months and years when these skills must be developing.

This idea seems quite consonant with much of the literature on early development in autism. The burgeoning literature on the early effects of experience on brain development may provide results with which to fill in the details in the Mundy and Crowson model. One implication of the model seems inconsistent with some of the intervention results: if social motivation (and attention to social input) is the fundamental deficit, and effectiveness of treatment depends on its ability to remediate this fundamental motivational deficit, one might expect that treatments focused on "wooing" the child into feeling more positive about interaction would be the most effective. However, although controlled, randomized studies of these types of intervention compared with more structured teaching approaches are sorely lacking, the available data suggest to us that more structured teaching of specific skills, including social skills, is generally more effective. It is possible that, at least for some children, the social motivation impairment is so severe and fundamental that merely making interactions as attractive as possible will not turn this impairment around. After all, social interaction between children and average parents is usually highly rewarding for the infant, and this interaction was not sufficient to engage the social motivation of the child. For children with autism, bypassing the engagement of the abnormal social motivation system and providing alternative motives, as in behavioral intervention where primary reinforcers and forceful prompting are initially used, may be necessary, at least in the early stages of intervention. In bypassing the abnormal motivation system and "forcing" social input as well as "forcing" the child to practice positive behaviors, the therapy may be leading to functional neural changes, which then leads the child to attach positive social–emotional valence to similar experiences. This would be parallel to treatment for dyslexia, in which motivating a dyslexic child to want to read may not change the way the brain processes reading material, but having them practice reading does (Temple *et al.*, 2003), which in turn may make them feel better about reading.

A second attempt to explain the possibility of recovery is that of Dawson and Zanolli (2003). They also suggest that poor social attention, especially attention to faces, is fundamental in the elaboration of autistic symptomatology. They speculate, based on the two-process theory of infant face perception by Morton and Johnson (1991), that face perception switches around 6 months of age from a subcortical to a cortical, "experience–expectant" system, which depends on substantial perceptual input about faces during a "sensitive period" for the development of an expert face processing system, which all normal humans possess. In support of this, congenital blindness from birth to 6 months permanently impairs the ability to process faces in a configural manner (Carey & Diamond, 1994). Dawson and Zanolli suggest that successful, behaviorally based intervention relies for its effectiveness on two processes. First, the attention to others' faces, and especially to others' eyes, which is a part of all behavioral intervention, promotes attention to social input. Second, the social feedback, such as praise, positive affect, and touching, provided by the therapist contingent on the child's social attention, serves to pair social stimuli with the primary reinforcers used in early stages of behavioral intervention. The social stimulation then comes to acquire secondary reinforcing value.

As with the Mundy and Crowson model (which is not inconsistent with that of Dawson and Zanolli), the overall idea is appealing, well supported by evidence outlined in their chapter, and consistent with the findings on early intervention. Two aspects of the theory seem to need addressing. First, if the sensitive period for face input is as early as the first 6 months of life, how could early intervention started as late as 3 years (which is still considered early for behavioral treatment) be successful? Perhaps the answer lies in the less than total disinterest of children with autism in others' faces. In some cases, the social disinterest appears to begin in the second year of life, perhaps allowing for the experience–expectant face processing system to get a good start. In other cases, the social disinterest may appear during the first year, but result in only a partial deprivation of experience, perhaps even prolonging the period of possible plasticity. The second point relates to the suggestion that adults in the environment of the child with austim acquire a secondary reinforcing value when paired with primary reinforcers. This does seem to be what happens in early treatment. However, once social rewards appear to be motivating for the child, most behavioral programs gradually withdraw the primary reinforcers. According to classic learning theory, this should result in a gradual extinction of the desired responses. Somehow, the social motivation has become functionally autonomous. We need a theory for how this comes about.

In addition to the promising suggestions of Mundy and Crowson (1997) and Dawson and Zanolli (2003), there are many possibilities for how early intervention might change brain functioning. Forcing the child to attend to social, language, and other inputs might allow these more complex, varied inputs to affect brain development as they are supposed to do. Perhaps suppression of interfering behaviors (which results in diminished attention to repetitive sensory and motor input) is the key for some children, allowing their attention to be captured by those stimuli important for social development. For some children, early forced normalization of inputs might be sufficient to normalize brain development to a greater or lesser extent. For others, abnormal brain development may be genetically fixed, but forcing the skill acquisition in a highly structured and bit-by-bit manner might allow the brain to find alternative pathways to relatively normal behavior. For yet others, the cognitive or motivational limitations inherent in their abnormal brain development will allow only limited progress. Understanding the probably varied etiologies for autism should shed light on which pathophysiologies are consistent with "recovery" and which ones limit progress even with the best intervention. Future research should also allow us to discover whether "recovered" children are behaviorally recovered but still share processing or structural similarities with those who remain autistic, or whether they are neurologically recovered as well.

REFERENCES

Abell, F., Krams, M., Ashburner, J., *et al.* (1999). The neuroanatomy of autism: A voxel-based whole brain analysis of structural scans. *Neuroreport*, **10**, 1647–51.

Akshoomoff, N., Lord, C., Lincoln, A. J., *et al.* (2004). Outcome classification of preschool children with autism spectrum disorders using MRI brain measures. *Journal of the American Academy of Child and Adolescent Psychiatry*, **43**, 349–57.

Alarcon, M., Cantor, R. M., Liu, J., Gilliam, T. C., & Geschwind, D. H. (2002). Evidence for a language quantitative trait locus on chromosome 7q in multiplex autism families. *American Journal of Human Genetics*, **70**, 60–71.

American Psychiatric Association. (2000). *Diagnostic and Statistical Manual of Mental Disorders –Text Revision*, 4th edn. Washington, DC: American Psychiatric Association.

Amir, R. E., Van den Veyver, I. B., Wan, M., *et al.* (1999). Rett syndrome is caused by mutations in X-linked MECP2 encoding methyl- CpG-binding protein 2. *Nature Genetics*, **23**, 185–9.

Aylward, E. H., Minshew, N. J., & Field, K. (2002). Effects of age on brain volume and head circumference in autism. *Neurology*, **59**, 175–83.

Bailey, A., le Couteur, A., Gottesman, I., *et al.* (1995). Autism as a strongly genetic disorder: Evidence from a British twin study. *Psychological Medicine*, **25**, 63–77.

Barton, M. & Volkmar, F. (1998). How commonly are known medical conditions associated with autism? *Journal of Autism and Developmental Disorders*, **28**, 273–8.

Bauman, M. L. & Kemper, T. L. (2005). Neuroanatomic observations of the brain in autism: A review and future directions. *International Journal of Developmental Neuroscience*, **23**, 183–7.

Bauminger, N. & Kasari, C. (2000). Loneliness and friendship in high-functioning children with autism. *Child Development*, **71**, 447–56.

Bolton, P., Macdonald, H., Pickles, A., *et al.* (1994). A case-control family history study of autism. *Journal of Child Psychology & Psychiatry*, **35**(5), 877–900.

Bolton, P., Murphy, M., & Macdonald, H. (1997). Obstetric complications in autism: Consequences or causes of the condition? *Journal of the American Academy of Child and Adolescent Psychiatry*, **36**(2), 272–81.

Bono, M. A., Daley, T., & Sigman, M. (2004). Relations among joint attention, amount of intervention and language gain in autism. *Journal of Autism and Developmental Disorders*, **34**, 495–505.

Bradford, Y., Haines, J., Hutcheson, H., *et al.* (2001). Phenotypic homogeneity provides increased support for linkage on chromosome 2 in autistic disorder. *American Journal of Medical Genetics*, **105**, 539–47.

Carey, S. and Diamond, R. (1994). Are faces perceived as configurations more by adults than by children? *Visual Cognition*, **1**, 253–74.

Casanova, M. F., Buxhoeveden, D. P., Switala, A. E., & Roy, E. (2002). Neuronal density and architecture (gray level index) in the brains of autistic patients. *Journal of Child Neurology*, **17**, 515–21.

Chakrabarti, S. & Fombonne, E. (2005). Pervasive developmental disorders in preschool children: Confirmation of high prevalence. *Archives of General Psychiatry*, **162**, 1133–41.

Charman, T. & Baird, G. (2002). Practitioner review: Diagnosis of autism spectrum disorder in 2- and 3-year-old children. *Journal of Child Psychology and Psychiatry*, **43**(3), 289–305.

Charman, T., Baron-Cohen, S., Swettenham, J., Cox, A., Baird, G., & Drew, A. (1998). An experimental investigation of social-cognitive abilities in infants with autism: Clinical implications. *Infant Mental Health Journal*, **19**, 260–75.

Charman, T., Swettenham, J., Baron-Cohen, S., Cox, A., Baird, G., & Drew, A. (1997). Infants with autism: An investigation of empathy, pretend play, joint attention and imitation. *Developmental Psychology*, **33**, 781–9.

Charman, T., Taylor, E., Drew, A., Cockerill, H., Brown, J. A., & Baird, G. (2005). Outcome at 7 years of children diagnosed with autism at age 2: Predictive validity of assessments conducted at 2 and 3 years of age and pattern of symptom change over time. *Journal of Child Psychology and Psychiatry*, **46**(5), 500–13.

Cohen, P. J., Paul, R., & Volkmar, F. (1987). Issues in the classification of PDD and associated conditions. In D. J. Cohen, A. M. Donnellan, & R. R. Paul (Eds.). *Handbook of Autism & Pervasive Developmental Disorders* (pp. 20–40). New York: Wiley.

Comings, D. & Comings, B. (1991). Clinical and genetic relationships between Autism pervasive developmental disorder and Tourette syndrome: A study of 19 Cases. *American Journal of Medical Genetics*, **39**, 180–91.

Cook, E. H. (2001). Genetics of autism. *Child and Adolescent Psychiatric Clinics of North America*, **10**(2), 333–50.

Courchesne, E., Carper, R., & Akshoomoff, N. (2003). Evidence of brain overgrowth in the first year of life in autism. *Journal of the American Medical Association*, **290**, 337–44.

Courchesne, E., Karns, C. M., Davis, H. R., *et al.* (2001). Unusual brain growth patterns in early life in patients with autistic disorder: An MRI study. *Neurology*, **57**, 245–54.

Cox, A., Klein, K., Charman, T., *et al.* (1999). Autism spectrum disorders at 20 and 42 months of age: Stability of clinical and ADI-R diagnosis. *Journal of Child Psychology and Psychiatry,* **40**, 719–32.

Dawson, G. (2008). Early behavioral intervention, brain plasticity, and the prevention of autism spectrum disorder. *Development and Psychopathology* **20**, 775–803.

Dawson, G. & Osterling, J. (1997). Early interevention in autism. In Guralnick, J. (Ed.). *The Effectivenss of Early Intervention* (pp. 307–26). Baltimore, MD: Brookes Publishing.

Dawson, G., Webb, S., Schellenberg, G., *et al.* (2002). Defining the broader phenotype of autism: Genetic, brain, and behavioral perspectives. *Development and Psychopathology*, **14**(3), 581–611.

Dawson, G. & Zanolli, K. (2003). Early intervention and brain plasticity in autism. In Novartis Foundation Symposium. *Autism: Neural Basis and Treatment Possibilities* (pp. 266–80). London: Wiley.

Dementieva, Y. A., Vance, D. D., Donnelly, S. L., *et al.* (2005). Accelerated head growth in early development of individual with autism. *Pediatric Neurology*, **32**, 102–8.

DeMyer, M. K., Barton, S., DeMyer, W. E., Norton, J. A., Allen, J., & Steele, R. (1973). Prognosis in autism: A follow-up study. *Journal of Autism and Childhood Schizophrenia*, **3**(3), 199–246.

Deutsch, C. K. & Joseph, R. M. (2003). Brief report: Cognitive correlates of enlarged head circumferences in children with autism. *Journal of Autism and Developmental Disorders*, **33**, 209–14.

Deykin, E. Y. & MacMahon, B. (1980). Pregnancy, delivery and neonatal complications among autistic children. *American Journal of Disabled Children*, **134**, 860–4.

Eaves, L. C. & Ho, H. H. (2004). The very early identification of autism: Outcome to age 4 ½ –5. *Journal of Autism and Developmental Disorders*, **34**(4), 367–78.

Egaas, B., Courchesne, E., & Saitoh, O. (1995). Reduced size of corpus callosum in autism. *Archives of Neurology*, **52**, 794–801.

Eikeseth, S., Smith, T., Jahr, E., & Eldevik, S. (2002). Intensive behavioral treatment at school for 4- to 7-year old children with autism: A 1-year comparison controlled study. *Behavior Modification*, **26**, 49–68.

Elia, M., Ferri, R., Musumeci, S. A., *et al.* (2000). Sleep in subjects with autistic disorder: A neuropsychological and psychological study. *Brain Development* **22**, 88–92.

Fecteau, S., Mottron, L., Berthiaume, C., & Burack, J. A. (2003). Developmental changes of autistic symptoms. *Autism*, **7**(3), 255–68.

Fein, D., Dixon, P., & Paul, J. (2005). Brief report: Pervasive developmental disorder can evolve into ADHD. Case illustrations. *Journal of Autism and Developmental Disorders*, **35**, 525–34.

Fein, D., Stevens, M., Dunn, M., *et al.* (1999). Subtypes of pervasive developmental disorder: Clinical characteristics. *Child Neuropsychology*, **5**, 1–23.

Filipek, P. A., Accardo, P. J., Baranek, G. T., *et al.* (1999). The screening and diagnosis of autistic spectrum disorder. *Journal of Autism and Developmental Disorders*, **29**(6), 439–84.

Finnegan, J. A. & Quarrington, B. (1979). Pre-, peri-, and neonatal factors and infantile autism. *Journal of Child Psychology and Psychiatry*, **20**, 119–28.

Folstein, S. (1999). Autism. *International Review of Psychiatry*, **11**(4), 269–77.

Folstein, S. & Mankoski, R. (2000). Invited editorial: Chromosome 7 q. Where autism meets language disorder? *American Journal of Human Genetics*, **67**, 278–81.

Folstein, S. & Rutter, M. (1977). Infantile autism: A genetic study of 21 twin pairs. *Journal of Child Psychology and Psychiatry*, **18**, 297–321.

Folstein, S. & Rutter, M. (1988). Autism: Familial aggregation and genetic implications. *Journal of Autism and Developmental Disorders*, **18**(1), 3–30.

Fombonne, E., Bolton, P., Prior, J., Jordan, H., & Rutter, M. (1997). A family study of autism: Cognitive patterns and levels in parents and siblings. *Journal of Child Psychology and Psychiatry*, **38**(6), 667–83.

Gillberg, C. (1990). Autism and pervasive developmental disorders. *Journal of Child Psychology and Psychiatry*, **31**, 99–119.

Gillberg, C. & Gillberg, I. C. (1983). Infantile autism: A total population study of reduced optimality in pre-, peri-, and neonatal period. *Journal of Autism and Developmental Disorders*, **13**(2), 153–66.

Gillberg, C. & Steffenburg, S. (1987). Outcome and prognostic factors in infantile autism and similar conditions: A population-based study of 46 cases followed through puberty. *Journal of Autism and Developmental Disorders*, **17**(2), 273–87.

Greenspan, S. I. & Wieder, S. (2000). A developmental approach to difficulties in relating and communicating in autism spectrum disorders and related syndromes. In E. Wetherby & B. Prizant (Eds.), *Autism Spectrum Disorders: A Transactional Developmental Perspective* (pp. 279–303). Baltimore: Paul H. Brooks.

Gustafsson, L. (1997). Inadequate cortical feature maps: A neural circuit theory of autism. *Biological Psychiatry*, **42**, 1138–47.

Gustafsson, L. (2004). Comment on "Disruption in the inhibitory architecture of the cell minicolumn: Implications for autism." *The Neuroscientist*, **10**, 189–91.

Gutstein, S. E. (2001). *Autism/Asperger's: Solving the Relationship Puzzle*. Arlington, TX: Future Horizons Press.

Gutstein, S. & Sheely, R. (2002a). *Relationship Development Intervention: Activities for Children, Adolescents, and Adults*. London: Jessica Kingsley Publications.

Gutstein, S. & Sheely, R. (2002b). *Relationship Development Intervention Activities for Young Children*. London: Jessica Kingsley Publications.

Happe, F., Ehlers, S., Fletcher, P., *et al.* (1996). 'Theory of mind' in the brain. Evidence from a PET scan study of Asperger syndrome. *Neuroreport: An International Journal for the Rapid Communication of Research in Neuroscience*, **8**, 197–201.

Harden, A. Y., Minshew, N. J., & Keshavan, M. S. (2000). Corpus callosum size in autism. *Neurology*, **55**, 1033–6.

Harris, S. L. & Handleman, J. S. (2000). Age and IQ at intake as predictors of placement for young children with autism: A four- to six-year follow-up. *Journal of Autism and Developmental Disorders*, **30**(2), 137–42.

Hashimoto, T., Tayama, M., Murakawa, K., *et al.* (1995). Development of the brainstem and cerebellum in autistic patients. *Journal of Autism and Developmental Disorders*, **25**, 1–18.

Helt, M., Kelley, E., Kinsbourne, M., *et al.* (2008). Can children with autism recover? If so, how? *Neuropsychology Review*, **18**, 339–66.

Herbert, M. R. (2005). Autism: A brain disorder, or a disorder that affects the brain? *Clinical Neuropsychiatry: Journal of Treatment Evaluation*, **2**, 354–79.

Herbert, M. R., Ziegler, D. A., Deutsch, C. K., *et al.* (2003). Dissociations of cerebral cortex, subcortical and cerebral white matter volumes in autistic boys. *Brain*, **126**, 1182–92.

Horwitz B., Rumsey, J. M., Grady, C. L., & Rapoport, S. I. (1988). The cerebral metabolic landscape in autism. *Archives of Neurology*, **45**, 749–55.

Howard, J., Sparkman, C., Cohen, H., Green, G., & Stanislaw, H. (2005). A comparison of intensive behavioral analytic and eclectic treatments for young children with autism. *Research in Developmental Disabilities*, **26**, 359–83.

Howlin, P., Good, S., Hutton, J., & Rutter, M. (2004). Adult outcome for children with autism. *Journal of Child Psychology and Psychiatry*, **45**(2), 212–29.

Howlin, P., Mawhood, L., & Rutter, M. (2000). Autism and developmental receptive language disorder – a follow-up comparison in early adult life. II: Social, behavioral, and psychiatric outcomes. *Journal of Child Psychology and Psychiatry*, **41**(5), 561–78.

Jones, M. & Szatmari, P. (1988). Stoppage rules and genetic studies of autism. *Journal of Autism and Developmental Disorders*, **18**(1), 31–40.

Just, M. A., Cherkassky, V. L., Keller, T. A., & Minshew, N. J. (2004). Cortical activation and synchronization during sentence comprehension in high-functioning autism: Evidence of underconnectivity. *Brain*, **127**, 1811–21.

Kanner, L. (1943). Autistic disturbances of affective contact. *Nervous Child*, **2**, 217–50.

Kelley, E., Fein, D., & Naigles, L. (2006). Language functioning in optimal outcome children with a history of autistic spectrum disorders. *Journal of Autism and Developmental Disorders*. **36**, 807–28.

Kim, J. A., Szatmari, P., Bryson, S. E., Streiner, D. L., & Wilson, F. J. (2000). The prevalence of anxiety and mood problems among children with autism and Asperger syndrome. *Autism*, **4** (2), 117–32.

Kjelgaard, M. M. & Tager-Flusberg, H. (2001). An investigation of language impairment in autism: Implications for genetic subgroups. *Language and Cognitive Processes*, **16**, 287–308.

Kobayashi, I. L., Murata, T., & Yoshinaga, K. (1992). A follow-up study of 201 children with autism in Kyushu and Yamaguchi areas, Japan. *Journal of Autism and Developmental Disorders*, **22**, 395–411.

Koegel, R. L., Koegel, L. K., & McNerney, E. K. (2001). Pivotal areas in intervention for autism. *Journal of Clinical Child Psychology*, **30**, 19–32.

Koegel, L. K., Koegel, R. L., Shoshan, Y., & McNerney, E. K. (1999). Pivotal response intervention II: Preliminary long-term outcomes data. *Journal of the Association for Persons with Severe Handicaps*, **24**, 186–98.

Kohler, F. W., Strain, P. S., Hoyson, M., & Jamieson, B. (1997). Merging naturalistic teaching and peer-based strategies to address the IEP objectives of preschoolers with autism: An examination of structural and child behavior outcomes. *Focus on Autism and Other Developmental Disabilities*, **12**, 196–206.

Konstantereas, M. M. & Homatidis, S. (1999). Chromosomal abnormalities in a series of children with autistic disorder. *Journal of Autism and Developmental Disorders*, **29**(4), 275–85.

Koshino, H., Carpenter, P. A., Minshew, N. J., Cherkassky, V. L., Keller, T. A., & Just, M. A. (2005). Functional connectivity in an fMRI working memory task in high- functioning autism. *Neuroimage*, **24**, 810–21.

Lainhart, J. E. (1999). Psychiatric problems in individuals with autism, their parents and siblings. *International Review of Psychiatry*, **11**, 278–98.

Lainhart, J. E. & Folstein, S. E. (1994). Affective disorders in people with autism: A review of published cases. *Journal Journal of Autism and Developmental Disorders*, **24**, 587–601.

Landa, R., Piven, J., Wzorek, M., Gayle, J. O., Chase, G. A., & Folstein, S. E. (1992). Social language use in parents of autistic individuals. *Psychological Medicine*, **2**, 245–54.

Landa, R., Wzorek, M., Piven, J., Folstein, S. E., & Isaacs, C. (1991). Spontaneous narrative discourse characteristics of parents of autistic individuals. *Journal of Speech and Hearing Research*, **34**, 1339–45.

Landry, R. & Bryson, S. E. (2004). Impaired disengagement of attention in young children with autism. *Journal of Child Psychology and Psychiatry*, **45**, 1115–22.

Lauritsen, M. B., Mors, O., Mortensen, P. B., & Ewald, H. (1999). Infantile autism and associated autosomal chromosome abnormalities: A register-based study and literature survey. *Journal of Child Psychology and Psychiatry*, **40**, 335–45.

Liss, M., Saulnier, C., Fein, D., & Kinsbourne, M. (2006). Sensory and attention abnormalities in Autistic Spectrum Disorders. *Autism*, **10**(2), 155–72.

Lockyer, L. & Rutter, M. (1969). A five- to fifteen-year follow-up study of infantile psychosis III. Psychological aspects. *British Journal of Psychiatry*, **115**, 865–82.

Lockyer, L. & Rutter, M. (1970). A five- to fifteen-year follow-up study of infantile psychosis: IV. Patterns of cognitive ability. *British Journal of Social and Clinical Psychology*, **9**, 152–63.

Lord, C. (1995). Follow-up of two-year-olds referred for possible autism. *Journal of Child Psychology and Psychiatry*, **36**, 1365–82.

Lord, C., Mulloy, C., Wendelboe, M., & Schopler, E. (1991). Pre- and perinatal factors in high-functioning females and males with autism. *Journal of Autism and Developmental Disorders*, **21**(2), 197–209.

Lord, C., Rutter, M., & le Couteur, A. (1994). Autism diagnostic interview-revised: A revised versions of a diagnostic interview for caregivers of individuals with possible pervasive developmental disorder. *Journal of Autism and Developmental Disorders*, **24**, 569–85.

Lord, C. & Schopler, E. (1989). Stability of assessment results of autistic and non- autistic language-impaired children from preschool years to early school age. *Journal of Child Psychology and Psychiatry*, **30**(4), 575–90.

Lord, C. & Venter, A. (1992). Outcome and follow-up studies of high-functioning autistic individuals. In E. Schopler & G. Mesibov (Eds.), *High Functioning Individuals with Autism* (pp. 187–198). New York: Plenum.

Lotter, V. (1974a). Social adjustment and placement of autistic children in Middlesex: A follow-up study. *Journal of Autism and Childhood Schizophrenia*, **4**, 11–32.

Lotter, V. (1974b). Factors related to outcome in autistic children. *Journal of Autism and Childhood Schizophrenia*, **4**(3), 263–77.

Lovaas, O. I. (1987). Behavioral treatment and normal educational and intellectual functioning in young autistic children. *Journal of Counseling and Clinical Psychology*, **55**, 3–9.

Maestrini, E., Paul, A., Monaco, A., & Bailey, A. (2000). Identifying autism susceptibility genes. *Neurons*, **28**, 19–24.

Manes, F., Piven, J., Vrancic, D., Nanclares, V., Plebst, C., & Starkstein, S. E. (1999). An MRI study of the corpus callosum and cerebellum in mentally retarded autistic individuals. *The Journal of Neuropsychiatry and Clinical Neurosciences*, **11**, 470–4.

McGovern, C. W. & Sigman, M. (2005). Continuity and change from early childhood to adolescence in autism. *Journal of Child Psychology and Psychiatry*, **46**(4), 401–17.

Mesibov, G. B., Shea, V., & Schopler, E. (2004). *The TEACCH Approach to Autism Spectrum Disorders*. New York: Springer.

Molloy, C. A., Keddache, M., & Martin, L. J. (2005). Evidence for linkage on 21q and 7q in subset of autism characterized by developmental regression. *Molecular Psychiatry*, **10**, 741–6.

Moore, V. & Goodson, S. (2003). How well does early diagnosis of autism stand the test of time? Follow-up study of children assessed for autism at age 2 and development of an early diagnostic service. *Autism*, **7**, 47–63.

Morrow, E. M., Yoo, S. Y., Flavell, S. W., *et al.* (2008). Identifying autism loci and genes by tracing recent shared ancestry. *Science*, **321**, 218–23.

Morton, J. & Johnson, M. (1991). CONSPEC and CONLERN: A two-process theory of infant face recognition. *Psychological Review*, **98**, 164–81.

Muhle, R., Trentacoste, S., & Rapin, I. (2004). The genetics of autism. *Pediatrics*, **114**, 472–86.

Mundy, P. (2003). Annotation: The neural basis of social impairments in autism. The role of the dorsal medial-frontal cortex and anterior cingulated system. *Journal of Child Psychology and Psychiatry*, **44**, 793–809.

Mundy, P. & Crowson, M. (1997). Joint attention and early social communication. *Journal of Autism and Developmental Disorder*, **27**, 653–76.

Mundy, P., Sigman, M., & Kasari, C. (1994). Joint attention, developmental level, and symptom presentation in young children with autism. *Development and Psychopathology*, **6**, 389–401.

Murakami, J. W., Courchesne, E., Press, R., & Yeung-Courchesne, R. (1989). Reduced cerebellar hemisphere size and its relationship to vermal hypoplasia in autism. *Archives of Neurology*, **46**, 689–94.

Newschaffer, C., Falb, M., & Gurney, J. (2005). National autism prevalence trends from United States special education data. *Pediatrics*, **115**, 277–82.

Nicolson, R. & Szatmari, P. (2003). Genetic and neurodevelopmental influences in Autistic Disorder. *Canadian Journal of Psychiatry*, **48**, 526–37.

Ozonoff, S. & Cathcart, K. (1998). Effectiveness of a home program intervention for young children with autism. *Journal of Autism and Developmental Disorders*, **28**, 25–32.

Palmen, S. J., Hulshoff, M. C., Pol, H. E., *et al.* (2005). Increased gray-matter volume in medication-naïve high-functioning children with autism spectrum disorder. *Psychological Medicine*, **35**, 561–70.

Palmen, S. J., van Engeland, H., Hof, P. R., & Schmitz, C. (2004). Neuropathological findings in autism. *Brain*, **127**, 2572–83.

Park, C. C. (1967). *The Siege: A Family's Journey Into the World of an Autistic Child*. Boston: Back Bay Books.

Pickles, A., Starr, E., & Kazak, S. (2000). Variable expression of the autism broader phenotype: Findings from extended pedigrees. *Journal of Child Psychology and Psychiatry*, **41**(4), 491–502.

Piven, J., Arndt, S., Bailey, J., & Andreasen, N. (1996a). Regional brain enlargement in autism: A magnetic resonance imaging study. *Journal of the American Academy of Child and Adolescent Psychiatry*, **35**, 530–6.

Piven, J., Bailey, J., Ranson, B. J., & Arndt, S. (1997c). An MRI study of the corpus callosum in autism. *American Journal of Psychiatry*, **154**, 1051–6.

Piven, J., Chase, G. A., Landa, R., *et al.* (1991). Psychiatric disorders in the parents of autistic individuals. *Journal of the American Academy of Child and Adolescent Psychiatry*, **30**, 471–8.

Piven, J., Gayle, J., Chase, J., *et al.* (1990). A family history study of neuropsychiatric disorders in the adult siblings of autistic individuals. *Journal of the American Academy of Child and Adolescent Psychiatry*, **29**, 177–83.

Piven, J., Harper, J., Palmer, P., & Arndt, S. (1996b). Course of behavioral change in autism: A retrospective study of higher-IQ adolescents and adults. *Journal of the American Academy of Child and Adolescent Psychiatry*, **35**(4), 523–9.

Piven, J. & Palmer, P. (1997). Cognitive deficits in parents from multiple-incidence autism families. *Journal of Child Psychology and Psychiatry*, **38**, 1011–22.

Piven, J., Palmer, P., Jacobi, D., Childress, D., & Arndt, S. (1997a). The broader autism phenotype: Evidence from a family history study of multiple-incidence autism families. *American Journal of Psychiatry*, **154**, 185–90.

Piven, J., Palmer, P., Landa, R., Santangelo, S., Jacobi, D., & Childress, D. (1997b). Personality and language characteristics in parents from multiple-incidence autism families. *American Journal of Medical Genetics (Neuropsychiatric Genetics)*, **74**, 398–411.

Piven, J., Simon, J., Chase, G. A., *et al.* (1993). The etiology of autism: Pre-, peri-, and neonatal factors. *Journal of the American Academy of Child and Adolescent Psychiatry*, **32**(6), 1256–63.

Piven, J., Wzorek, M., Landa, R., *et al.* (1994). Personality characteristics of parents of autistic individuals. *Psychological Medicine*, **24**(3), 783–95.

Polleux, F. & Lauder, J. (2004). Toward a developmental neurobiology of autism. *Mental Retardation and Developmental Disabilities*, **10**, 303–17.

Prizant, B. M., Wetherby, A. M., & Rydell, P. J. (2000). Communication intervention issues for young children with autism spectrum disorders. In E. Wetherby & B. Prizant (Eds.), *Autism Spectrum Disorders: A Transactional Developmental Perspective* (193–224). Baltimore: Paul H. Brooks.

Ramachandran, V. S. & Oberman, L. M. (2006, November). Broken Mirrors: A Theory of Autism. *Scientific American*, 62–9.

Risch, N., Spiker, D., Lotspeich, L., *et al.* (1999). A genomic screen of autism: Evidence for a multilocus etiology. *American Journal of Human Genetics*, **65**(2), 493–507.

Ritvo, E. R., Freeman, B. J., & Mason-Brothers, A. (1985). Concordance for the syndrome autism in 40 pairs of afflicted twins. *American Journal of Psychiatry*, **142**(1), 74–7.

Ritvo, E. R., Freeman, B. J., Pingree, C., *et al.* (1989). The UCLA- University of Utah epidemiologic survey of autism: Prevalence. *American Journal of Psychiatry*, **146**(2), 194–9.

Rodier, P. M. (2002). Converging evidence for brain stem injury in autism. *Development and Psychopathology*, **14**, 537–57.

Rogers, S. (1998). Empirically supported treatment for young children with autism. *Journal of Clinical Child Psychology*, **27**, 168–79.

Rogers, S. J. & DiLalla, D. L. (1991). A comparative study of the effects of a developmentally based instructional model on young children with autism and young children with other disorders of behavior and development. *Topics in Early Childhood Special Education*, **11**, 29–47.

Ruble, L. A. & Dalrymple, N. J. (1996). An alternative view of outcome in Autism. *Focus on Autism and Other Developmental Disabilities*, **11**(1), 3–14.

Rumsey, J. M. & Ernst, M. (2000). Functional neuroimaging of autistic disorders. *Mental Retardation and Developmental Disabilities Research Reviews* **6**(3), 171–9.

Rutter, M. (1970). Psychological development: Predictions of infancy. *Journal of Child Psychology and Psychiatry*, **11**(1), 49–62.

Rutter, M., Greenfeld, D., & Lockyer, L. (1967). A five to fifteen year follow-up study of infantile psychosis: II. Social and behavioral outcome. *British Journal of Psychiatry*, **113**, 1183–99.

Rutter, M., Silberg, J., & O'Connor, T. (1999). Genetics and child psychiatry: II. Empirical research findings. *Journal of Child Psychology and Psychiatry*, **40**(1), 19–55.

Sallows, G. O. & Graupner, T. D. (2005). Intensive behavioral treatment for children with autism: Four-year outcome and predictors. *American Journal on Mental Retardation*, **6**, 417–38.

Sansosti, F. J., Powell-Smith, K. A., & Kincaid, D. (2004). A research synthesis of social story interventions for children with autism spectrum disorders. *Focus on Autism and Other Developmental Disabilities*, **19**, 194–204.

Santangelo, S. & Folstein, S. (1999). Autism: A genetic perspective. In H. Tager-Flusberg (Ed.), *Neurodevelopmental Disorders* (pp. 431–447). Cambridge, MA: The MIT Press.

Schultz, R., Gauthier, I., Klin, A., *et al.* (2000). Abnormal ventral temporal cortical activity during face discrimination among individuals with autism and Asperger's syndrome. *Archives of General Psychiatry*, **57**, 331–40.

Schultz, R. T. & Robins, D. L. (2005). Functional neuroimaging studies of autism spectrum disorders. In F. Volkmar, A. Klin, & R. Paul (Eds.), *Handbook of Autism and Pervasive Developmental Disorders*, 3rd edn (pp. 515–33). New York: John Wiley and Sons.

Sears, L. L., Vest, C., Mohamed, S., Bailey, J., Ranson, B. J., & Piven, J. (1999). An MRI study of the basal ganglia in autism. *Progress in Neuro-Psychopharmacology & Biological Psychiatry*, **23**, 613–24.

Sebat, J., Lakshmi, B., Malhotra, D., *et al.* (2007). Strong association of de novo copy number mutations with autism. *Science*, **316**, 445–9.

Sigman, M. & Ruskin, E. (1999). Continuity and change in social competence of children with autism, Down Syndrome, and developmental delays. *Monographs of the Society for Research in Child Development*, **64**, 1–114.

Smalley, S. (1998). Autism and tuberous sclerosis. *Journal of Autism and Developmental Disorders*, **28**(5), 407–14.

Smith, T., Groen, A. D., & Wynn, J. W. (2000). Randomized trial of intensive early intervention for children with pervasive developmental disorder. *American Journal on Mental Retardation*, **105**, 269–85.

Sparks, B. F., Friedman, S. D., Shaw, D. W., *et al.* (2002). Brain structural abnormalities in young children with autism spectrum disorder. *Neurology*, **59**, 184–92.

Starr, E., Szatmari, P., Bryson, S., & Zwaigenbaum, L. (2003). Stability and change among high-functioning children with pervasive development disorders: A 2-year outcome study. *Journal of Autism and Developmental Disorders*, **33**(1), 15–22.

Steffenburg, J., Gillberg, C., Hellgren, L., *et al.* (1989). A twin study of autism in Denmark, Finland, Iceland, Norway, and Sweden. *Journal of Child Psychology and Psychiatry*, **30**(3), 405–16.

Stevens, M. C., Fein, D. A., Dunn, M., *et al.* (2000). Subgroups of children with autism by cluster analysis: A longitudinal examination. *Journal of the American Academy of Child and Adolescent Psychiatry*, **39**(3), 346–52.

Stone, W. L., Ousley, O. Y., Hepburn, S. L., Hogan, K. L., & Brown, C. S. (1999). Patterns of adaptive behavior in very young children with autism. *American Journal of Mental Retardation*, **104**(2), 187–99.

Strain, P. S. & Hoyson, M. (2000). The need for longitudinal, intensive social skill intervention: LEAP follow-up outcomes for children with autism. *Topics in Early Childhood Special Education*, **20**, 116–22.

Sundberg, M. L. & Partington, J. W. (1998). *The Assessment of Basic Language and Learning Skills (the ABLLS)*. Davie, FL: Behavior Analysts, Inc.

Sutera, S., Pandey, J., Esser, E., *et al.* (2007). Predictors of optimal outcome in toddlers diagnosed with autism spectrum disorders. *Journal of Autism and Developmental Disorders*, **37**, 98–107.

Swettenham, J., Baron-Cohen, S., Charman, T., *et al.* (1998). The frequency and distribution of spontaneous attention shifts between social and non-social stimuli in autistic, typically developing and non-autistic developmentally delayed infants. *Journal of Child Psychology and Psychiatry*, **39**, 747–54.

Szatmari, P., Bryson, S. E., Boyle, M. H., Streiner, D. L., & Duku, E. (2003). Predictors of outcome among high functioning children with autism and Asperger syndrome. *Journal of Child Psychology and Psychiatry*, **44**(4), 520–8.

Szatmari, P., Bryson, S. E., Streiner, D. L., Wilson, F., Archer, L., & Ryerse, C. (2000). Two-year outcome of preschool children with autism or Asperger's syndrome. *American Journal of Psychiatry*, **157**(12), 1980–7.

Szatmari, P., Jones, M. B., Tuff, L., Bartolucci, G., Fisman, S., & Mahoney, W. (1993). Lack of cognitive impairment in first-degree relatives of children with pervasive developmental disorders. *Journal of the American Academy of Child and Adolescent Psychiatry*, **32**, 1264–73.

Szatmari, P., Jones, M. B., Zwaigenbaum, L., & Maclean, J. E. (1998). Genetics of autism: Overview and new directions. *Journal of Autism and Developmental Disabilities*, **28**(5), 351–69.

Tager-Flusberg, H., Joseph, R., & Folstein, S. (2001). Current directions in research on autism. *Mental Retardation and Developmental Disabilities*, **7**, 21–9.

Temple, E., Deutsch, G. K., Poldrack, R. A., *et al.* (2003). Neural deficits in children with dyslexia ameliorated by behavioral remediation: Evidence from functional MRI. *Proceedings of the National Academy of Sciences of the United States of America*, **100**, 2860–5.

Trevathan, E. (2004). Seizures and epilepsy among children with language regression and autistic spectrum disorders. *Journal of Child Neurology*, **19**, 49–57.

Tsai, L. (1992). Diagnostic issues in high-functioning autism. In E. Schopler & G. Mesibov (Eds.), *High-Functioning Individuals with Autism* (pp. 11–40). New York: Plenum Press.

Vargas, D., Nascimbene, C., Krishnan, C., Zimmerman, A., & Pardo, C. (2005). Neuroglial activation and neuroinflammation in the brain of patients with autism. *Annals of Neurology*, **57**, 67–81.

Volkmar, F. & Nelson, D. (1990). Seizure disorders in autism. *Journal of the American Academy of Child and Adolescent Psychiatry*, **29**, 127–9.

Waterhouse, L. & Fein, D. (1984). Longitudinal trends in cognitive skills for children diagnosed as autistic and schizophrenic. *Child Development*, **55**, 236–48.

Wassink, T. H., Brzustowicz, L. M., Bartlett, C. W., & Szatmari, P. (2004). The search for autism disease genes. *Mental Retardation and Developmental Disabilities*, **10**, 272–83.

Weidmer-Mikhail, E., Sheldon, S., & Ghaziuddin, M. (1998). Chromosomes in autism and related pervasive developmental disorders: A cytogenic study. *Journal of Intellectual Disability Research*, **42**(1), 8–13.

Williams, P., Sears, L., & Allard, A. (2004). Sleep problems in children with autism. *Journal of Sleep Research*, **13**, 265–8.

Williams, J., Waiter, G., Gilchrist, A., Perrett, D., Murray, A., & Whiten, A. (2006). Neural mechanisms of imitation and 'mirror neuron' functioning in autistic spectrum disorder. *Neuropsychologia*, **44**, 610–21.

Wing, L. & Gould, J. (1979). Severe impairments of social interaction and associated abnormalities in children: Epidemiology and classification. *Journal of Autism and Developmental Disorders*, **8**, 79–97.

Wolf, L. & Goldberg, B. (1986). Autistic children grow up: An eight to twenty-four year follow-up study. *Canadian Journal of Psychiatry*, **31**, 550–6.

Zwaigenbaum, L., Bryson, S., Rogers, T., Roberts, W., Brian, J., & Szatmari, P. (2005). Behavioral manifestations of autism in the first year of life. *International Journal of Developmental Neuroscience*, **23**, 143–52.

3

Development in spina bifida: Neurobiological and environmental factors

Marcia A. Barnes, Heather B. Taylor, Susan B. Landry,
and Lianne H. English

Introduction

Spina bifida myelomeningocele (SBM) is one of the world's most common disabling birth defects, yet, until recently, its genetic, neural, and cognitive phenotypes have been less systematically investigated than those of other neurogenetic disorders, including several of those featured in this volume. This chapter describes the findings from a large-scale multi-site study of more than 260 children with SBM between the ages of 7 and 16 years and over 160 children with SBM and their typically developing peers followed from infancy into school age that involves collaboration between the University of Texas Health Science Center at Houston, the University of Houston, and the Toronto Hospital for Sick Children.

The material is organized as follows: (1) What is SBM?; (2) The SBM genotype; (3) Relations between genotype and physical and neural phenotypes; (4) The SBM behavioral phenotype in relation to lesion level and environmental factors: intelligence, academic skills, and adaptive function; (5) Theoretical questions about typical and atypical development generated from studies of the SBM phenotype; (6) Longitudinal development in SBM from infancy through childhood and into adult life; and (7) Clinical care and intervention issues.

What is SBM?

SBM, a neural tube defect that affects the development of both spine and brain, arises in the third to fourth week of embryogenesis, and results in a failure of neural tube closure. The physical phenotype includes paraplegia of the lower limbs and neurogenic bladder and bowel function (Charney, 1992). SBM affects between

The work reported in this chapter was supported by grants from the Canadian Institutes of Health Research to the first author and from NIH (P01 HD35946) and NINDS (R01HD046609 – 04). We also thank Maureen Dennis for her editorial comments and Kimberly Raghubar for editorial assistance.

0.1 to 0.2 live births in North America, and globally, over 300,000 children are born each year with this defect (March of Dimes, 2006). The Chiari II hindbrain malformation, which occurs in almost all cases of SBM, results in downward displacement of the cerebellar vermis into the cervical spinal canal with elongation of the brainstem and obliteration of the fourth ventricle (Barkovich, 2000). The resulting hydrocephalus typically requires a diversionary shunt.

While the spinal lesion repair occurs shortly after birth in most individuals, a more recent option involves repair in utero. To date, some 400 such surgeries have been conducted (Sutton, 2008), with a randomized control trial (Management of Myelomeningocele Study, MOMS) under way to evaluate ambulatory and developmental outcomes in the first 3 years.

The SBM genotype

The origins of spina bifida are multifactorial: its prevalence differs across countries, largely in relation to genetic and environmental factors (reviewed in Northrup & Volcik, 2000). Population-based studies show that the incidence of SBM varies with ethnicity; in the United States, for example, persons of Hispanic (i.e., Mexican-American) origin are at higher risk for SBM than are Caucasians who are at higher risk than African Americans. There is also an increased risk of the disorder in siblings of those born with SBM.

Several genetic pathways have been implicated in SBM. The methylenetetrahydrofolate reductase (MTHFR) gene is involved in folate metabolism. Specific genotype studies of the genes involved in folate metabolism have shown that the maternal C677T MTHFR mutant genotype is a risk factor, in particular, for upper level spinal lesions in Hispanic populations (Volcik *et al.*, 2000) and the findings fit with a model of multi-site neural tube closure specifying two initiation sites for closure in spinal development (van Allen *et al.*, 1993).

The introduction of folic acid supplementation to the North American wheat flour supply in the 1990s is credited with reducing the incidence of neural tube defects in the United States and Canada (Williams *et al.*, 2005). In northern China, which had the highest prevalence of SBM in the world in the mid-1990s, the incidence of neural tube defects dropped from 6 to 1 per 1000 births after a large trial of folic acid supplementation (March of Dimes, 2006). Similar reductions in neural tube defects from pre- to post-folic acid supplementation have been reported elsewhere (March of Dimes, 2006). However, fortification has not led to equal increases in folic acid uptake in all racial/ethnic groups; in the United States, Black and Mexican-American women of child-bearing age have less folic acid uptake than White women (Bentley *et al.*, 2006).

Although more research is needed, a recent adequately powered genotyping study suggests that single nucleotide polymorphisms on some of the genes associated with glucose metabolism and obesity (LEPR, GLUTI, & HK1) may be associated with increased risk for SBM (Davidson *et al.*, 2008). These findings are consistent with the hypothesis that hyperglycemia produces excessive apoptosis or cell death, resulting in disruptions to neural tube formation. They also fit with epidemiological findings that there is an increased risk of SBM in women who are obese and/or who have type 2 diabetes, and with evidence from animal studies showing that high glucose levels affect the expression of those genes involved in regulating embryonic development, including formation of the neural tube (reviewed in Davidson *et al.*, 2008).

In sum, there is evidence for considerable genetic contribution to SBM, but the pathways may be multi-factorial and interact with specific environmental variables; of particular interest to connecting the study of genetics with that of brain and behavioral development are the findings that the level of spinal lesion is related to the MTHFR gene in Hispanic mothers of children with SBM (Volcik *et al.*, 2000). These findings are discussed below.

Relations between genotype and physical and neural phenotypes

Findings from the large-scale study on SBM (led by J. M. Fletcher at University of Houston and M. Dennis at University of Toronto; http://www.uh.edu/~sandi/) have resulted in a better understanding of how spinal lesion level is related to neural and cognitive heterogeneity (Fletcher *et al.*, 2004, 2005). In particular, this study has considered other sources of potential variance between upper and lower spinal lesions groups (e.g., birthweight, perinatal complications, presence of hydrocephalus, shunt revisions, seizures, and so forth) that may have produced inconsistent results across smaller descriptive studies.

Children with lower level lesions (lumbar–sacral) and those with upper level lesions (thoracic) were compared, but also analyzed with respect to ethnicity, which in this study was not only connected to the genetics of the disorder (e.g., greater incidence of upper level lesions in the Hispanic cohort), but also to socio-economic disadvantage. Magnetic resonance imaging of the brain was carried out. In terms of the neural phenotype, upper level lesions were associated with greater magnetic resonance imaging abnormalities in the tectum, posterior fossa, pons, falx, and the splenium of the corpus callosum. For quantitative magnetic resonance imaging measures, the upper lesion group had smaller brain volumes (less gray and white matter), smaller cerebellar volumes (less gray and white matter), and smaller area of the corpus callosum. Greater detail on lesion level group differences for qualitative abnormalities and quantitative analyses of the neural structures can be found in Fletcher *et al.* (2005).

How do the brains of children with SBM compare to those of typically developing individuals? In a recent study by Juranek *et al.* (2008) comparing children with

SBM to age-matched controls, there was no difference between the groups in overall cerebral volume. Children with SBM had a reduction in white matter volumes compared to controls, increased cerebrospinal fluid, and no difference in gray matter volumes. Interestingly, parts of the frontal cortex were thicker in the group with SBM. The normal developmental pattern involves a decrease in cortical thickness of the frontal polar region (O'Donnell *et al.*, 2005) and regional-specific increases in white matter volume with increasing age, which suggests that there is considerable disruption and reorganization of brain development in SBM. How these findings are related to neurocognitive development is currently under investigation.

The SBM behavioral phenotype in relation to lesion level and environmental factors: Intelligence, academic skills, and adaptive function

To understand relations between genetic, neural, and behavioral variability *within* SBM, we have considered how spinal lesion level and its neural correlates influence broad neurobehavioral outcomes (intellectual function, academic achievement, motor abilities, and adaptive behaviors) (Fletcher *et al.*, 2004, 2005). Because ethnicity and socio-economic status (SES) are related, the clearest comparisons are those between upper and lower level lesion subgroups within ethnicity. Upper level lesions are associated with greater impairment in intellectual function (Fletcher *et al.*, 2005). Interestingly, the commonly reported profile of higher verbal IQ than performance IQ that has been found in many studies (Dennis *et al.*, 1981; Donders *et al.*, 1990; Fletcher *et al.*, 1992; Wills, 1993) is observed only for the children in the lower lesion non-Hispanic group, who form the majority of participants in most previous studies in the literature. In our population-based study of individuals with SBM from Ontario and Texas, nonverbal IQ is better than verbal IQ in both upper and lower lesion Hispanic groups, pointing to the importance of the environment in moderating developmental outcomes in children with neurogenetic disorders (also see Dennis *et al.*, 2006).

Another way to look at intellectual function in neurogenetic disorders is to take a categorical/diagnostic approach by determining the incidence of intellectual disability. Intellectual disability is identified when both IQ scores and measures of adaptive function are significantly below the population mean. In our sample, we defined intellectual disability when both IQ (Stanford Binet-4 composite) and adaptive behavior (Scales of Independent Behavior) scores were 2 or more standard deviations below the test means of 100. This results in the highest rate of intellectual disability in the Hispanic upper level lesion group compared to the Hispanic lower level lesion group (59% vs. 23%); the incidence of intellectual disability in upper and lower level lesion groups in the non-Hispanic cohort does not differ (about 17% in both groups).

For broad academic outcomes, reading (word decoding and reading comprehension) and math (pencil and paper calculation) are also poorer in upper lesion groups, although these academic skills are also lower in the Hispanic children. This underscores the main effects of socio-economic disadvantage on academic outcomes in children with neurogenetic disorders, even in the absence of mental retardation. Between 50 and 60% of the sample meet criteria for learning disabilities (defined using low achievement cut points, below the 25th percentile and no mental retardation). Upper level lesions in the Hispanic cohort (although not in non-Hispanic groups) are associated with a greater rate of learning disabilities than lower level lesions.

For both Hispanic and non-Hispanic groups, lesion level affects functional outcomes, including mobility and motor function, whether considered categorically (can or cannot walk) or from an adaptive perspective, reflecting variability in functional independence related to both fine and gross motor functioning. Upper level lesions have a negative effect on personal living skills such as self-care and hygiene. In contrast, social interaction/communication skills and community living skills (e.g., time and punctuality, knowing the value of money, and so forth) are lower in the upper lesion group only for Hispanic children. Upper spinal lesions disrupt functional outcomes that involve motor and physical abilities regardless of environmental influences; in contrast, there is an interaction of biological and environmental factors for functional outcomes that involve language and communication.

Neurobehavioral functioning in SBM is multi-factorial, and lesion level provides a link between the genetic, neural, and cognitive aspects of SBM. While upper level lesions are a marker for greater brain dysmorphology, which is related to poorer motor, cognitive, and adaptive outcomes, environmental factors such as SES are also important for accounting for variability in outcomes in SBM.

Theoretical questions about typical and atypical development generated from studies of the SBM phenotype

Core deficits

Studies of SBM inform brain–behavior models of specific neurocognitive functions. In contrast to the broad neurocognitive outcomes discussed above, an approach currently used in several studies of neurogenetic disorders is to look for core cognitive deficits derived from cognitive models that might be more closely related to specific brain anomalies or dysfunction. We have proposed that SBM involves core deficits in movement, timing, and attention orienting that contribute to a broader set of functional outcomes across many domains from behavior regulation to memory and reading comprehension (Dennis *et al.*, 2006). These core deficits emerge in infancy, before formal education and persist throughout the life span; are demonstrable across a range of general cognitive abilities; are weakly related to other core deficits, but strongly related to specific congenital brain dysmorphologies; and produce deficits similar to those produced by an acquired lesion in the same brain region in adults. Our review of a model of neurocognitive outcome over the life span in SBM that discusses core deficits and functional assets and deficits in greater detail can be found in Dennis *et al.*, 2006. In the section below, we discuss two core deficits: timing and attention orienting.

Timing

Individuals with SBM have core deficits in timing. They are unable to discriminate brief auditory temporal intervals (around 400 ms), even though they accurately discriminate pitch, and they have deficits in the temporal processes involved in production of rhythmic movement (Dennis *et al.*, 2004). Dennis and colleagues have suggested that timing deficits in children with SBM produce a temporal disconnection between sensation and movement, resulting in asynchrony of feed-forward processes that encode the sensory consequences of motor acts, as well as a central processing disruption of the brain mechanisms for rhythm, which may involve deficient timing and rhythm generators that produce problems in movement regulation.

Variability in timing is related in principled ways to the neural phenotype in SBM. Perceptual timing is related to cerebellar volume measures in both children with SBM and their age-matched controls, and motor timing is related to cerebellar measures in children with SBM. These findings suggest that deficits in timing are a core deficit in SBM, because they are found in children with SBM who are not intellectually deficient, their relation to brain structure is specific rather than general, and the deficits parallel those found in adults with acquired cerebellar lesions.

Attention orienting

From one-quarter to one-third of children with SBM are rated as inattentive (Burmeister *et al.* 2005; Fletcher *et al.*, 2005; Holmbeck *et al.*, 2003). Cognitive–behavioral evidence of poor attention has also been reported (Brewer *et al.*, 2001; Loss *et al.*, 1998; Rose & Holmbeck, 2007).

Recent systematic comparisons of SBM and other attention disorders (Dennis *et al.*, 2008) have suggested that children with SBM are inattentive but not hyperactive, and have difficulties primarily with the stimulus orienting aspect of attention, in contrast to children with ADHD, who are often inattentive and who have difficulties primarily with the response control component of attention.

The way in which attention has been approached in SBM has been to use brain–behavior models to investigate those aspects of attention that could reasonably be expected to be deficient in SBM compared to those that might show relative sparing. Attention orienting and disengagement have been studied in individuals with SBM at school age and in infancy (Dennis *et al.*, 2005a,b; Taylor *et al.*, submitted). These aspects of attention are of particular interest because they are associated with areas of brain (midbrain, posterior cortex) that are abnormally developed in SBM.

Attention orienting involves the ability of the organism to orient to information that is either salient or interesting. It typically involves automatic shifts of attention to environmentally salient information. It can be covert (internal shifts of attention) or overt (moving the eyes or the body).

In SBM, difficulties in attention orientation involving attention to and disengagement from salient environmental stimuli are present from infancy using habituation paradigms (Taylor *et al.*, submitted). At 18 months of age, infants with SBM take significantly longer to shift their attention from a blinking light to a face stimulus projected on a screen (attention orienting) than typically developing infants. In contrast, there is no difference in these infants' ability to habituate to a familiar stimulus when compared to typically developing infants. Thus, while infants with SBM have difficulty in attention orienting, once they attend to a stimulus, they learn about (habituate to) that stimulus at a rate comparable to their typically developing peers.

At school age, children with SBM are slower to orient to salient sensory information (exogenous orienting) as well as to interesting cognitive cues (endogenous orienting). They also have significant difficulties in disengaging from salient sensory information and show attenuated inhibition of return compared to typically developing controls, meaning that they are more likely to return their attention sooner to just previously attended-to locations (Dennis *et al.*, 2005b). Difficulties in attention orienting and inhibition of return are related to midbrain dysmorphology in SBM, and problems in disengaging attention are related to posterior cortex white matter volumes (Dennis *et al.*, 2005a, b).

In individuals with SBM, deficits in attention are selective, discernible early in life and persist across development, present in individuals who are not intellectually deficient, and related to specific aspects of brain dysmorphology in SBM parallel to those in adults with acquired lesions (Posner *et al.*, 1984; reviewed in Klein, 2000). In accordance with the model of neurocognitive function discussed earlier (Dennis *et al.*, 2006), attention orienting is a core deficit for individuals with SBM.

Associative vs. assembled processing

One common approach in cognitive studies of neurogenetic disorders is to find cognitive strengths in an overall context of intellectual disability (e.g., Down syndrome, Williams syndrome); another is to find cognitive deficits in the context of broadly average intellectual function (Turner syndrome, SBM). Although the combination of upper level lesions and socio-economic disadvantage is associated with intellectual disability, most children with SBM have broadly normal intellectual function. However, SBM is associated with a cognitive phenotype that shows variability both across cognitive domains (e.g., word reading is better developed than math calculations) and also within domains (e.g., word reading is better developed than reading comprehension).

To understand the profile of cognitive and academic strengths and weaknesses in this disorder, Dennis *et al.*, (2006) propose that individuals with SBM have intact stipulated or associative processing and deficient assembled processing. The former is largely data- or stimulus-driven and reliant on associative learning. The latter requires the assembly and integration of information, including the suppression of irrelevant information and the updating and selection of relevant information contingent on the context. This classification scheme represents a change from an earlier focus on content domains (e.g., language vs. visual perception) to an emphasis on cognitive processes.

Classifications are central to understanding psychological phenomena because they allow larger sets of entities to be grouped into smaller more homogeneous subgroups based on hypothesized key similarities between entities within the group and key differences in the things that belong to different groups (Fletcher *et al.*, 2007). Valid and reliable classifications can facilitate communication between scientists and clinicians, are useful for making predictions both within and across disorders, and may be pertinent to thinking about interventions (Fletcher *et al.*, 2007).

We have used the distinction between associative and assembled processing to capture cognitive assets and deficits between domains (e.g., reading vs. math), but also to explain and predict assets and deficits within domains of function traditionally thought to be categorically impaired in SBM. Visual perception is one such example. Visual perception can be preserved or deficient, depending on whether associative or assembled processing is required and is best illustrated by comparing face and object perception to spatial perception. Children with SBM have relatively preserved categorical perception involving faces and objects (Dennis *et al.*, 2002), a form of processing related to a ventral occipital–temporal pathway (see Haxby *et al.*, 1991, for discussion of two visual processing pathways). In contrast, their poorer performance on tasks requiring location-based processing relies on a more action-based "where" visual processing system that is reliant on the dorsal occipital–parietal pathway known to be more compromised in SBM (Dennis *et al.*, 2002). This model of associative vs. assembled processing has also been applied to explain assets and deficits in memory, language, academics, and behavior (see Dennis *et al.*, 2006). In the following section, this cognitive processing classification is used to explain and organize previous findings on the cognitive phenotype of reading in SBM and to predict new findings.

Reading

Many studies of SBM in samples of largely middle class children and adolescents have found that their ability to read words accurately is similar to, and sometimes better than, their age peers, although reading comprehension is less well developed (Barnes & Dennis, 1992; Barnes *et al.*, 2004a,b; Friedrich *et al.*, 1991; Mayes & Calhoun, 2006; Wills *et al.*, 1990). We have investigated the sources of reading comprehension difficulties in SBM to tell us more about how and why comprehension breaks down in this disorder, but also to test cognitive models of comprehension difficulty. We have been particularly interested in how models of comprehension difficulty might be constrained by comparisons across groups with a similar behavioral phenotype of good decoding/less skilled comprehension, but who differ with respect to etiological origins of those difficulties (e.g., frank brain injury and disorder in SBM vs. neurologically normal adults and children with comprehension difficulties). In a similar approach, Murphy, Mazzocco, and McCloskey (Chapter 7) use neurogenetic disorders as pathways to understanding mathematical learning disabilities.

We first discuss our population-based study of comprehension difficulties. Then we review studies using cognitive models of text and discourse comprehension to investigate the integrity of comprehension processes in SBM and similarities and differences between populations with good decoding/less skilled comprehension (Barnes *et al.*, 2007a,b).

Our large-scale study of SBM has allowed us to look at rates of learning disabilities in reading comprehension and listening comprehension. Difficulties in reading comprehension are presumed to reflect general problems in comprehension that also occur in listening comprehension whether at the level of individual word meanings or at the level of text or discourse (Fletcher *et al.*, 2007). We used a low achievement definition of learning disabilities (below the 25th percentile for reading decoding, reading comprehension, and listening comprehension measures with an absence of intellectual disability) to identify disability. One-third of the sample has a disability in reading comprehension (Barnes *et al.*, 2007b), and this is greater than the rate of word reading disability (Fletcher *et al.*, 2004). Reading comprehension difficulties are most apparent on the reading comprehension test that requires more inferential and global (thematic) comprehension than on a cloze task involving shorter texts and more local inferences. Unlike measures of word decoding, reading comprehension measures may produce different results depending on their processing demands. Similarly, on the measure of listening comprehension (Listening Comprehension from the Test of Language Competence-E, Wiig & Secord, 1989), which taps the ability to make inferences, nearly half of the children meet the low achievement definition of disability.

Even when children and adults with SBM do not have achievement-defined disabilities in reading comprehension, their reading comprehension is often significantly lower than their word decoding, a pattern not observed in their typically developing controls (Barnes *et al.*, 2004a,b). The pattern of good decoding/less skilled comprehension may be found in children without frank neurological impairment (Muter *et al.*, 2004; Oakhill *et al.*, 2003) at rates between 5 and 10% in United Kingdom and European samples (Cornoldi *et al.*, 1996; Yuill & Oakhill, 1991), although these specific reading comprehension disabilities are not typically diagnosed until after third grade (Leach *et al.*, 2003). Because the pattern of good decoding/less skilled comprehension is quite common in children with SBM and because SBM is diagnosed before or at birth, this neurogenetic disorder provides a model for studying the development of comprehension abilities and disabilities.

Although comparisons of rates of comprehension disabilities across groups are of some interest, understanding the specific cognitive processes that lead to better or worse comprehension outcomes in SBM and other groups requires the use of models and paradigms from cognitive theories of comprehension ability and disability. Comprehension models distinguish between surface-level, text-based, and situation model representations (Clifton & Duffy, 2001; Kintsch, 1988; Schmalhofer *et al.*, 2002). We have considered whether the comprehension difficulties of children with SBM involve problems in building representations at these various levels, and whether associative and assembled processing are required to build these representations.

Accessing meaning from the surface code requires accurate and sufficiently fast word reading, comprehension of individual words, comprehension of syntax or sentence structure, and understanding stipulated or fixed meanings, such as common or frozen idioms (e.g., *Let me give you a hand.*). In relation to our neuro-cognitive model of SBM, some comprehension models propose that a passive semantic process activates stored word meanings regardless of context; that is, accessing word meanings in text relies, at least initially, on data-driven associative or semantic processes in which simply reading a word causes the reader to access its meaning(s) (Gernsbacher, 1990; Schmalhofer *et al.*, 2002). Some models of figurative language comprehension also propose that the meanings of frozen idioms are retrieved in idiom format or as a lexicalized unit, not as individual words (Gibbs, 1986). And models of syntactic comprehension suggest that many grammatical structures are rapidly activated from stored knowledge (MacDonald *et al.*, 1994). Problems in accessing the meaning of surface level representations, including understanding the meaning of words and syntax, contribute to comprehension disabilities in some, but not all, children with comprehension difficulties (reviews in Cain & Oakhill, 2007; Johnston *et al.*, 2008).

Surface level representations of written text and oral discourse are intact in children with SBM. They read words accurately as discussed above, and at the single word level, children with hydrocephalus, many with SBM, read individual words and nonwords as quickly as typically developing peers (Barnes *et al.*, 2001). Vocabulary knowledge and production approximate population means at the pre-school period, at school age, and in young adulthood (Barnes *et al.*, 2004a,b; 2005; Horn *et al.*, 1985). Even though children with SBM are similar to typically developing children when it comes to knowing what words mean on vocabulary tasks, they could have difficulties in rapidly accessing word meanings as they are reading, what is referred to as *on-line* processing. In on-line comprehension tasks, processes such as accessing word meanings are studied as the person is reading and comprehending. As assessed by using on-line measures that tap the ability to accurately and rapidly access word meanings during reading, children with SBM access word meanings similarly to typically developing peers. They quickly access both meanings of ambiguous words regardless of context less than half a second after reading them (e.g., the card and tool meanings of *spade*). These findings are taken as evidence for a passive semantic process that initially activates all word meanings when a word is read (Barnes *et al.*, 2004b; see Chapter 4 for an example of the use of this same paradigm in autism). Syntactic skills are also intact in school-age children with SBM: they comprehend sentences with different syntactic constructions (Dennis *et al.*, 1987), and they produce sentences that are as syntactically complex as their typically developing peers in narrative reproduction tasks (Barnes & Dennis, 1998; Dennis *et al.*, 1994). Children with hydrocephalus, most with SBM, also do not differ from controls in accessing the meanings of formulaic expressions or common idioms (Barnes & Dennis, 1998). All of these data suggest that children with SBM are intact in their ability to access surface-level information during text and discourse comprehension.

In contrast to data-driven associative processing that is required to access the meaning of the surface structure of text, the construction of text-based representations often requires two forms of assembled processing: the use of context to suppress context-irrelevant meanings over time (Gernsbacher, 1990), and the making of bridging inferences that link two propositions within a text (Albrecht & O'Brien, 1993). We have studied meaning suppression and bridging inference processes in on-line reading comprehension tasks in SBM (Barnes *et al.*, 2004b).

Suppression of irrelevant word meaning requires assembled processing, because it involves the ability to update and revise meaning contingent on the sentence context; for example, using the context in *The man dug with the spade* to select the *tool* meaning of spade and to suppress the *card* meaning of spade. One second after reading a sentence (e.g., *The man dug with the spade*), typically developing children use context to suppress irrelevant meanings (their representations of the text no longer contain the *card* meaning of *spade*, only the *tool* meaning), while children with SBM continue to show interference from irrelevant meanings (their representations still contain both the *card* and *tool* meanings of spade a full second after having read the sentence about the man digging with the spade). The result is that the text-based representation of the child with SBM is likely "cluttered" with conflicting or irrelevant information that is not useful for specifying meaning and that may actually interfere with the construction of the intended meaning of the text. These findings are similar to those for neurologically intact adults with poor comprehension (Gernsbacher & Faust, 1991).

Bridging inferences require the assembly of meaning through the integration of ideas that appear at different places in the text. The ability to make bridging inferences can be tested by varying the textual distance over which two sentences must be integrated to specify meaning. For example, it might be necessary to integrate information about a child having had a large lunch and his later refusal of extra cake at a birthday party. While children with SBM can make bridging inferences accurately over smaller and larger segments of text, they are slower than peers to integrate information over larger text segments (Barnes *et al.*, 2004b). In other words, they are as accurate, but slower, than age peers to maintain ongoing semantic coherence. Similar difficulties in integration have been reported for neurologically intact children who are good decoders/less skilled comprehenders (Cain *et al.*, 2004; and see reviews in Cain & Oakhill, 2007; Johnston *et al.*, 2008).

The presence of deficient suppression and sluggish bridging inference-making suggests that children with SBM lack efficiency in the building of text-based representations, which could cause *bottlenecks* in comprehension as they read increasingly longer texts requiring them to continuously derive meaning from text and update their text-based representations. Comprehension processes that require resource-heavy meaning revision and text integration are deficient in SBM, in keeping with the hypothesis that increased assembled processing demands will tax comprehension in SBM.

Individuals construct mental models of the situation described by the text (Zwaan & Radvansky, 1998) by making inferences about space, time, causality, and character goals and emotions. Situation models are interesting to test in relation to our model of neurocognitive processing in SBM because the models can vary in the amount of assembled processing that is needed and the type of information that must be assembled. Situation models can be built at the single sentence level or may need to be built across several sentences. Thus, situation model experiments allow one to test whether cognitive resource requirements make a difference to situation model building and whether situation models requiring some kinds of inferences are more difficult than constructing models requiring other types of inferences for individuals with SBM. As suggested earlier, the utility of a new classification system is not only to organize previous findings but also to predict new findings. To this end, we used our neurocognitive processing model to make predictions about the integrity of situation model building in SBM, hypothesizing intact ability to build models at the single sentence level, particularly for affective information, but difficulties building models requiring the integration of information across sentences (see Barnes *et al.*, 2007a,b).

Children with SBM can build simple spatial and affective situation models from single sentences (Barnes *et al.*, 2007a). Like age peers, they show a false recognition effect (Bransford & Franks, 1972) incorrectly saying they had read the sentence *Three turtles rested on a floating log and a fish swam beneath it*, when they had actually previously read a target sentence such as *Three turtles rested on a floating log and a fish swam beneath them*, which changes the wording, but preserves the spatial mental model (both children with SBM and controls are able to say they did not read *Three turtles rested on a floating log and a fish swam beside them*, which does change the spatial mental model). Furthermore, they make inferences about emotions and inferences about space equally well.

Children with SBM do experience difficulty relative to controls when they must build spatial situation models across several sentences (Barnes *et al.*, 2007a). In our study, they listened to a 4-sentence description of a spatial layout and decided if a test sentence was true. Sometimes the test sentence was the same as one of the sentences explicitly read in the description, sometimes it represented a spatial relationship between objects that was not explicitly mentioned in any of the presented sentences, but which was a true inference, and sometimes it represented a spatial relationship between objects that could not be true given the description in the sentences (false inference). Although children with SBM perform above chance when the spatial relationship had been explicitly presented in the sentence, they are inaccurate at recognizing true inferences and false inferences compared to controls.

To our knowledge, similar experiments on the building of spatial situation models at the single vs. multi-sentence level have not been conducted with neurologically intact children who are good word readers/less skilled comprehenders. However, we have used the same paradigm in good word readers/less skilled comprehenders with and without SBM to test the ability to build situation models that require the integration of world knowledge with ongoing text to derive meaning. In these experiments, we taught children a new knowledge base about a make believe planet, had them learn the new knowledge to perfect criterion, and then had them read or listen to a multi-episode story in which they had to integrate their new knowledge with the text in order to understand the events as they unfolded. In comparison to good comprehenders, both the children with SBM (Barnes & Dennis, 1998) and neurologically intact good decoders/less skilled comprehenders (Cain *et al.*, 2001) had difficulty making these knowledge-based inferences, although inference-making was improved when the situation required fewer cognitive resources (the inference using the new knowledge base could be made when the pertinent sentence from the text was presented in isolation; Cain *et al.*, 2001).

To summarize, children with SBM access the surface code of the text as well as age peers, suggesting they are both accurate and fluent in deriving meaning at this level. In contrast, when the construction of meaning involves text-based representations or mental models of the situation described by the text, their comprehension is deficient. The difficulty may not be so much in constructing a text-based representation or a situation model per se as in the processing requirements related to assembling meaning across longer chunks of text, and between knowledge and ongoing texts. In terms of our model of neurocognitive function in SBM, access to stipulated meanings or associative processing for meaning is intact, but assembled meanings are deficient, particularly as the cognitive resource or working memory requirements needed for assembly become greater (Barnes *et al.*, 2007a,b). In keeping with these ideas, it has been shown that children with SBM have difficulty understanding idioms whose meaning requires them to be integrated with context (Huber-Okrainec *et al.*, 2005).

What do these model-driven cognitive studies of reading comprehension in SBM tell us, beyond their relevance to a broader model of neurocognitive function in SBM? First, they show that SBM does not impair all aspects of reading comprehension–information that broad measures of achievement in reading comprehension cannot provide. For example, vocabulary, syntax, passive semantic activation processes (also see Yeates & Enrile, 2005), and even mental model construction at the single sentence level are intact, yet difficulties arise as comprehension demands integration with context, between sentences, and between knowledge and text. This presents a more nuanced view of reading comprehension in SBM that is only possible when attention to cognitive models of the skill are employed to guide investigation. Second, just as has been the case for other aspects of neurocognitive function in SBM such as those reviewed above, model-driven investigations of cognitive and academic skills are also more likely to have a clearer link to brain function than omnibus standardized tests. For example, Huber-Okrainec *et al.* (2005) tested several aspects of idiom comprehension in SBM using models of figurative language and showed that more extensive damage to corpus callosum structures was related to difficulties in understanding figurative expressions requiring integration of the context or the suppression of the literal meaning of the figurative expression. Third, they demonstrate that the type of representation may be less important for understanding individual differences in comprehension than are the processes that go into building those representations. This conclusion is largely consistent with findings from studies of adults with acquired lesions in which comprehension breaks down at the level of surface structure such as syntax due to limitations in cognitive resources such as working memory (Caplan & Waters, 2006). Fourth, the overlap in the profiles of intact and deficient comprehension processes in good word readers/less skilled comprehenders with and without frank brain injury is substantial, which points to core difficulties across populations in suppression/revision processes (not activation processes), and difficulties in inference and text integration (not vocabulary or syntax) (Cain *et al.*, 2001, 2004; Gernsbacher & Faust, 1991). Such findings, using identical experimental tasks across populations (also see Chapter 4), provide converging evidence for a finite set of key comprehension processes that account for many individual differences in comprehension. Constraints on cognitive models are important for explaining the existing research base, for the posing of new research questions, and for targeting interventions.

Longitudinal development in SBM from infancy through childhood and into adult life

We now consider how SBM has been used in longitudinal and life-span studies to more comprehensively investigate the sources of environmental risk on the outcomes of children with SBM and to understand the developmental course of cognitive skills. Longitudinal investigations of children with neurogenetic disorders are informative for several reasons and have been employed in other populations described in this volume (Chapters 7 and 8). If the modal cognitive profile or phenotype at school age for a disorder is known, children can be followed from birth to ask questions about developmental trajectories of skills as well as early precursors of later developing assets and deficits. Longitudinal and life-span approaches also allow one to consider how biological and environmental factors and their potential interactions produce better or worse outcomes across motor, cognitive, academic, and social–emotional and adaptive domains.

Environmental risk and protective factors in the development of children with SBM

Consistent with the findings from the large school-age sample of SBM reviewed earlier, our longitudinal studies of children with SBM between 6 and 36 months (led by S. Landry) show that SES is related to growth in language and cognition. Although children from lower SES backgrounds exhibited slower growth in infancy and toddlerhood (both the children with SBM and their typically developing controls), having spina bifida affected growth in language and cognition above the impact of SES (Lomax-Bream *et al.*, 2007a). In our model of neurocognitive outcomes in SBM, environmental factors can infer risk or protection and we see them as moderating the impact of the injury to the developing brain on the development of many, although likely not all cognitive, academic, and adaptive outcomes (Dennis *et al.*, 2006). In our longitudinal studies, we have sought to go beyond general markers of environment such as SES and investigate the impact of environmental factors on development at a more microgenetic level. Why is this important? SES is an omnibus measure in much the same way that standardized cognitive and academic tests are and the same critiques apply: a better understanding of environmental factors requires a theoretically motivated investigation of environmental mechanisms and interventions are more likely to be effective if appropriate targets for environmental change are identified.

One important aspect of environment for child outcomes has to do with parenting style and quality. Parenting style has been associated with better or worse outcomes in children at high biological and environmental risk (Collins *et al.*, 2003) and may be a particularly potent predictor of outcomes for children with special needs (Landry *et al.*, 1997, 2006, 2008a). We looked at the impact of parenting style and parenting quality on child outcomes (Lomax-Bream *et al.*, 2007b). A responsive parenting style is used to describe parental behaviors that involve accurate perception of their child's needs consistent with their developmental level and the current context as well as responses to their child that are contingent on those needs. Because children with SBM may experience difficulties in gaining autonomy at many points in development due to their gross and fine motor and cognitive limitations, a responsive parenting style may be particularly important for supporting learning at the same time as providing the child with some control over their environment (Holmbeck *et al.*, 2006; Landry *et al.*, 2008b).

Important components of a responsive parenting style are those parenting behaviors that provide emotional/affective support and that provide cognitive support, including language input and maintaining of the focus of attention. For children with SBM who have difficulties in components of attention, being able to maintain attentional focus may be very important for learning, and when focused, these children do learn at a rate comparable to their peers (Taylor *et al.*, submitted). The parents' ability to support their child to maintain focus may help the infant with SBM to use limited attentional and cognitive capacity to process information about objects of interest (Landry *et al.*, 2008b). Knowing about how parenting style affects growth in infants with SBM is particularly relevant in light of research on how characteristics of a child at risk for developmental delays can disrupt positive mother–child interactions (Goldberg, 1978; Kogan, 1980) and also given that mothers from low SES backgrounds are more likely to believe that their actions have little effect on their infants, regardless of medical status (Hess & Shipman, 1965).

In our longitudinal studies of the impact of parenting on the development of cognitive, language, and daily living or adaptive skills, 165 children were followed from infancy to 3 years of age (91 with SBM and their controls). Higher levels and faster growth in cognitive skills, including language, were found for children with SBM whose mothers used higher levels of maintaining behaviors, even after controlling for SES and motor development (Lomax-Bream *et al.*, 2007b). These intriguing findings suggest that the physical and cognitive disabilities associated with SBM might not alter the parenting factors that predict cognitive and language growth in typically developing children and other high-risk populations.

Life-span and longitudinal investigations of mathematical cognition in SBM

Like some of the other neurogenetic disorders in this volume (Turner syndrome, fragile X), SBM is associated with a high prevalence of math disabilities (Fletcher *et al.*, 1995; Wills, 1993). Disabilities in math not accompanied by disabilities in reading were present in 29% of our population-based sample, and this is much higher than the estimated rate of specific math disability in children without neurodevelopmental disorder (Shalev *et al.*, 2000). In contrast to this high rate of specific math disability, only 2% had specific reading disability (Fletcher *et al.*, 2005) and another 26% had disabilities in both math and reading. In short, over 50% of children with SBM and no intellectual disability have learning disabilities that almost always affect math, either absolutely or relative to reading (Barnes *et al.*, 2002, 2006). We now consider the value of studying a skill such as math from a life-span perspective in neurogenetic disorders and some of the benefits of longitudinal studies of skill development in disorders that are discernible from before or after birth (also see Chapter 8).

As early as 36 months of age, toddlers with SBM differ from their typically developing controls on early measures of mathematical abilities that have some predictive value for later mathematical outcomes (Gersten *et al.*, 2005). They are less skilled at demonstrating knowledge of counting principles such as one-to-one correspondence, at rote counting, and matching based on quantity (Barnes *et al.*, 2005). At this early age, fine motor dexterity and speed are related to counting skills, whereas visual–spatial abilities are related to quantity matching, suggesting that different early mathematical skills may draw on somewhat different general cognitive abilities. As children with SBM have difficulties in both fine motor and some visual–spatial domains, it will be important to better understand whether these cognitive competencies are actually implicated in growth in math abilities across the preschool years both in SBM and in other populations.

By school age, children with SBM and math disabilities look very similar to children with math disabilities and no neurological impairment (Geary *et al.*, 2000; Jordan *et al.*, 2003). They are inaccurate and slow at single-digit arithmetic, and they use more counting strategies such as counting sum (for 5 + 2 = ? 1,2,3,4,5 and 6,7) and counting up or min (for 5 + 2 = ? 5 and 6,7) and less direct retrieval (just knowing that 5 + 2 = 7) than typically developing children (Barnes *et al.*, 2006). They make procedural errors in multi-digit arithmetic (e.g., problems in borrowing from zero), reflecting delays in understanding base ten concepts and in learning algorithms for solving problems (Ayr *et al.*, 2005; Barnes *et al.*, 2002, 2006), and make similar types of errors as do children with developmental math disabilities (Raghubar *et al.*, 2009). Despite their difficulties with visual–spatial processing, these children do not make more errors than their typically developing peers in reading or writing numbers, and they do not crowd their written work, misread signs, or have difficulty keeping numbers aligned in columns (Ayr *et al.*, 2005; Barnes *et al.*, 2006), which contrasts with the profile sometimes seen in adults with lesions associated with visual–spatial dyscalculia (Hartje, 1987; Roselli & Ardila, 1989; and Chapter 7).

Although math is an academic area of considerable difficulty for individuals with SBM, they show a profile of relative assets and deficits within the broader domain of mathematics. Children with SBM without co-occurring reading disabilities take longer to consolidate procedural math knowledge. For example, by middle childhood, they have consolidated procedures for the first operations taught, i.e., addition and subtraction, although later-taught multi-digit multiplication and division remain weaker (Barnes *et al.*, 2002). In comparison to their better-developed skills in arithmetic computation and numeration (e.g., ordering numbers, understanding units, rational numbers), geometry, word problem solving, and estimation are considerably less well developed areas of math for children and adolescents with SBM, even for those children who do not have identified math disabilities (Barnes *et al.*, 2002). Consistent with the model of neurocognitive function in SBM discussed earlier, those aspects of math that depend more on associative processing, such as the learning of math facts in single-digit arithmetic (Geary, 1993) and procedures in multi-digit arithmetic (also see Colvin *et al.*, 2003; Dennis *et al.*, 2006; Edelstein *et al.*, 2004; Salman *et al.*, 2006; Taylor *et al.*, submitted; for papers on intact procedural learning in other domains), are relatively better developed than those requiring assembled processing. The latter includes skills such as integrating different sources of quantitative information for comparison purposes in estimation and using the language context and mathematical relations expressed in it to come up with an arithmetic solution in word problems.

In young and middle adulthood, reading remains stronger than math, and math, but not reading, is related to functional independence (Barnes *et al.*, 2004a; Dennis & Barnes, 2002). Young adults have difficulties, not only with math computations, but also with functional numeracy, involving skills needed for everyday activities such as making change, balancing a bank account, under-standing graphical and numerical information presented in newspapers, and the like. Although there is controversy over whether deficits in working memory are causally related to math disability (Berch, 2008; Butterworth & Regiosa, 2007; Geary *et al.*, 2007; Swanson, 2007), experimental studies in adults employing dual task methodology have shown that working memory is implicated in the performance of many mathematical tasks, including math computations (reviewed in LeFevre *et al.*, 2005). Consistent with these studies, Dennis and Barnes (2002) found that numerical working memory predicted math outcomes in adults with SBM. Some of the adults in the study by Dennis and Barnes (2002) were tested as children, and those who had lower arithmetic skills in childhood continued to have difficulties with arith-metic in adulthood. As with disabilities in reading (Shaywitz *et al.*, 1999), disabilities in math in SBM persist across the life span and have consequences for full participation in society (Dennis & Barnes, 2002).

Because the prevalence of math disabilities is known in SBM, one promising route for understanding the origins of math disabilities in SBM and perhaps in other groups as well is to test whether level and growth in candidate cognitive skills in infancy and early childhood are related to math outcomes at school age. In our longitudinal studies of SBM, we have used models of math disabilities and mathematical development to propose candidate developmental precursors of later mathematical ability. One of these is working memory, which is related to math in children with math disabilities (Geary *et al.*, 2007; Swanson & Jerman, 2006); to specific math outcomes at particular ages in typically devel-oping preschoolers, school-age children, and adolescents (e.g., Bisanz *et al.*, 2005; Holmes & Adams, 2006); to single- and multi-digit exact arithmetic and estimation in adult dual task studies (reviewed in LeFevre *et al.*, 2005; Kalaman & LeFevre, 2007); and to growth in math in the early primary grades (Bull *et al.*, 2008). We looked at level and growth in working memory between 12 and 26 months of age in children with SBM and their typically developing peers using a delayed response task (Diamond & Doar, 1989) that assesses working memory/inhibitory control. Level and/or growth in working memory/inhibitory control are related to some math outcomes at 5 and 7 to 8 years of age over and above the impact of SES (English *et al.*, 2009). We have much still to learn about the developmental precursors of mathematical ability and dis-ability, but the examples above illustrate the type of model-driven longitudinal investigation that is possible in neurogenetic disorders. From a theoretical perspective, knowing about the early developmental precursors of later emerg-ing math disabilities in SBM could be informative for studying these precursors in other samples at risk for math disability.

Clinical care and intervention issues

The current state of knowledge on the neurocognitive phenotype in SBM and of the relations between genotype, and neural and behavioral phenotypes has implications for clinical care and intervention for this neurogenetic condition. We now discuss what some of these implications might be for some of the domains of function reviewed in the chapter.

It has been claimed that locomotion and training in gross motor abilities improve visual–spatial skills and nonverbal intelligence (e.g., Rendeli *et al.*, 2002). However, these studies have generally confounded spinal lesion level with both motor and cognitive outcomes. The findings from our large-scale study of SBM show that gross motor skills are strongly tied to spinal lesion level, which itself is strongly related to greater brain dysmorphology, including those parts of brain that support a number of visual–spatial processes tapped by tests of nonverbal intelligence. We also note that environmental factors do not seem to moderate these motor outcomes in infants, toddlers, or school-age children. Although these findings suggest that interventions to improve locomotion in children with upper level lesions may be unsuccessful, it is possible that interventions and accommodations that improve the children's ability to navigate through and explore their environment and the objects in it early in life (without actually improving the child's ability to walk) could improve visual–spatial processing and those aspects of cognition related to reaching and object manipulation (Thelen & Smith, 1994). Parent–child interventions that show parents how to direct and sustain the child's attention to objects (Landry *et al.*, 2008b) in combination with accommodations for poor upper limb control and fine motor function could represent promising avenues for early interventions.

Findings from the longitudinal studies of children with SBM and their typically developing peers have several practical implications. Knowing what contributes to better or worse outcomes allows for appropriately timed and targeted prevention and intervention. For example, the same parenting quality factors predict cognitive and language growth in both typically developing children and children with SBM. Such findings hold promise for interventions with young children with SBM and their parents, particularly in those subgroups that are at highest biological and environmental risk. For example, if particular parenting behaviors in infancy predict later cognitive and social development in children with SBM, then early parent–child interventions found to work in other populations at high biological and/or environmental risk might also be helpful for promoting growth in young children with neurogenetic disorders.

Model-driven investigations of cognitive processes and academic skills in neurogenetic disorders are important for how we think about cognitive and academic deficits from a clinical perspective. Evidence-based clinical practice incorporates neurobiological and cognitive developmental models of the disorder. Clinical assessment and intervention models that are not based on the evidence will limit what is assessed, how it is assessed, what is considered to be the appropriate target for intervention, and even whether intervention is thought to be worthwhile. For example, the comprehension difficulties of children with neurogenetic and other childhood disorders affecting the brain are often characterized as those having to do with problems in understanding abstract vs. concrete language. For SBM, such views might limit which aspects of comprehension are assessed as well as assessment of those cognitive skills that support comprehension processes such as text integration. Erroneous assumptions about the sources of comprehension problems in these children will also affect the type of comprehension intervention used and/or the accommodations and compensatory strategies that are recommended.

One of the important findings to emerge from our studies is that the cognitive processing phenotypes of disabilities in comprehension and mathematics look remarkably similar to those in neurologically normal children with learning disabilities. In the absence of evidence to the contrary, the interventions that work for children with disabilities in comprehension and mathematics ought to be good candidate interventions for children with SBM (Barnes *et al.*, 2007b; Fletcher *et al.*, 2007).

In adults with SBM, knowing the neurobiological, medical, cognitive, and social/environmental predictors of morbidity associated with aging can inform models of cognitive aging/reserve in individuals who are born with central nervous system anomalies and injury (Dennis *et al.*, 2000). This information could also have important clinical implications for continuum of care guidelines and prevention of difficulties associated with aging in neurogenetic disorders. The latter is particularly relevant given that, in this newer era of shunt diversion, individuals with SBM have begun to live longer lives, yet mortality and morbidity increase greatly in adulthood (Bowman *et al.*, 2001). It has been recognized that, in order to reduce early mortality in adulthood, the *medical/surgical* needs of this developmental disorder require a multi-disciplinary framework and follow-up approach similar to that used in childhood (McDonnell & McCann, 2000). Yet the *cognitive* and *psychosocial* needs of this growing adult population with SBM are largely unexplored (Hetherington *et al.*, 2006). For example, although psychosocial functioning in late childhood and early adolescence has been studied using sophisticated explanatory models (Coakley *et al.*, 2006), less is known about quality of life and psychosocial functioning in adults (Hetherington *et al.*, 2006; Lemelle *et al.*, 2006), including the relation of factors such as unmanaged pain and social isolation to depression (Oddson *et al.*, 2006). The recent report of increased prospective memory deficits in older but not younger adults with SBM (Dennis *et al.*, 2009) has implications for their ability to plan medical visits, take medication, and to live independently. Deficits in memory functioning over time that affect independence and quality of life and their relation to medical and biological factors have only recently begun to be studied (Dennis *et al.*, 2007).

Conclusions

SBM is a neurogenetic disorder associated with considerable variability in genotype, and neural and cognitive phenotypes. We have exploited this variability to better understand relations between genes, brain, and behavior, and have investigated how cognitive outcomes show significant moderation by the environment. Considerable advances in understanding of neurogenetic and developmental disorders can be made using such interdisciplinary approaches (Fletcher *et al.*, 2007), particularly when neurocognitive models are used to guide studies of brain–behavior relations, cognitive and academic outcomes, and development over time and across the life span. Fruitful areas for future research include the linking of neural processes, such as developmental changes in brain regions of interest, with cognitive- and social-affective development using newer neuroimaging and analysis techniques (Juranek *et al.*, 2008) and the use of the current multi-disciplinary knowledge base to design interventions for infants and their parents, and for children and adults with SBM (Fletcher *et al.*, 2008).

REFERENCES

Albrecht, J. E. & O'Brien, E. J. (1993). Updating a mental model: Maintaining both local and global coherence. *Journal of Experimental Psychology: Learning, Memory, and Cognition*, **19**, 1061–70.

Ayr, L. K., Yeates, K. O., & Enrile, B. G. (2005). Arithmetic skills and their cognitive correlates in children with acquired and congenital brain disorder. *Journal of the International Neuropsychological Society*, **11**, 249–62.

Barkovich, A. J. (2000).Congenital malformations of the brain and skull / Congenital anomalies of the spine. In: Barkovich AJ, editor. *Pediatric Neuroimaging* (pp. 330–7). Philadelphia: Lippincott Williams & Wilkins.

Barnes, M. A. & Dennis, M. (1992). Reading in children and adolescents after early-onset hydrocephalus and in normally developing peers: Phonological analysis, word recognition, word comprehension, and passage comprehension skill. *Journal of Pediatric Psychology*, **17**, 445–65.

Barnes, M. A. & Dennis, M. (1998). Discourse after early-onset hydrocephalus: Core deficits in children of average intelligence. *Brain and Language*, **61**, 309–34.

Barnes, M. A., Dennis, M., & Hetherington, R. (2004a). Reading and writing skills in young adults with spina bifida and hydrocephalus. *Journal of the International Neuropsychological Society*, **10**, 655–63.

Barnes, M. A., Faulkner, H. J., & Dennis, M. (2001). Poor reading comprehension despite fast word decoding in children with hydrocephalus. *Brain and Language*, **76**, 35–44.

Barnes, M. A., Faulkner, H., Wilkinson, M., & Dennis, M. (2004b). Meaning construction and integration in children with hydrocephalus. *Brain and Language*, **89**, 47–56.

Barnes, M. A., Huber, J., Johnston, A. M., & Dennis, M. (2007a). A model of comprehension in spina bifida meningomyelocele: Meaning activation, integration, and revision. *Journal of the International Neuropsychological Society. Special Issue: Reviews*, **13**, 854–64.

Barnes, M. A., Johnston, A. M., & Dennis, M. (2007b). Comprehension in a neurodevelopmental disorder, spina bifida myelomeningocele. In K. Cain & J. Oakhill (Eds.), *Children's Comprehension Problems in Oral and Written Language: A Cognitive Perspective. Challenges in Language and Literacy* (pp. 193–217). New York: Guilford Press.

Barnes, M. A., Pengelly, S., Dennis, M., Wilkinson, M., Rogers, T., & Faulkner, H. (2002). Mathematics skills in good readers with hydrocephalus. *Journal of the International Neuropsychological Society*, **8**, 72–82.

Barnes, M. A., Smith-Chant, B., & Landry, S. H. (2005). Number processing in neurodevelopmental disorders: Spina bifida. In J. I. D. Campbell (Ed.), *Handbook of Mathematical Cognition* (pp. 299–313). New York: Psychology Press.

Barnes, M. A., Wilkinson, M., Khemani, E., Boudesquie, A., Dennis, M., & Fletcher, J. M. (2006). Arithmetic processing in children with spina bifida: Calculation accuracy, strategy use, and fact retrieval fluency. *Journal of Learning Disabilities*, **39**, 174–87.

Bentley, T. G., Willett, W. C., Weinstein, M. C., & Kuntz, K. M. (2006). Population-level changes in folate intake by age, gender, and race/ethnicity after folic acid fortification. *American Journal of Public Health*, **96**(11), 2040–7.

Berch, D. B. (2008). Working memory and mathematical cognitive development: Limitations of limited-capacity resource models. *Developmental Neuropsychology*, **33**, 427–46.

Bisanz, J., Sherman, J. L., Rasmussen, C., & Ho, E. (2005). Development of arithmetic skills and knowledge in preschool children. In J. I. D. Campbell (Ed.), *Handbook of Mathematical Cognition* (pp. 143–162). New York: Psychology Press.

Bowman, R. M., McLone, D. G., Grant, J. A., Tomita, T., & Ito, J. A. (2001). Spina bifida outcome: A 25-year prospective. *Pediatric Neurosurgery*, **34**, 114–20.

Bransford, J. D. & Franks, J. J. (1972). The abstraction of linguistic ideas: A review. *Cognition*, **1**, 211–49.

Brewer, V. R., Fletcher, J. M., Hiscock. M., & Davidson, K. C. (2001). Attention processes in children with shunted hydrocephalus versus attention deficit-hyperactivity disorder. *Neuropsychology*, **15**, 185–98.

Bull, R., Espy, K. A., & Wiebe, S. A. (2008). Short-term memory, working memory, and executive functioning in preschoolers: Longitudinal predictors of mathematical achievement at 7 years. *Developmental Neuropsychology*, **33**, 205–28.

Burmeister, R., Hannay, H. J., Copeland, K., Fletcher, J. M., Boudousquie, A., & Dennis, M. (2005). Attention problems and executive functions in children with spina bifida and hydrocephalus. *Child Neuropsychology*, **11**, 265–83.

Butterworth, B. & Reigosa, V. (2007). Information processing deficits in dyscalculia. In D. B. Berch & M. M. M. Mazzocco (Eds.), *Why Is Math so Hard for Some Children? The*

Nature and Origins of Mathematical Learning Difficulties and Disabilities (pp. 107–20). Baltimore: Paul H. Brookes Publishing Co.

Cain, K. & Oakhill, J. (2007). Reading comprehension difficulties: Correlates, causes, and consequences. In K. Cain & J. Oakhill (Eds.), *Children's Comprehension Problems in Oral and Written Language: A Cognitive Perspective. Challenges in language and literacy* (pp. 41–75). New York: Guilford Press.

Cain, K., Oakhill, J., Barnes, M. A., & Bryant, P. E. (2001). Comprehension skill, inference making ability and their relation to knowledge. *Memory & Cognition*, **29**, 850–9.

Cain, K., Oakhill, J., & Lemmon, K. (2004). Individual differences in the inference of word meanings from context: The influence of reading comprehension, vocabulary knowledge, and memory capacity. *Journal of Educational Psychology*, **96**, 671–81.

Caplan, D. & Waters, G. (2006). Language disorders in aging. In E. Bialystok & F. I. M. Craik (Eds.), *Life Span Cognition: Mechanisms of Change*. Oxford, UK: Oxford University Press.

Charney, E. (1992). Neural tube defects: Spina bifida and meningomyelocele. In M. Batshaw & Y. Perret (Eds.), *Children with Disabilities: A Medical Primer* 3rd edn. (pp. 471–88). Baltimore: Paul H. Brookes.

Clifton, C., Jr. & Duffy, S. A. (2001). Sentence and text comprehension: Roles of linguistic structure. *Annual Review of Psychology*, **52**, 167–96.

Coakley, R. M., Holmbeck, G. N., & Bryant, F. B. (2006). Constructing a prospective model of psychosocial adaptation in young adolescents with spina bifida: An application of optimal data analysis. *Journal of Pediatric Psychology*, **31**, 1084–99.

Collins, W. A., Maccoby, E. E., Steinberg, L., Hetherington, E. M., & Bornstein, M. H. (2003). Contemporary research on parenting: The case for nature and nurture. In M. E. Hertzig & E. A. Farber (Eds.), *Annual Progress in Child Psychiatry and Child Development* (pp. 125–54). New York: Routledge.

Colvin, A. N., Yeates, K. O., Enrile, B. G., & Coury, D. L. (2003). Motor adaptation in children with myelomeningocele: Comparison to children with ADHD and healthy siblings. *Journal of the International Neuropsychological Society*, **9**, 642–52.

Cornoldi, C., De Beni, R., & Pazzaglia, F. (1996). *Profiles of Reading Comprehension Difficulties: An Analysis of Single Cases*. Mahwah, NJ: Erlbaum.

Davidson, C. M., Northrup, H., King, T. M., *et al.* (2008). Genes in glucose metabolism and association with spina bifida. *Reproductive Sciences*, **15**, 51–8.

Dennis, M. & Barnes, M. A. (2002). Numeracy skills in adults with spina bifida. *Developmental Neuropsychology*, **21**, 141–56.

Dennis, M., Edelstein, K., Copeland, K., et al. (2004). Neurobiology of timing in children with spina bifida in relation to cerebellar volume. *Brain*, **127**, 1292–301.

Dennis, M., Edelstein, K., Copeland, K., *et al.* (2005a). Covert orienting to exogenous and endogenous cues in children with spina bifida. *Neuropsychologia*, **43**, 976–87.

Dennis, M., Edelstein, K., Copeland, K., *et al.* (2005b). Space-based inhibition of return in children with spina bifida. *Neuropsychology*, **19**, 456–65.

Dennis, M., Fletcher, J. M., Rogers, T., Hetherington, R., & Francis, D. J. (2002). Object-based and action-based visual perception in children with spina bifida and hydrocephalus. *Journal of the International Neuropsychological Society*, **8**, 95–106.

Dennis, M., Fritz, C. R., Netley, C. T., *et al.* (1981). The intelligence of hydrocephalic children. *Archives of Neurology*, **38**, 607–15.

Dennis, M., Hendrick, E. B., Hoffman, H. J., & Humphreys, R. P. (1987). Language of hydrocephalic children and adolescents. *Journal of Clinical and Experimental Neuropsychology*, **9**, 593–621.

Dennis, M., Jacennik, B., & Barnes, M. A. (1994). The content of narrative discourse in children and adolescents after early-onset hydrocephalus and in normally developing age peers. *Brain and Language*, **46**, 129–65.

Dennis, M., Jewell, D., Drake, J., *et al.* (2007). Prospective, declarative, and non-declarative memory in young adults with spina bifida. *Journal of the International Neuropsychological Society*, **13**, 312–23.

Dennis, M., Landry, S. H., Barnes, M., & Fletcher, J. M. (2006). A model of neurocognitive function in spina bifida over the life span. *Journal of the International Neuropsychological Society*, **12**, 285–96.

Dennis, M., Nelson, R., & Fletcher, J. M. (2009). Prospective memory in younger and older adults with spina bifida. Poster presentation, Rotman Research Institute 14th Annual Conference "Cognitive Aging," Toronto ON 8–9 March 2009, Toronto Ontario.

Dennis, M., Sinopoli, K. J., Fletcher, J. M., & Schachar, R. (2008). Puppets, robots, critics, and actors within a taxonomy of attention for developmental disorders. *Journal of the International Neuropsychological Society*, **14**, 673–90.

Dennis, M., Spiegler, B. J., & Hetherington, R. (2000). New survivors for the new millennium: Cognitive risk and reserve in adults with childhood brain insults. *Brain and Cognition*, **42**, 102–5.

Diamond, A. & Doar, B. (1989). The performance of human infants on a measure of frontal cortex function, the delayed response task. *Developmental Psychobiology*, **22**, 271–94.

Donders, J., Canady, A. I., & Rourke, B. P. (1990). Psychometric intelligence after infantile hydrocephalus: A critical review and reinterpretation. *Child's Nervous System*, **6**, 148–54.

Edelstein, K., Dennis, M., Copeland, K., *et al.* (2004). Motor learning in children with spina bifida: Dissociation between performance level and acquisition rate. *Journal of the International Neuropsychological Society*, **10**, 877–87.

English, L. H., Barnes, M. A., Taylor, H. B., & Landry, S. H., (2009). Mathematical development in spina bifida. *Developmental Disabilities Research Reviews*, **15**, 28–34.

Fletcher, J. M., Bohan, T. P., Brandt, M. E., *et al.* (1992). Cerebral white matter and cognition in hydrocephalic children. *Archives of Neurology*, **49**, 818–24.

Fletcher, J. M., Brookshire, B. L., Bohan, T. P., Brandt, M. E., & Davidson, K. C. (1995). Early hydrocephalus. In B. P. Rourke (Ed.), *Syndrome of Nonverbal Learning Disabilities: Neurodevelopmental Manifestations* (pp. 206–238). New York: Guilford.

Fletcher, J. M., Copeland, K., Frederick, J., *et al.* (2005). Spinal lesion level in spina bifida meningomyelocele: A source of neural and cognitive heterogeneity. *Journal of Neurosurgery*, **102**, 268–79.

Fletcher, J. M., Dennis, M., Northup, H., *et al.* (2004). Spina bifida: Genes, brain, and development. In L. M. Glidden, (Ed.), *Handbook of Research on Mental Retardation* (Vol. 28, pp. 63–117). San Diego: Academic Press.

Fletcher, J. M., Lyon, G. R., Fuchs, L. S., & Barnes, M. A. (2007). *Learning Disabilities: From Identification to Intervention*. New York: The Guilford Press.

Fletcher, J. M., Ostermaier, K. K., Cirino, P. T., & Dennis, M. (2008). Neurobehavioral outcomes in spina bifida: Processes versus outcomes. *Journal of Pediatric Rehabilitation Medicine: An Interdisciplinary Approach*, **1**, 311–24.

Friedrich, W. N., Lovejoy, M. C., Shaffer, J., Shurtleff, D. B., & Beilke, R. L. (1991). Cognitive abilities and achievement status of children with myelomeningocele: A contemporary sample. *Journal of Pediatric Psychology*, **16**, 423–8.

Geary, D. C. (1993). Mathematical disabilities: Cognitive, neuropsychological, and genetic components. *Psychological Bulletin*, **114**, 345–62.

Geary, D. C., Hamson, C. O., & Hoard, M. K. (2000). Numerical and arithmetical cognition: A longitudinal study of process and concept deficits in children with learning disability. *Journal of Experimental Child Psychology*, **77**, 236–63.

Geary, D. C., Hoard, M. K., Byrd-Craven, J., Nugent, L., & Numtee, C. (2007). Cognitive mechanisms underlying achievement deficits in children with mathematical learning disability. *Child Development*, **78**, 1343–59.

Gernsbacher, M. A. (1990). *Language Comprehension as Structure Building*. Hillsdale, NJ: Lawrence Erlbaum.

Gernsbacher, M. A. & Faust, M. E. (1991). The mechanism of suppression: A component of general comprehension skill. *Journal of Experimental Psychology: Learning, Memory, and Cognition*, **17**, 245–62.

Gersten, R., Jordan, N. C., & Flojo, J. R. (2005). Early identification and interventions for students with mathematics difficulties. *Journal of Learning Disabilities*, **38**, 293–304.

Gibbs, R. W. (1986). Skating on thin ice: Literal meaning and understanding idioms in conversation. *Discourse Processes*, **9**, 17–30.

Goldberg, S. (1978). Prematurity: Effects on parent-infant interaction. *Journal of Pediatric Psychology*, **3**, 137–44.

Hartje, W. (1987). The effect of spatial disorders on arithmetical skills. In G. Deloche & X. Seron (Eds.), *Mathematical Disabilities: A Cognitive Neuropsychological Perspective* (pp. 121–35). Hillsdale, NJ: Erlbaum.

Haxby, J. V., Grady, C. L., Horwitz, B., *et al.* (1991). Dissociation of object and spatial visual processing pathways in human extrastriate cortex. *Proceedings of the National Academy of Sciences of the United States of America*, **88**(5), 1621–5.

Hess, R. D. & Shipman, V. C. (1965). Early experience and the socialization of cognitive modes in children. *Child Development*, **36**, 869–86.

Hetherington, R., Dennis, M., Barnes, M., Drake, J., & Gentilli, F. (2006). Functional outcome in young adults with spina bifida and hydrocephalus. *Child's Nervous System*, **22**, 117–24.

Holmbeck, G. N., Greenley, R. N., Coakley, R. M., Greco, J., & Hagstrom, J. (2006). Family functioning in children and adolescents with spina bifida: An evidence-based review of research and interventions. *Journal of Developmental and Behavioral Pediatrics*, **27**(3), 249–77.

Holmbeck, G. N., Westhoven, V. C., Phillips, W. S., *et al.* (2003). A multimethod, multi-informant, and multi-dimensional perspective on psychosocial adjustment in preadolescents with spina bifida. *Journal of Consulting and Clinical Psychology*, **71**, 782–96.

Holmes, J. & Adams, J. W. (2006). Working memory and children's mathematical skills: Implications for mathematical development and mathematical curricula. *Educational Psychology*, **26**, 339–66.

Horn, D. G., Lorch, E. P., Lorch, R. F., & Culatta, B. (1985). Distractibility and vocabulary deficits in children with spina bifida and hydrocephalus. *Developmental Medicine and Child Neurology*, **27**, 713–20.

Huber-Okrainec, J., Blaser, S. E., & Dennis, M. (2005). Idiom comprehension deficits in relation to corpus callosum agenesis and hypoplasia in children with spina bifida meningomyelocele. *Brain and Language*, **93**, 349–68.

Johnston, A. M., Barnes, M. A., & Desrochers, A. (2008). Reading comprehension: Developmental processes, individual differences, and interventions. *Canadian Psychology*, **49**, 125–32.

Jordan, N. C., Hanich, L. B., & Kaplan, D. (2003). A longitudinal study of mathematical competencies in children with specific mathematics and reading difficulties. *Child Development*, **74**, 834–50.

Juranek, J., Fletcher, J. M., Hasan, K. M., *et al.* (2008). Neurocortical reorganization in spina bifida. *Neuroimage*, **40**, 1516–22.

Kalaman, D. A. & LeFevre, J. (2007). Working memory demands of exact and approximate addition. *European Journal of Cognitive Psychology*, **19**, 187–212.

Kintsch, W. (1988). The role of knowledge in discourse comprehension: A construction-integration model. *Psychological Review*, **95**, 163–82.

Klein, R. M. (2000). Inhibition of return. *Trends in Cognitive Sciences*, **4**, 138–47.

Kogan, K. L. (1980). Interaction systems between preschool handicapped or developmentally delayed children and their parents. In T. Field, S. Goldberg, D. Stern, & A. M. Sostek (Eds.), *High-risk Infants and Children: Adult and Peer Interactions* (pp. 227–47). New York: Academic Press, Inc.

Landry, S. H., Denson, S. E., & Swank, P. R. (1997). Effects of medical risk and socioeconomic status on the rate of change in cognitive and social development for low birth weight children. *Journal of Clinical and Experimental Neuropsychology*, **19**, 261–74.

Landry, S. H., Smith, K. E., & Swank, P. R. (2006). Responsive parenting: Establishing early foundations for social, communication, and independent problem-solving skills. *Developmental Psychology*, **42**, 627–42.

Landry, S. H., Smith, K. E., Swank, P. R., & Guttentag, C. (2008b). A responsive parenting intervention: The optimal timing across early childhood for impacting maternal behaviors and child outcomes. *Developmental Psychology*, **44**, 1335–53.

Landry, S. H., Taylor, H. B., Guttentag, C., & Smith, K. E. (2008a). Responsive parenting: Closing the learning gap for at-risk children. In L. Glidden (Ed.), *International Review of Research in Mental Retardation* (Vol. 36 pp. 27–60). Burlington: Academic Press.

Leach, J. M., Scarborough, H. S., & Rescorla, L. (2003). Late-emerging reading disabilities. *Journal of Educational Psychology*, **95**, 211–24.

LeFevre, J., DeStefano, D., Coleman, B., & Shanahan, T. (2005). Mathematical cognition and working memory. In J. I. D. Campbell (Ed.), *The Handbook of Mathematical Cognition* (pp. 361–78). New York: Psychology Press.

Lemelle, J.L., Guillemin, F., Aubert, D., Guys, J.M., Lottmann, H., Lortat-Jacob, S., Mouriquand, P., Ruffion, A., Moscovici, J., & Schmitt, M. (2006). Quality of life and continence in patients with spina bifida. *Quality of Life Research*, **15**, 1481–92.

Lomax-Bream, L. E., Barnes, M., Copeland, K., Taylor, H. B., & Landry, S. H. (2007a). The impact of spina bifida on development across the first 3 years. *Developmental Neuropsychology*, **31**, 1–20.

Lomax-Bream, L. E., Taylor, H. B., Landry, S. H., Barnes, M. A., Fletcher, J. M., & Swank, P. (2007b). Role of early parenting and motor skills on development in children with spina bifida. *Journal of Applied Developmental Psychology*, **28**, 250–63.

Loss, N., Yeates, K. O., & Enrile, B. G. (1998). Attention in children with myelomeningocele. *Child Neuropsychology*, **4**, 7–20.

MacDonald, M. C., Pearlmutter, N. J., & Seidenberg, M. S. (1994). Lexical nature of syntactic ambiguity resolution. *Psychological Review*, **101**, 676–703.

March of Dimes (2006). *Global Report on Birth Defects: The Hidden Toll of Dying and Disabled Children*. White Plains, NY: March of Dimes.

Mayes, S. D. & Calhoun, S. L. (2006). Frequency of reading, math, and writing disabilities in children with clinical disorders. *Learning and Individual Differences*, **16**, 145–57.

McDonnell, G. V. & McCann, J. P. (2000). Issues of medical management in adults with spina bifida. *Child's Nervous System*, **16**, 222–7.

Muter, V., Hulme, C., Snowling, M. J., & Stevenson, J. (2004). Phonemes, rimes, vocabulary, and grammatical skills as foundations of early reading development: Evidence from a longitudinal study. *Developmental Psychology*, **40**, 665–81.

Northrup, H. & Volcik, K. A. (2000). Spina bifida and other neural tube defects. *Current Problems in Pediatrics*, **30**, 317–32.

Oakhill, J. V., Cain, K., & Bryant, P. E. (2003). Dissociation of single-word reading and text comprehension skills. *Language and Cognitive Processes*, **18**, 443–68.

Oddson, B. E., Clancy, C. A., & McGrath, P. J. (2006). The role of pain in reduced quality of life and depressive symptomology in children with spina bifida. *Clinical Journal of Pain*, **22**, 784–9.

O'Donnell, S., Noseworthy, M. D., Levine, B., & Dennis, M. (2005). Cortical thickness of the frontopolar area in typically developing children and adolescents. *Neuroimage*, **24**, 948–54.

Posner, M. I., Walker, J. A., Friedrich, F. J., & Rafal, R. D. (1984). Effects of parietal injury on covert orienting of attention. *Journal of Neuroscience*, **4**, 1863–74.

Raghubar, K. P., Cirino, P. T., Barnes, M. A., Ewing-Cobbs, L., Fletcher, J. M., & Fuchs, L. (2009). Errors in multi-digit arithmetic and behavioral inattention in children with math difficulties. *Journal of Learning Disabilities* 42, 356–71.

Rendeli, C., Salvaggio, E., Cannizzaro, G. S., Bianchi, E., Caldarelli, M., & Guzzetta, F. (2002). Does locomotion improve the cognitive profile of children with meningomyelocele? *Child's Nervous System*, **18**, 231–4.

Rose, B. M. & Holmbeck, G. N. (2007). Attention and executive functions in adolescents with spina bifida. *Journal of Pediatric Psychology*, **32**, 983–94.

Roselli, M. & Ardila, A. (1989). Calculation deficits in patients with right and left hemisphere damage. *Neuropsychologia*, **27**, 607–17.

Salman, M. S., Blaser, S., Sharpe, J. A., & Dennis, M. (2006). Cerebellar vermis morphology in children with spina bifida and Arnold Chiari Type II malformation. *Child's Nervous System*, **22**, 385–93.

Schmalhofer, F., McDaniel, M. A., & Keefe, D. (2002). A unified model for predictive and bridging inferences. *Discourse Processes*, **33**, 105–32.

Shalev, R. S., Auerbach, J., Manor, O., & Gross-Tsur, V. (2000). Developmental dyscalculia: Prevalence and prognosis. *European Child and Adolescent Psychiatry*, **9**, II58–II64.

Shaywitz, S. E., Fletcher, J. M., Holahan, J. M., *et al.* (1999). Persistence of dyslexia: The Connecticut Longitudinal Study at adolescence. *Pediatrics*, **104**, 1351–9.

Sutton, L. N. (2008). Fetal surgery for neural tube defects. *Best Practice & Research Clinical Obstetrics and Gynaecology*, **22**, 175–88.

Swanson, H. L. (2007). Commentary on Part I, Section II: Cognitive aspects of math disabilities. In D. B. Berch & M. M. M. Mazzocco (Eds.), *Why Is Math so Hard for Some Children? The Nature and Origins of Mathematical Learning Difficulties and disabilities* (pp. 133–44). Baltimore: Paul H. Brookes Publishing Co.

Swanson, H. L. & Jerman, O. (2006). Math disabilities: A selective meta-analysis of the literature. *Review of Educational Research*, **76**, 249–74.

Taylor, H. B., Landry, S. H., Barnes, M., Cohen, L., Swank, P., & Fletcher, J. (submitted). Early information processing among infants with and without spina bifida. *Infant Behavior and Development*.

Thelen, E. & Smith, L. B. (1994). *A Dynamic Systems Approach to the Development of Cognition and Action*. Cambridge, MA: MIT Press.

van Allen, M. I., Kalousek, D. K., Chernoff, G. F., *et al.* (1993). Evidence for multi-site closure of the neural tube in humans. *American Journal of Medical Genetics*, **47**, 723–43.

Volcik, K. A., Blanton, S. H., Tyerman, G. H., *et al.* (2000). Methylenetetrahydrofolate reductase and spina bifida: Evaluation of level of defect and maternal genotypic risk in Hispanics. *American Journal of Medical Genetics*, **95**, 21–7.

Wiig, E. H. & Secord, W. (1989). *Test of Language Competence — Expanded Edition (TLC-E)*. San Antonio, TX: The Psychological Corporation.

Williams, L. J., Rasmussen, S. A., Flores, R. S., Kirby, R. S., & Edmunds, L. D. (2005). Decline in the prevalence of spina bifida and anencephaly by race/ethnicity: 1995–2002. *Pediatrics*, **116**, 580–6.

Wills, K. E. (1993). Neuropsychological functioning in children with spina bifida and/or hydrocephalus. *Journal of Clinical Child Psychology*, **22**, 247–65.

Wills, K. E., Holmbeck, G. N., Dillon, K., & McClone, D. G. (1990). Intelligence and achievement in children with myelomeningocele. *Journal of Pediatric Psychology*, **15**, 161–76.

Yeates, K. O. & Enrile, B. G. (2005). Implicit and explicit memory in children with congenital and acquired brain disorder. *Neuropsychology*, **19**, 618–28.

Yuill, N. & Oakhill, J. (1991). Children's problems in text comprehension: An experimental investigation. *Cambridge Monographs and Texts in Applied Psycholinguistics*. New York: Cambridge University Press.

Zwaan, R. A. & Radvansky, G. A. (1998). Situation models in language comprehension and memory. *Psychological Bulletin*, **123**, 162–85.

Genetic disorders and models of neurocognitive development

Language and communication in autism spectrum disorders

Susan Ellis Weismer

Introduction

Language and communication deficits are a hallmark of autism, constituting one of its major diagnostic features (ICD-10, World Health Organization, 1993; DSM-IV, American Psychiatric Association, 2000). Problems with pragmatic aspects of verbal and nonverbal communication are common, as might be expected given the social impairments that also characterize autism. Contemporary research has shifted away from concentrating primarily on pragmatics to considering linguistic features of autism more broadly, including phonological, lexical, and grammatical abilities. This shift in focus has served, at least in part, as an impetus for investigators to explore further the overlap between language difficulties seen in autism and those observed in other types of developmental language disorders. Investigating these potential overlaps has theoretical implications relative to dimensional vs. distinct category accounts of language disorder, as well as practical ramifications for early differential diagnosis. Current research in the area of autism has also expanded beyond classic autistic disorder to include children diagnosed with PDD-NOS/atypical autism and Asperger disorder, with these three pervasive developmental disorders referred to as autism spectrum disorders (ASD) (Charman & Baird, 2002; Lord *et al.*, 2000; and see Chapter 2).

Several new and exciting lines of inquiry have been made possible by recent advances in early clinical diagnosis, as well as the application of new technologies in brain imaging and developments in human genetics research. These recent research endeavors involve attempts to characterize early language development, identify predictors of later outcomes, and elucidate the nature of language processing in mature language users on the autism spectrum. Additionally, investigators

Support for the preparation of this chapter was provided by the National Institutes of Health, NIDCD grant R01 DC0371, "Linguistic Processing in Specific Language Delay" (Ellis Weismer, PI, Evans & Chapman, Co-PIs) and NIDCD/NICHD grant R01DC007223, "Early Language Development within the Autism Spectrum" (Ellis Weismer, PI, Gernsbacher, Co-PI).

have examined phenotypic and etiologic overlap between ASD and language disorders in an effort to better understand the link between these conditions, their causes, and their treatment. The purpose of the present chapter is to provide a brief overview of each of these respective topics. In the first section, early language profiles and predictors of outcomes are described. Follow-up studies, including those exploring the overlap between ASD and language disorders are considered in the second section of the chapter. The third section deals with language processing in adults and adolescents with ASD and language disorders. The fourth section focuses on behavioral and neural phenotypes of ASD and language disorders and their genetic bases. Finally, conclusions and future directions for research are presented.

Early language profiles and predictors of language outcomes

Recent research has begun to provide a picture of early language and communication abilities in children with ASD. Charman *et al.* (2003) assessed language development through the use of a parent report measure, the MacArthur-Bates Communicative Development Inventory (CDI) – Words and Gestures form. Their sample was composed of 134 preschoolers with ASD (116 boys, 18 girls). The mean age was 3 years, 2 months, but ages ranged widely from 18 months to just over 7 years. Results revealed that the ASD group was significantly delayed compared to the CDI normative sample. Despite significant delays in comprehension and production for both a chronological age and nonverbal mental age analysis, language skills for ASD children showed clear developmental trends across age levels. Findings for the ASD group were similar to typical developmental patterns in a number of ways, yet differed in certain respects from the typical pattern. Children on the autism spectrum exhibited considerable variability in language development: word comprehension was ahead of production in absolute terms, gesture production served as a "bridge" between word comprehension and production (i.e., gestures were used as a means of making the transition from understanding the meaning of a word to being able to express that concept verbally), and the broad pattern of word category acquisition followed the typical pattern with respect to common nouns, predicates, and closed class words. However, two findings for the ASD sample were unlike the typical developmental pattern. First, the comprehension level of children with ASD was delayed relative to production, that is, there was less of a gap in favor of production than is typically observed. Second, production of early gestures (e.g., sharing reference) was delayed relative to later gestures (e.g., use of objects). Few differences in language profiles were noted according to diagnosis within the autism spectrum. When controlling for nonverbal IQ, the only significant difference was that children with autism produced fewer early gestures than the PDD subgroup.

Another investigation conducted by Eaves and Ho (2004) focused exclusively on toddlers with ASD. The mean age at which parents first reported being concerned about these children's development was 13 months; loss of words prior to 2 years, 6 months (2;6) was reported for 28% of the cases. According to testing completed at 2;6, 70% of the toddlers scored below 12 months in expressive and receptive language, while 24% scored between 12 and 24 months in terms of language levels. Nearly half of the toddlers with ASD did not use spoken words at 2;6. Although the vast majority of the participants in this study demonstrated significant early language deficits, 3 toddlers (out of 49) had language skills that were roughly within normal range. Eaves and Ho speculate that children who are identified quite early, as in the case of their sample, tend to be lower functioning relative to the autism population at large. This assertion appears to be supported when comparing the overall level of functioning of the toddlers in the Eaves and Ho (2004) study to that of the somewhat older sample in the Charman *et al.* (2003) investigation, although it is also possible that overestimation of children's abilities on the parent report measure used by Charman and colleagues was a factor in the differences in ability levels.

Ellis Weismer and colleagues characterized early language abilities and outcomes in a large, representative sample of children with ASD (Ellis Weismer *et al.*, 2005a). In a prior project, a sample of 170 children on the autism spectrum had been assembled by Gernsbacher and colleagues (Gernsbacher *et al.*, 2008); this sample captured 75% of all autism cases reported by the Department of Public Instruction within a defined age range (4–16 years) and geographical area (Dane County, Wisconsin). Profiles of language skills at 2 to 3 years of age were identified from retrospective, landmark-based parent interviews. These language profiles were confirmed through analysis of historic home videotape for selected cases. Children's language production from the videotapes was transcribed and analyzed using Systematic Analysis of Language Transcripts (SALT, Miller & Chapman, 2000). Analyses of retrospective data were conducted to determine the types of language profiles exhibited by toddlers who were subsequently diagnosed with ASD. The distribution of these early language profiles was then examined relative to current autism diagnoses in order to better understand the range of language variation within diagnostic categories. Ellis Weismer *et al.* (2005a) identified four profiles of early language skills in toddlers on the autism spectrum: (1) normal vocabulary skills (ASD: Normal Vocabulary), 27% of the sample; (2) delays in vocabulary but production of at least 10 spoken words, similar to that of late talkers who are not on the spectrum (ASD: Late Talker), 35% of the sample; (3) no talking or sporadic use of fewer than 10 spoken words (ASD: Severe Delay), 26% of the sample; and (4) loss of more than 10 spoken words or the ability to combine words prior to age 3;0 (ASD: Regression), 12% of the sample. Three of the four early language profiles (ASD: Normal Vocabulary; ASD: Late Talker; and ASD: Regression) were associated with a range of current day DSM-IV diagnoses (as classified by community practitioners), including autism, Asperger's, and PPD-NOS. While a subset of children who reportedly exhibited normal vocabulary development at 2–3 years of age had a current diagnosis of Asperger's (25%), the remainder of the ASD: Normal Vocabulary profile had diagnoses of PDD-NOS (45%) or autism (30%). Furthermore, children with Asperger diagnoses also comprised a small proportion of the early language profiles that involved late talking (12%) or regression (5%). These findings are consistent with other research that has questioned traditional diagnostic criteria for Asperger's, including normal language development (Howlin, 2003; Mayes *et al.*, 2001). Those children who had presented an early profile of ASD: Severe Delay either had current day diagnoses of autism (75%) or PDD-NOS (25%).

Language outcomes in 113 children were also examined by Ellis Weismer *et al.* (2005a). In this sample, 82% of the children were reported to have persistent language problems ranging from continuing delays to no functional spoken language. The same pattern was observed for younger children whose parents reported early outcomes (at 4–8 years) as for older children (at 9–16 years); therefore, the outcome data were collapsed across age ranges. Children with an early ASD: Normal Vocabulary profile had the best outcome across the four profiles; however, 57% (12/21) of the ASD: Normal Vocabulary toddlers had subsequent language difficulties. The vast majority, 89% (34/38), of children with an early ASD: Late Talker profile displayed persistent language problems, although 11% had moved into the normal range. Children with a regression profile fared somewhat better than the late talker subgroup, with 78% (14/18) having poor language outcomes and 22% demonstrating normal range language skills later in development. The children who had an early pattern of severe delay had the worst outcomes: 92% (33/36) had poor language outcomes, with only 8% in normal limits. Although none of the 36 toddlers with severe delays moved into normal limits by 8 years of age, 3 were reported to have normal language at later outcomes (9–16 years). In summary, more than half of the toddlers with good early language abilities did not continue on a typical developmental trajectory. Nearly 90% of the late talkers on the autism spectrum had persistent language delay, which is the reverse of the outcome pattern observed for late talkers without autistic features (Ellis Weismer, 2007). Finally, these findings suggest that severe early language delay is a poor prognostic sign but that good early language skills may not be associated with positive language outcomes.

A number of investigations have sought to identify predictors of language outcomes in children on the autism spectrum. Several studies have reported that onset of spoken language prior to 5 years of age is a positive prognostic indicator for later language and social abilities in autism (Ballaban-Gil *et al.*, 1996; Rutter, 1970; Venter *et al.*, 1992). Variables that have been examined specifically with respect to prediction of *language* outcomes include early language and cognitive abilities, joint attention, imitation skills, and amount of intervention. Charman *et al.* (2005) investigated the predictive validity of autism symptom severity, cognitive, and language performance during toddlerhood (2 and 3 years) for outcomes at 7 years. In a sample of 26 children with ASD, they found that performance on standard assessments at 3 years, but not 2 years, predicted outcomes at age 7. Although standard assessments were not predictive at the earliest time point, an informal measure of the rate of nonverbal communicative acts during interactive play-based assessment at age 2 was found to be predictive of language, communication, and social outcomes. Findings by Eaves and Ho (2004) indicated that children with higher nonverbal IQ and milder autistic symptoms at age 2 displayed the greatest gains in verbal skills at age 4. Similarly, Charman *et al.* (2003) found that a PDD diagnosis at 20 months was associated with better receptive and expressive language abilities at 42 months than an autism diagnosis. Based on a 2-year follow-up investigation of children who received an autism spectrum diagnosis at 2 years of age, Stone and Yoder (2001) found that a composite measure of expressive language was significantly correlated across time points (r=0.72); that is, early expressive skills predicted subsequent productive language abilities. A study of later outcomes for ASD children conducted by Sigman and Ruskin (1999) reported significant associations between language scores at 4 years and 13 years, both for receptive language (r=0.61) and expressive language (r=0.51).

Various investigations have explored the role of joint attention, imitation, and/or intervention in language outcomes for children on the autism spectrum. Mundy and colleagues found that joint attention was a significant predictor of language development in young children with autism across a 13-month follow-up period (Mundy *et al.*, 1990). Receptive language outcome at 42 months has been reported to be positively associated with stronger joint attention and imitation abilities at 20 months in children with ASD (Charman *et al.*, 2003). Results from a study conducted by Bono *et al.* (2004) revealed that language gains were associated with better initial language abilities, higher cognitive abilities, and better joint attention in children aged 31 to 64 months. In that study, joint attention was found to moderate the relationship between amount of intervention and language gains. That is, children with stronger joint attention skills demonstrated greater increases in language scores with more intervention.

Some negative findings have also been reported in the literature regarding the predictive role of joint attention or amount of intervention. Stone and Yoder (2001) reported that better motor imitation skills and higher number of hours of language therapy predicted better expressive language outcomes; however, when controlling for expressive language at age 2, joint attention was not correlated with expressive language outcomes. Another study that examined performance on three measures of joint attention found that joint attention was not correlated with vocabulary development in children with autism (Morgan *et al.*, 2003). With respect to intervention, results of the study by Eaves and Ho (2004) indicated that the amount of time a child spent in intervention was not a significant predictor of gains in language or other areas of development. They conducted a separate analysis of outcomes for 21 children within their sample who participated in intensive applied behavior analysis programs (i.e., 10–40 hours/week). This analysis similarly revealed no significant difference in improvement in performance IQ or verbal IQ compared to the rest of the sample. Thus, there are mixed findings regarding the role of joint attention or intervention in predicting ASD language outcomes. While there are relatively few studies examining imitation as a predictor of later language abilities, the findings appear to be promising.

Follow-up studies: Overlap in ASD and language disorders

Researchers have examined the overlap between ASD and language disorders through follow-up studies to determine the extent to which similar outcomes are observed. There are several issues that have motivated this line of research. To begin with, a deficit in communicative use of language is one of the key features of an autism diagnosis. Children who have language disorders may also develop secondary social problems (Rice *et al.*, 1991; Whitehurst & Fischel, 1994). Furthermore, a portion of children with language disorders have pragmatic difficulties involving reciprocal social interaction that are similar to those observed in ASD (Bishop, 2000; Botting & Conti-Ramsden, 1999 , 2003). Therefore, there is interest in these comparisons for the purpose of establishing behavioral phenotypes and developing models of language disorder.

Rutter and colleagues have conducted a long-term follow-up study of two groups of 7- to 8-year-olds with normal range IQs, one with autism and the other with severe receptive language disorder (Bartak *et al.*, 1975, 1977; Cantwell *et al.*, 1989; Mawhood *et al.*, 2000). In the most recent report of these individuals when they were young adults (Mawhood *et al.*, 2000), they displayed problems in sustaining conversations and produced unusual prosodic patterns. These language difficulties were more evident in the language disorders group than they had been at earlier time points, but were still less notable than in the autism group. The language disorders group was also reported to have social difficulties, although they were not as severe as those of the autism group. Social difficulties noted in the young adults in the language disorders group consisted of impoverished social relationships, narrow interests, and routinized behavior patterns.

Other follow-up studies have also addressed this issue of the overlap between ASD and language disorders (Beitchman *et al.*, 1996; Conti-Ramsden *et al.*, 2001; Michelotti *et al.*, 2002). Beitchman and colleagues (1996) reported that a subset of children with mixed expressive and receptive language delays at age 5 had social difficulties at 12 years of age. Results from a study by Conti-Ramsden *et al.* (2001) indicated that 4% (10/242) of children attending language units in the United Kingdom at 7 years, displayed behaviors associated with ASD at age 11. Michelotti and colleagues (2002) conducted a follow-up study of 18 children who presented severe receptive/expressive language delay and some autistic features in preschool (but who did not meet criteria for an autism diagnosis). Contrary to their expectations, features of autism in these children did not dissipate with improvements in language abilities. Severity of social communication impairments and repetitive behaviors at age 4 was found to be associated with severity of autism symptoms and pragmatic abilities at age 8. In particular, results from the Michelotti *et al.* study suggest that the presence of restricted, repetitive, and stereotyped behaviors is a negative prognostic sign. This same finding regarding early repetitive behaviors being indicative of a poor prognosis has also been reported by Lord (2005).

Language processing in ASD and language disorders

Recent research has shed light on language processing in mature language users with ASD (Just *et al.*, 2004; Norbury, 2005). Just and colleagues used functional magnetic resonance imaging to examine brain activation in adults with high-functioning autism compared to verbal IQ-matched controls during a sentence (reading) comprehension task. Behavioral findings indicated that participants with autism responded faster but somewhat less accurately than controls. Imaging data results showed group differences in the distribution of activation across major cortical language areas and differences in functional connectivity. Compared with controls, adults with autism displayed significantly more activation in Wernicke's area (left superior temporal gyrus), which has been implicated in lexical processing, and displayed significantly less activation is Broca's area (left inferior frontal gyrus), which has been implicated in syntactic processing, semantic processing, and working memory. These findings were interpreted as suggesting that individuals with autism engage in more extensive processing of individual words while directing less processing toward integrating meanings of single words into coherent semantic/syntactic structures. The second main finding regarding reduced functional connectivity was obtained by calculating the correlation between the activation time series data of two brain regions. Adults with autism demonstrated consistently lower functional connectivity than controls, suggesting reduced levels of cortical synchronization and coordination.

Based on their findings, Just and colleagues (2004) have proposed the "under-connectivity theory" of autism. According to this theory, underfunctioning integrative circuitry impedes integration of information at neural and cognitive levels. That is, autism is thought to involve a disruption of complex information processing, particularly in the face of increased levels of computational demand. The underconnectivity theory is postulated to account for a variety of behavioral characteristics of autism beyond language processing. For example, Just *et al.* claim that theory of mind deficits (Baron-Cohen *et al.*, 1985) observed in autism may be the outcome of a deficiency in integrating social and cognitive processing. In terms of previous theories of autism, the underconnectivity theory is most closely aligned with the weak central coherence theory (Frith, 1989), which posits that individuals with autism focus on details at the expense of creating more integrated representations. Underconnectivity theory differs from the weak central coherence theory in that it attempts to specify neurobiological phenomena associated with deficits in mental processes, views coherence as an emergent property of collaboration among brain regions, and postulates that cortical centers corresponding to components of the cognitive system are tuned to be more highly specialized and operate more autonomously in autism.

The interpretation of the findings by Just *et al.* (2004) raises a number of questions. To begin with, it is not clear how to reconcile the behavioral findings with the group differences for the imaging data. Just and colleagues assume that differences in activation patterns across groups reflect language processing deficiencies in autism. Some individuals with high-functioning autism do have language problems. However, in this study, the tendency for the autism group to perform less accurately than the cognitive-matched control group was not statistically significant, but the individuals with high-functioning autism did perform significantly faster than controls. Therefore, the extent to which the observed neural underconnectivity can be viewed as accounting for "deficits" in language processing is questionable in this case. Furthermore, it remains to be seen whether this same pattern of findings would be obtained across the full autism spectrum (including individuals with more severe autistic symptoms) and whether similar results would extend to areas of cognitive functioning other than language processing. If the underconnectivity theory is posited to account for autism generally, then it will be important to establish that it applies broadly to children with classic autistic disorder, as well as those with high-functioning autism, and to determine that lack of neural connectivity characterizes performance on social tasks or other deficit areas associated with this diagnosis.

There is some evidence that the imaging results in the Just *et al.* study may be more closely related to differential language processing than to autism per se. Similar to the findings of Just *et al.* (2004), a functional magnetic resonance imaging investigation by Ellis Weismer *et al.* (2005b) revealed significantly less activation in the insular portion of the left inferior frontal gyrus in adolescents with SLI than controls with normal language development during the word recognition phase of a verbal working memory task (as well as significantly less activation of the left parietal lobule and the precentral sulcus during spoken sentence comprehension; however, SLI adolescents did not demonstrate significantly greater activation than controls in any of the regions of interest). Ellis Weismer and colleagues also observed that the SLI adolescents exhibited atypical coordination of activation across cortical regions for both encoding and recognition phases of the task, with some indication of underconnectivity relative to controls during word recognition. If future neuroimaging studies confirm that children with language impairment who do not have autism also exhibit underconnectivity, then the explanatory basis of the underconnectivity theory relative to the condition of autism is called into question.

An investigation by Norbury (2005) sought to establish whether deficiency in contextual processing during a language comprehension task is related to autism or language impairment. Participants in this study (9–17 years of age) composed four groups, including participants with ASD who had language impairment, participants with ASD who had normal range language abilities, participants with SLI, and typically developing controls. Norbury examined predictions of the weak central coherence theory of autism by assessing these groups' ability to integrate information during comprehension. She used a version of a task developed by Gernsbacher *et al.* (1990), based on the structure building framework, to explore contextual facilitation and suppression of irrelevant meanings during processing of lexical ambiguity. According to this framework, as a mental representation is built up during language comprehension, activations of related meanings are enhanced while unrelated meanings are suppressed. Results revealed that all groups displayed contextual facilitation such that they responded faster and more accurately to biased contexts than to neutral contexts ("He *fished* from the bank" vs. "He *ran* from the bank," accompanied by a picture of "river"). However, the two groups with language impairment used context less efficiently than the groups without language impairment. Similarly, performance on the suppression condition reflected poorer contextual processing for the two groups with language impairment ("He stole from the *bank*," accompanied by a picture of "river"). These findings challenge the predictions of the weak central coherence theory in that deficits in contextual processing were not observed across the autism spectrum. Instead, children with language impairment–with and without autism–displayed deficits in integrating information in context (the same paradigm has been used in other neurogenetic disorders, see Chapter 3). Additional research employing the type of design used by Norbury (2005) is needed. In particular, investigations that also incorporate a functional imaging component (functional magnetic resonance imaging) would provide further insight into integrative cognitive processes and their associated neural circuitry in autism relative to other populations with communication and language deficits.

Examination of phenotypic and etiologic overlap between ASD and language disorders

Overlap in behavioral phenotypes

The contemporary view of the nature of language and communication impairments in ASD is that there is a certain degree of overlap between language difficulties observed within the autism spectrum and those observed in children without autism (Gernsbacher *et al.*, 2005). In particular, there is empirical evidence of phenotypic overlap with respect to language and communication challenges of children with ASD and those with SLI (Barrett *et al.*, 2004; Bishop & Norbury, 2002 , 2005; Kjelgaard & Tager-Flusberg, 2001; Tager-Flusberg & Joseph, 2003), pragmatic language impairment (PLI) (Bishop & Norbury, 2002 , 2005; Botting & Conti-Ramsden, 2003), and early language delay (Charman *et al.*, 2003).

SLI involves a significant language deficit in the absence of developmental disabilities or other identifiable causes (e.g., hearing loss, frank neurological deficits, motor problems). Children with SLI exhibit a variety of profiles with respect to lexical–semantic, morphosyntactic, and pragmatic areas of language comprehension and use. In the 1980s, a "semantic–pragmatic" subtype of SLI was proposed (Bishop & Rosenbloom, 1987; Rapin & Allen, 1983). More recently, this profile of language difficulties has been referred to as "pragmatic language impairment" (Bishop, 2000; Bishop & Norbury, 2002; Conti-Ramsden & Botting, 1999). PLI (or semantic–pragmatic subtype of SLI) is characterized by fluent and grammatically complex expressive language, but difficulties with the use of language in context (i.e., pragmatic aspects of language). Children identified as having PLI do not display socially appropriate conversational language, they have problems understanding and producing connected discourse, and may exhibit use of stereotyped phrases or utterances.

A debate has existed in the literature regarding the diagnosis of PLI (semantic–pragmatic category) and its relation to ASD. Some researchers have claimed that this category simply reflects the language and communicative abilities in high-functioning autism (Gagnon *et al.*, 1997; Shields *et al.*, 1996). However, there is evidence to indicate that at least some children with PLI display no autistic features (Bishop, 1998; Bishop & Norbury, 2002; Botting & Conti-Ramsden, 2003).

Bishop and Norbury (2002) conducted two studies to assess the claim that PLI is synonymous with autism or PDD-NOS. They proposed three scenarios: (1) PLI is equivalent to autistic disorder; (2) PLI is equivalent to PDD-NOS; or (3) PLI exists in children who are not on the autism spectrum. In Study 1, 21 children (6 to 9 years old) were categorized based on their performance on the Children's Communication Checklist (Bishop, 1998) as PLI (n = 13) or typical SLI (n = 8). Autistic features were evaluated in these children using two parental report measures (ADI-R, Lord, Rutter, & Le Couteur, 1994; Social Communication Questionnaire, SCQ, Berument, Rutter, Pickles, Lord, & Bailey, 1999) and one direct assessment instrument (Autism Diagnostic Observation Schedule, ADOS, Lord *et al.*, 2000). In Study 2, autistic features were examined using the SCQ and ADOS in 18 children with PLI, 11 children with typical SLI, and 11 children with high-functioning autism. Overall results revealed good diagnostic agreement for the parent report measures (ADI-R and SCQ), but poor agreement between parent report and ADOS diagnoses such that the ADOS appeared to result in several false positives (e.g., two children who scored within the range for PDD-NOS on the ADOS did not meet criteria by parental report). Findings supported scenario 3 in that not all PLI cases were diagnosed as having autistic features (although a number of PLI cases did exhibit autism or autistic features). Children with PLI who did not have ASD were characterized as social and communicative with normal nonverbal communication, but were noted to use stereotyped language with atypical prosodic characteristics. Bishop and Norbury (2002) conclude that pragmatic difficulties often co-occur with autistic symptoms, but that not all children with PLI meet criteria for autism or an autism spectrum diagnosis. They further suggest that there is no clear dividing line between SLI – PLI – ASD and contend that these findings support a dimensional rather than categorical view of communicative disorders (Bishop, 2000).

Other researchers have also been interested in the extent to which it is possible to differentiate autism, PLI, and SLI, given that differential diagnosis of these conditions would have implications for genetic studies and for tailoring treatment approaches. Botting and Conti-Ramsden (2003) examined whether autism, PLI, and SLI could be distinguished using psycholinguistic markers. They focused on psycholinguistic markers that have been used to identify children with SLI. These markers included nonword repetition (Children's Non-Word Repetition, Gathercole & Baddeley, 1990), sentence repetition (Clinical Evaluation of Language Fundamentals-Revised, Semel *et al.*, 1987), and past tense knowledge (Past Tense Task, Marchman *et al.*, 1999). School-age children with ASD, PLI, or SLI who had performance IQs above 70 participated in this study. Because preliminary findings indicated that there was a bimodal distribution of performance for the PLI group, this group was subdivided into PLIpure (no autistic features) and PLIplus (some autistic features). Group comparisons revealed that the nonword repetition scores were significantly lower for the SLI group than other groups. Past tense knowledge and sentence repetition were low for all groups except PLIplus. With respect to sensitivity and specificity, sentence repetition was the most discriminating marker overall, followed by past tense knowledge. Nonword repetition was poor at differentiating individuals within the various groups except for SLI vs. PLIplus. Considering all measures, PLIplus could be distinguished from SLI and PLIpure with 80% accuracy. Less reliable classification was found for PLIplus vs. ASD and SLI vs. ASD (around 70% accuracy). Children with PLIpure could not be reliably distinguished from SLI or ASD. Botting and Conti-Ramsden conclude that, although classification accuracy levels were not sufficiently high for clinical diagnosis by themselves, these psycholinguistic markers may assist in differentiating subgroups with communication deficits.

Research by Tager-Flusberg and colleagues (Kjelgaard & Tager-Flusberg, 2001; Tager-Flusberg & Joseph, 2003) has highlighted similarities in language and cognitive profiles between children with ASD and those with SLI. Kjelgaard and Tager-Flusberg (2001) compared phonological, lexical, grammatical, and nonword repetition skills in 89 children with ASD (mean age of 7 years). They divided the sample on the basis of vocabulary scores (Peabody Picture Vocabulary Test-Revised, Dunn & Dunn, 1997) into normal (>85), borderline (70–85), and impaired (<75) levels of functioning. Findings indicated that vocabulary skills were higher than grammatical abilities and that language skills were sometimes independent of cognitive abilities in children with autism. Kjelgaard and Tager-Flusberg concluded that these cognitive and language profiles significantly overlapped with those observed in SLI. Similarly, Tager-Flusberg and Joseph (2003) have presented evidence for two subtypes of autism involving features of language overlap with SLI or uneven (verbal < nonverbal) cognitive profiles. In contrast to the dimensional views of communication disorders, they contend that there is a qualitatively distinct subtype of autism that is characterized by the same type of structural language difficulties observed in SLI. Furthermore, Tager-Flusberg and Joseph speculate there is a common etiology in autism and SLI such that the same genes that cause SLI also result in this particular subtype of autism when inherited along with other risk genes.

Overlap in neural phenotypes

Recent research has revealed common morphometric features in the brains of individuals with autism and SLI. Two neuroanatomical markers have been identified both in school-age boys with autism and school-age boys with language impairment: brain and radiate white matter enlargement (Herbert *et al.*, 2003a,b, 2004) and asymmetry in language cortex and higher-order association areas (de Fosse *et al.*, 2004; Herbert *et al.*, 2005). Herbert and colleagues (2005) conducted a whole-brain magnetic resonance imaging morphometric study of asymmetry in boys with high-functioning autism, developmental language impairment, and age-matched typically developing controls. Results showed that the children with autism and language impairment exhibited remarkably similar patterns of asymmetry throughout the cerebral cortex (at the level of cortical parcellation units); both groups displayed a rightward bias, whereas the reverse pattern was observed in the typically developing control group. The asymmetry differences across groups were most pronounced in higher-order association cortex. Herbert *et al.* suggest that higher-order association areas may be particularly vulnerable to connectivity abnormalities associated with white matter enlargement. These findings are consistent with the view that there is considerable overlap in the brain-based phenotypic features of autism and language impairment (e.g., Rapin & Dunn, 2003).

A study by de Fosse *et al.* (2004) compared asymmetry patterns in language-association cortex in autism and SLI. This investigation provides unique insights into the nature of the phenotypic overlap between these groups because, unlike other studies, it included autistic children with and without language impairment. Based on prior research, de Fosse and colleagues predicted group differences in volumetric asymmetry in language-related regions, namely, inferior lateral frontal cortex (Broca's area) and posterior superior temporal cortex. Findings revealed reversed asymmetry in frontal language cortex for the autism group with language impairment and the SLI group. That is, frontal language cortex was larger on the right hemisphere for both groups with language impairment, whereas this region was larger on the left hemisphere for both groups without language impairment (the group with autism who had normal language and the control group). These results add further evidence of neural phenotypic overlap between SLI and a subtype of autism, while also suggesting that Broca's area asymmetry reversal is more closely associated with language impairment than an autism diagnosis.

Etiological overlap

Although there is considerable evidence for behavioral and neural phenotypic overlap, the evidence for etiological overlap between autism and SLI is mixed. In this context, the term "etiology" is used to refer to genetic and environmental factors which produce these disorders or predispose an individual toward them. On the positive side, various studies of family members of children with autism have reported elevated rates of language deficits (Bailey *et al.*, 1998; Folstein *et al.*, 1999; Szatmari *et al.*, 2000). Investigations of twins have revealed that co-twins discordant for autism exhibit high rates of language problems that are similar to the patterns seen in SLI (Folstein & Rutter, 1977; Le Couteur *et al.*, 1996). Tomblin *et al.* (2003) found that the prevalence of autism in siblings of a population-based sample of children with SLI were significantly higher than estimates for the general population; similarly, Folstein and Mankoski (2000) have reported increased risk of SLI for siblings of children with autism. Finally, findings from molecular genetic investigations provide some support for etiological overlap between autism and SLI in that linkage signals to sites on chromosomes 2q or 7q and 13q are strengthened when both probands have autism with language deficits (Bradford *et al.*, 2001; Shao *et al.*, 2002).

On the other hand, Bishop (2003) has pointed out evidence against the notion of overlapping etiologies; she notes that there is a substantial minority of children with autism who do not display language deficits similar to those seen in SLI and that difficulties in speech sound production that are common in preschoolers with SLI are not typical of verbal children with autism. There are also conflicting findings regarding the extent to which relatives of individuals with autism actually have a heightened prevalence of language and literacy problems. Although autism family members routinely report more language difficulties than controls, direct testing has not necessarily confirmed these self-reported ratings (Fombonne *et al.*, 1997; Piven *et al.*, 1997). Additionally, molecular genetic findings have failed to reveal overlap in loci that show linkage to SLI and those that show linkage to autism (Barnby & Monaco, 2003).

In a recent investigation, Bishop and colleagues (2004) addressed the issue of etiological overlap between autism and SLI in a large sample of children participating in the Western Australia Family Study of Autism Spectrum Disorders. They examined whether phonological processing deficits, often thought to be a hallmark of SLI, are part of the broad autism phenotype. A current etiological view of autism espouses that individual components of the broader autism phenotype are inherited separately (such as social reticence, obsessiveness, or language impairment) and that these components are manifested independently in non-autistic family members (Folstein *et al.*, 1999). Two phonological processing tasks were administered to 80 probands with autistic disorder or PDD-NOS (index cases) and to 59 typically developing controls, as well as their parents and siblings. The phonological processing measures consisted of nonword repetition and nonsense passage reading. Findings revealed that probands with ASD were significantly impaired on both phonological processing measures (spoken and written) compared to controls. These results are consistent with other findings of deficits in nonword repetition in children with autism (Kjelgaard & Tager-Flusberg, 2001). However, index relatives performed similarly to control relatives on both phonological measures. Verbal IQ was the only measure that showed familiality within the index group. Furthermore, there was not a significant difference in reported history of language and literacy difficulties for the index parents and control parents. Although those categorized as cases of the broad autism phenotype reported more language and literacy problems than other index parents, current testing (phonological measures) did not confirm verbal difficulties. Based on these findings, Bishop and colleagues (2004) conclude that phonological processing deficits are not part of the broad autism phenotype. They suggest that the similarities in structural language observed in SLI and autism may be phenocopies, rather than reflecting a common underlying etiology. That is, while Bishop *et al.* found overlap in the structural language deficits in SLI and autism, they propose that the types of phonological problems that characterize SLI are not part of the heritable phenotype observed in autism. As noted below, it seems that further investigation of this issue is warranted using measures other than phonological processing.

Summary

There is considerable behavioral evidence for overlap in the language phenotypes in autism and SLI. There are also neural commonalities with respect to white matter enlargement and reversed brain asymmetry in these groups. Whereas there are definite similarities in phenotypic expression, it is less clear that the etiological bases of autism overlap with those of language impairment.

Conclusions and future directions

Recent research on language and communication deficits observed in the autism spectrum has begun to provide a broader characterization of functioning across various linguistic domains, extending beyond the well-documented pragmatic problems to include phonological, lexical, and grammatical skills. Whereas pragmatic deficits are pervasive among individuals with autism, there appears to be more individual variation with respect to abilities in other linguistic domains; therefore, further investigation of early performance in these aspects of language functioning may reveal useful predictors of language outcomes. It would be worthwhile to examine these linguistic variables within the context of extralinguistic variables, such as imitation skills, joint attention, and amount of intervention, that have also been identified by prior studies as possible predictors of language and communication outcomes. Large-scale, longitudinal studies of early language development in young children on the autism spectrum are needed to chart language growth, characterize linguistic profiles, and conduct detailed studies of learning patterns that may assist with tailoring intervention efforts to children with differing linguistic profiles.

Studies have just begun to provide insights into the neural bases of language processing deficits associated with autism. As this work continues, it will be important to link behavioral and neuroimaging data, examine the extent to which similar patterns are observed across the entire autism spectrum, and distinguish between findings that are attributable to language impairment more generally rather than being specific to an autism spectrum diagnosis.

There is considerable evidence for phenotypic overlap between those with autism and other populations with language and communication deficits, particularly children with SLI. It would be useful to determine if similarities in language phenotypes are also apparent at early stages of development in late talking toddlers with and without ASD. Further research is needed to establish whether the observed overlaps in language abilities are best conceptualized according a dimensional account of language ability/disability or as a qualitatively distinct subtype of autism that has commonalities with developmental language impairment. Questions regarding etiologic overlap between autism and SLI or other types of language delay remain to be explored beyond the domain of phonological processing. Advances in behavioral assessments, neuroimaging, and genetics hold great promise for providing additional insights into the nature and origin of language and communication deficits in individuals with autism.

REFERENCES

American Psychiatric Association. (2000). *Diagnostic and Statistical Manual of Mental Disorders*, 4th edn. Text Revision. Washington, DC: American Psychiatric Association.

Bailey, A., Palferman, S., Heavey, L., & Le Couteur, A. (1998). Autism: The phenotype in relatives. *Journal of Autism and Developmental Disorders*, **28**, 369–92.

Ballaban-Gil, K., Rapin, I., Tuchman, R., & Shinnar, S. (1996). Longitudinal examination of the behavioral, language, and social changes in a population of adolescents and young adults with autistic disorder. *Pediatric Neurology*, **15**, 217–23.

Barnby, G. & Monaco, A. P. (2003). Strategies for autism candidate gene analysis. *Novartis Foundation Symposium*, **251**, 48–63.

Baron-Cohen, S., Leslie, A. M., & Frith, U. (1985). Does the autistic child have a 'theory of mind'? *Cognition*, **21**, 37–46.

Barrett, S., Prior, M., & Manjiviona, J. (2004). Children on the borderlands of autism. *Autism*, **8**, 61–87.

Bartak, L., Rutter, M., & Cox, A. (1975). A comparative study of infantile autism and specific developmental receptive language disorder. I. The children. *British Journal of Psychiatry*, **126**, 127–45.

Bartak, L., Rutter, M., & Cox, A. (1977). A comparative study of infantile autism and specific developmental receptive language disorder. III. Discriminant function analysis. *Journal of Autism and Childhood Schizophrenia*, **7**, 383–96.

Beitchman, J., Wilson, B., Brownlie, E., Walters, H., Inglis, A., & Lancee, W. (1996). Long-term consistency in speech/language profiles: II. behavioral, emotional, and social outcomes. *Journal of the American Academy of Child & Adolescent Psychiatry*, **35**, 815–25.

Berument, S. K., Rutter, M., Lord, C., Pickles, A., & Bailey, A. (1999). Autism screening questionnaire: Diagnostic validity. *British Journal of Psychiatry*, **175**, 444–451. Published as the Social Communication Questionnaire by Western Psychological Services.

Bishop, D. (1998). Development of the children's communication checklist (CCC): A method of assessing qualitative aspects of communicative impairment in children. *Journal of Child Psychology and Psychiatry*, **39**, 879–91.

Bishop, D. (2000). Pragmatic language impairment: A correlate of SLI, a distinct subgroup, or part of the autistic continuum? In D. Bishop & L. Leonard (Eds.), *Speech and Language Impairments in Children: Causes, Characteristics, Intervention and Outcome*. The Hove: Psychology Press.

Bishop, D. (2003). Autism and specific language impairment: Categorical distinction or continuum? *Novartis Foundation Symposium*, **251**, 213–26.

Bishop, D. V., Maybery, M., Wong, D., Maley, A., Hill, W., & Hallmayer, J. (2004). Are phonological processing deficits part of the broad autism phenotype? *American Journal of Medical Genetics. Part B, Neuropsychiatric Genetics*, **128**, 54–60.

Bishop, D. & Norbury, C. (2002). Exploring the borderlands of autistic disorder and specific language impairment: A study using standardized diagnostic instruments. *Journal of Child Psychology and Psychiatry*, **37**, 391–403.

Bishop, D. & Norbury, C. (2005). Executive functions in children with communication impairments, in relation to autistic symptomatology I: Generativity. *Autism*, **9**, 7–27.

Bishop, D. & Rosenbloom, L. (1987). Classification of childhood language disorders. In W. Yule & M. Rutter (Eds.), *Language Development and Disorders. Clinics in Developmental Medicine* (pp. 101–102). London: Mac Keith Press.

Bono, M., Daley, L., & Sigman, M. (2004). Relations among joint attention, amount of intervention and language gain in autism. *Journal of Autism and Developmental Disorders*, **34**, 495–505.

Botting, N. & Conti-Ramsden, G. (1999). Pragmatic language impairment without autism: The children in question. *Autism*, **3**, 371–96.

Botting, N. & Conti-Ramsden, G. (2003). Autism, primary pragmatic difficulties and specific language impairment: Can we distinguish them using psycholinguistic markers? *Developmental Medicine and Child Neurology*, **45**, 515–45.

Bradford, Y., Haines, J., Hutcheson, H., *et al.* (2001). Incorporating language phenotypes strengthens evidence of linkage to autism. *American Journal of Medical Genetics*, **105**, 539–47.

Cantwell, D., Baker, L., Rutter, M., & Mawhood, L. (1989). Infantile autism and developmental receptive dysphasia: A comparative follow-up into middle childhood. *Journal of Autism and Developmental Disorders*, **19**, 19–31.

Charman, T. & Baird, G. (2002). Practitioner review: Diagnosis of autism spectrum disorders in 2- and 3-year-old children. *Journal of Child Psychology and Psychiatry*, **43**, 289–305.

Charman, T., Drew, A., Baird, C., & Baird, G. (2003). Measuring early language development in preschool children with autism spectrum disorder using the MacArthur Communicative Development Inventory (Infant Form). *Journal of Child Language*, **30**, 213–36.

Charman, T., Taylor, E., Drew, A., Cockerill, H., Brown, J., & Baird, G. (2005). Outcome at 7 years of children diagnosed with autism at age 2: Predictive validity of assessments conducted at 2 and 3 years of age and pattern of symptom change over time. *Journal of Child Psychology and Psychiatry*, **46**, 500–13.

Conti-Ramsden, G. & Botting, N. (1999). Classification of children with specific language impairment: Longitudinal considerations. *Journal of Speech, Language, and Hearing Research*, **42**, 1195–204.

Conti-Ramsden, G., Botting, N., & Faragher, B. (2001). Psycholinguistic markers for SLI. *Journal of Child Psychology and Psychiatry*, **42**, 741–8.

de Fosse, L., Hodge, S., Makris, N., et al. (2004). Language-association cortex asymmetry in autism and specific language impairment. *Annals of Neurology*; **56**, 757–66.

Dunn, L. & Dunn, L., (1997). *Peabody Picture Vocabulary Test*, 3rd edn. Circle Pines, MN: American Guidance Service.

Eaves, L. & Ho, H. (2004). The very early identification of autism: Outcome to age 4 1/2-5. *Journal of Autism and Developmental Disorders*, **34**, 367–78.

Ellis Weismer, S. (2007). Typical talkers, late talkers, and children with specific language impairment: A language endowment spectrum? In R. Paul (Ed.), *Language Disorders and Development From a Developmental Perspective: Essays in Honor of Robin S. Chapman* (pp. 83–101). Mahwah, NJ: Lawrence Erlbaum Associates.

Ellis Weismer, S., Gernsbacher, M. A., Sauer, S., *et al.* (2005a). Characterizing early language profiles and language outcomes for children on the autism spectrum. Poster presented at the Symposium on Research in Child Language Disorders, Madison, WI.

Ellis Weismer, S., Plante, E., Jones, M., & Tomblin, B. (2005b). A functional magnetic resonance imaging investigation of verbal working memory in adolescents with specific language impairment. *Journal of Speech, Language, and Hearing Research*, **48**, 405–25.

Folstein, S. E., & Mankoski, R. E. (2000). Chromosome 7q: Where autism meets language disorder? *American Journal of Human Genetics*, **67**, 278–81.

Folstein, S. & Rutter, M. (1977). Infantile autism: A genetic study of 21 twin pairs. *Journal of Child Psychology and Psychiatry*, **18**, 297–321.

Folstein, S. E., Santangelo, S. L., Gilman, S. E., *et al.* (1999). Predictors of cognitive test patterns in autism families. *Journal of Child Psychology & Psychiatry & Allied Disciplines*, **40**, 1117–28.

Fombonne, E., Bolton, P., Prior, J., Jordan, H., & Rutter, M. (1997). A family study of autism: Cognitive patterns and levels in parents and siblings. *Journal of Child Psychology & Psychiatry & Allied Disciplines*, **38**, 667–83.

Frith, U. (1989). *Autism: Explaining the Enigma*. Oxford: Basil Blackwell.

Gagnon, L., Mottron, L., & Joanette, Y. (1997). Questioning the validity of the semantic-pragmatic syndrome diagnosis. *Autism*, **1**, 37–55.

Gathercole, S. & Baddeley, A. (1990). Phonological memory deficits in language disordered children: Is there a causal connection? *Journal of Memory and Language*, **29**, 336–360.

Gernsbacher, M., Geye, H., & Ellis Weismer, S. (2005). Profiles of early language development among children on the autism spectrum: A retrospective study. In P. Fletcher & J. Miller (Eds.), *Language Disorders and Developmental Theory*. Philadelphia: John Benjamins.

Gernsbacher, M., Sauer, E., Geye, H., Schweigert, E., & Goldsmith, H.H. (2008). Infant and toddler oral- and manual-motor skills predict later speech fluency in autism. *Journal of Child Psychology and Psychiatry*, **49**, 43–50.

Gernsbacher, M., Varner, K., & Faust, M. (1990). Investigating differences in general comprehension skill. *Journal of Experimental Psychology: Learning, Memory, and Cognition*, **16**, 430–45.

Herbert, M. R., Ziegler, D. A., Deutsch, C. K, *et al.* (2005). Brain asymmetries in autism and developmental language disorder: A nested whole-brain analysis. *Brain*, **128**, 213–26.

Herbert, M. R., Ziegler, D. A., Deutsch, C. K., *et al.* (2003a). Dissociations of cerebral cortex, subcortical and cerebral white matter volumes in autistic boys. *Brain*, **126**, 1182–92.

Herbert, M. R., Ziegler, D. A., Makris, N., *et al.* (2003b). Larger brain and white matter volumes in children with developmental language disorder. *Developmental Science*, **6**, F11–F22.

Herbert, M. R., Ziegler, D. A., Makris, N., *et al.* (2004). Localization of white matter volume increase in autism and developmental language disorder. *Annals of Neurology*, **55**, 530–40.

Howlin, P. (2003). Outcome in high-functioning adults with autism and without early language delays: Implications for the differentiation between autism and Asperger syndrome. *Journal of Autism and Developmental Disorders*, **33**, 3–13.

Just, M. A., Cherkassky, V. L., Keller, T. A., & Minshew, N. J. (2004). Cortical activation and synchronization during sentence comprehension in high-functioning autism: Evidence of underconnectivity. *Brain*, **127**, 1811–21.

Kjelgaard, M. & Tager-Flusberg, H. (2001). An investigation of language impairment in autism: Implications for genetic subgroups. *Language and Cognitive Processes*, **16**, 287–308.

Le Couteur, A., Bailey, A., Goode, S., *et al.* (1996). A broader phenotype of autism: The clinical spectrum in twins. *Journal of Child Psychology & Psychiatry & Allied Disciplines*, **37**, 785–801.

Lord, C. (March, 2005). Early diagnosing of children with autism spectrum disorders. Invited talk to the Waisman Center MRDDRC Brown Bag Seminar, Madison, WI.

Lord, C., Risi, S., Lambrecht, L., Cook, E., *et al.* (2000). The Autism Diagnostic Observation Schedule-Generic: A standard measure of social and communication deficits association with the spectrum of autism. *Journal of Autism and Developmental Disorders*, **30**, 205–23.

Lord, C., Rutter, M., & Le Couteur, A. (1994). Autism Diagnostic Interview –Revised. A revised version of a diagnostic interview for caregivers of individuals with possible pervasive developmental disorders. *Journal of Autism and Developmental Disorders*, **24**, 659–85.

Marchman, V. A., Wulfeck, B., & Ellis Weismer, S. (1999). Morphological productivity in children with normal language and SLI: A study of the English past tense. *Journal of Speech, Language, and Hearing Research*, **42**, 206–19.

Mawhood, L., Howlin, P., & Rutter, M. (2000). Autism and developmental language disorder – a comparative follow-up in early adult life: I. Cognitive and language outcomes. *Journal of Child Psychology and Psychiatry and Allied Disciplines*, **41**, 547–59.

Mayes, S., Calhoun, S., & Crites, D. (2001). Does DSM-IV Asperger's disorder exist? *Journal of Abnormal Child Psychology*, **29**, 263–71.

Michelotti, J., Charman, T., Slonims, V., & Baird, G. (2002). Follow-up of children with language delay and features of autism from preschool years to middle childhood. *Developmental Medicine and Child Neurology*, **44**, 812–9.

Miller, J. & Chapman, R. (2000). *SALT: Systematic Analysis of Language Transcripts* [Computer software]. Language Analysis Laboratory. University of Wisconsin-Madison: Waisman Center.

Morgan, B., Maybery, M., & Durkin, K. (2003). Weak central coherence, poor joint attention, and low verbal ability: Independent deficits in early autism. *Developmental Psychology*, **39**, 646–56.

Mundy, P., Sigman, M., & Kasari, C. (1990). A longitudinal study of joint attention and language development in autistic children. *Journal of Autism and Developmental Disorders*, **22**, 115–27.

Norbury, C. (2005). Barking up the wrong tree: Lexical ambiguity resolution in children with language impairments and autism spectrum disorders. *Journal of Experimental Child Psychology*, **90**, 142–71.

Piven, J., Palmer, P., Landa, R., Santangelo, S., Jacobi, D., & Childress, D. (1997). Personality and language characteristics in parents from multiple-incidence autism families. *American Journal of Medical Genetics*, **74**, 398–411.

Rapin, I. & Allen, D. (1983). Developmental language disorders: Nosologic considerations. In U. Kirk (Ed.),*Neuropsychology of Language, Reading, and Spelling* (pp. 158–184). New York: Academic Press.

Rapin, I. & Dunn, M. (2003). Update on the language disorders of individuals on the autistic spectrum. *Brain Development*, **25**, 166–72.

Rice, M. L., Sell, M. A., & Hadley, P. A. (1991). Social interactions of speech and language impaired children. *Journal of Speech and Hearing Research*, **34**, 1299–1307.

Rutter, M. (1970). Autistic children: Infancy to adulthood. *Seminars in Psychiatry*, **2**, 435–50.

Semel, E. M., Wiig, E. H., & Secord, W. (1987). *Clinical Evaluation of Language Fundamentals – Revised*. San Antonio, Texas: Psychological Corporation.

Shao, Y., Raiford, K. L., Wolpert, C. M., et al, (2002). Phenotypic homogeneity provides increased support for linkage on chromosome 2 in autistic disorder. *American Journal of Human Genetics*, **70**, 1058–61.

Shields, J., Varley, R., Broks, P., & Simpson, A. (1996). Social cognition in developmental language disorders and high-level autism. *Developmental Medicine and Child Neurology*, **38**, 487–95.

Sigman, M. & Ruskin, E. (1999). Change and continuity in the social competence of children with Autism, Down syndrome, and developmental delays. *Monograph of the Society for Research in Child Development*. London: Blackwell.

Stone, W. & Yoder, P. (2001). Predicting spoken language level in children with autism spectrum disorders. *Autism*, **5**, 341–61.

Szatmari, P., MacLean, J. E., Jones, M. B., *et al.* (2000). The familial aggregation of the lesser variant in biological and nonbiological relatives of PDD probands: A family history study. *Journal of Child Psychology and Psychiatry*, **41**, 579–86.

Tager-Flusberg, H. & Joseph, R. (2003). Identifying neurocognitive phenotypes in autism. *Philosophical Transactions of the Royal Society*, **358**, 303–14.

Tomblin, J. B., Hafeman, L. L., & O' Brien, M. (2003). Autism and autistic behaviors in siblings of children with language impairment. *International Journal of Language and Communication Disorders*, **38**, 235–50.

Venter, A., Lord, C., & Schopler, E. (1992). A follow-up study of high functioning autistic children. *Journal of Child Psychology and Psychiatry*, **33**, 489–507.

Whitehurst, G. & Fischel, J. (1994). Practitioner review: Early developmental language delay: what, if anything, should the clinician do about it? *Journal of Child Psychology and Psychiatry*, **35**, 613–48.

World Health Organization. (1993). *International Classification of Diseases*, 10th rev. Geneva, Switzerland: World Health Organization.

5

Language development in children with Williams syndrome: New insights from cross-linguistic research

Stavroula Stavrakaki

Introduction

Williams syndrome (WS) is a genetically based neurodevelopmental disorder, which is caused by a microdeletion of chromosome 7, more specifically, at the region of chromosome 7q11.23 (Doll & Grzeschik, 2001; Ewart *et al.*, 1993; Korenberg *et al.*, 2000). Due to its uneven cognitive profile, WS has recently been the focus of scientific research in the field of developmental cognitive neuroscience (Clahsen & Almazan, 1998; Clahsen & Temple, 2003; Jordan *et al.*, 2002; Thomas *et al.*, 2001). Impaired visuo-spatial cognition, planning, and problem solving co-occur with relatively spared abilities in the domain of language, social cognition, and face processing (Bellugi *et al.*, 1988; Karmiloff-Smith, 1998; Karmiloff-Smith *et al.*, 1997; Mervis *et al.*, 2000; Tager-Flusberg *et al.*, 2003; Tager-Flusberg & Sullivan, 2000).

There is much controversy surrounding the status and development of the relatively spared cognitive abilities in WS, especially language. More specifically, some researchers argue that language development in WS (and other developmental disorders) reflects the abnormal development of the entire cognitive system (Karmiloff-Smith, 1998; Thomas *et al.*, 2001; Thomas & Karmiloff-Smith, 2002). Consequently, the developmental pattern in WS is expected to be qualitatively different from typical development. If this is the case, then there should not be selective preservation of cognitive abilities in WS while the rest of the system develops abnormally. In other words, there should be no evidence for "residual normality" in WS (Thomas & Karmiloff-Smith, 2002). Therefore, according to Karmiloff-Smith and collaborators (Thomas & Karmiloff-Smith, 2002; Thomas

I am grateful to all the children who participated in this study and their families for their collaboration. Many thanks also go to E. Darili, E. Lefkou, K. Thomaidis, and G. Varlamis and the late child cardiologist G. Darilis for introducing the children with WS and their families to me and supporting my work on WS subjects. Part of this research was supported by the Greek State Scholarship Foundation (IKY).

et al., 2001) the linguistic performance on the surface, good or poor, is simply the outcome of abnormal functions in the underlying cognitive mechanisms.

In comparison, other researchers argue that language development in WS, or at least aspects of language development, follows the pattern of typical development. However, there is no consensus among these researchers with respect to (1) which language abilities follow the normal path of development and (2) to what extent those abilities follow the normal path of development. On the one hand, Mervis and colleagues suggest that the whole process of language development in WS is delayed but normal (Mervis *et al.*, 2004). Despite language abilities in WS being below those of typically developing (TD) children matched for chronological age (CA), they are still at the expected level for overall IQ performance. Furthermore, Mervis *et al.* (2004) argue that, whereas language abilities in WS are linked to all aspects of cognition, they are more dependent on verbal memory than on aspects of conceptual cognition.

On the other hand, Clahsen and colleagues (Clahsen & Almazan, 1998; Clahsen *et al.* 2004) suggest that only particular aspects of language in WS fall within the normal range: whereas the computational (rule-based) system for language is select-ively spared, lexical representations and/or their access are impaired (Clahsen & Almazan, 1998; Clahsen & Temple, 2003; Clahsen *et al.*, 2004). It is, therefore, expected that, although aspects of the computational component of language, that is, phonology, morphology, and syntax, should be completely intact, aspects of lexical abilities should be problematic.

This chapter addresses the question of how language develops in WS adopting a cross-linguistic perspective, which enables abstraction away from language-particular characteristics and provides a novel insight into the language abilities of WS subjects. In particular, the syntactic abilities of children with WS are focused on by splitting the chapter into two parts. In the first part, current cross-linguistic studies on the syntactic abilities in WS in terms of methodological and theoretical issues are discussed. In the second part, new data from the Greek language con-cerning sentence comprehension abilities in WS, with particular emphasis on the issue of (normal or abnormal) developmental processes involved in WS, are presented. Overall, this chapter aims to show how cross-linguistic research on WS can provide us with a better understanding of WS language abilities.

Syntax in Williams syndrome

The study of syntactic abilities has received remarkable attention in recent years and has sparked diverse explanations for the status and development of language abilities in WS.

Bellugi *et al.* (1988) were the first to report that WS subjects have well-preserved syntactic abilities and produce complex syntactic structures in their spontaneous speech. Because spontaneous speech data do not always constitute a reliable way of assessing grammatical abilities, a number of experimental studies, which tested specific linguistic variables, followed.

Karmiloff-Smith *et al.* (1998) studied syntactic comprehension in WS using different off- and on-line tasks. They argued that the performance of individuals with WS is significantly lower than that of normal controls on off-line sentence interpretation and is characterized by selective deficits in on-line processing of structures violating subcategory constraints. Based on those findings, Karmiloff-Smith and colleagues suggested first that the WS participants showed difficulties with syntax, and second that the WS participants performed similarly to second-language learners. This is due to problems that both individuals with WS and second-language learners encounter with identifying subcategory violations in sentence processing (see Gleitman, 1990).

Lower performance of WS individuals compared to that of their TD peers matched for CA has also been reported in a study by Mervis *et al.* (2004). After assessing the grammatical abilities of the WS individuals using a number of measures (e.g., spontaneous speech, Test for Reception of Grammar: TROG; Bishop, 1989), Mervis and colleagues proposed that the grammatical abilities of individuals with WS were in fact predictable from their general level of cognitive ability.

Similarly, Volterra and colleagues (1996, 2001) identified specific language problems in Italian WS children. Testing on the basis of receptive language measures (e.g., TROG) revealed lexical and grammatical errors indicating difficulties with different levels of language processing and not exclusive difficulties with grammar per se. As the authors pointed out, considerable dissociations were found within the linguistic domain. In particular, aspects of Italian morphology carrying out a semantic function were found to be more vulnerable in WS grammar than other aspects of morphology (Voltera *et al.* 2001).

Detailed investigations of the syntactic abilities of WS subjects were carried out by Clahsen and Almazan (1998) who tested the interpretation of passive sentences and syntactic binding of four WS subjects and their mental age (MA) -matched controls. In terms of linguistic theory (Chomsky, 1981), verbal passive formation includes noun phrase (NP) movement from the object to subject position (A-movement), while syntactic binding includes syntactic dependencies formed between reflexives and pronouns and their antecedents. Interestingly, the WS children showed error-free performance on the interpretation of syntactic binding and adult level performance on the interpretation of passive sentences. Based on those results, Clahsen and Almazan (1998) concluded that the computational component in WS language appears to be intact. In contrast, the lexical component of language was considered to be selectively impaired as the WS children produced lexical errors (Temple *et al.*, 2002) and showed selective problems with the irregular past tense (Clahsen & Alamazan 1998; Clahsen *et al.*, 2004), which has been assumed to be part of the lexicon (Pinker, 1999).

Further evidence for normal syntactic abilities in WS was provided by Bartke (2004) who studied the interpretation of passives by German speaking children with WS. She showed that both WS subjects and TD children performed better on irreversible vs. reversible passives and produced reversal theta-role errors. Quantitative differences, however, were found, but only between the younger WS subjects and their MA-matched controls, with the former performing lower than the latter.

Evidence for advanced grammatical abilities in WS was provided by Stavrakaki (2004) who studied Greek WS children's ability to produce wh-questions. Two out of three WS children that participated in her study showed ceiling performance on both subject and object wh-questions, whereas one child performed better on the production of who-object than on who-subject questions. The better performance on object than subject wh-questions was interpreted as overuse of grammatical processes and rules required for object wh-questions, in particular A-bar in terms of linguistic theory (Chomsky, 1981).

In addition, Zukowski (2001, 2004, 2009) argued that children with WS make errors in grammar that are "developmental" in nature; hence, they do not show evidence for a deviant pattern of language development in terms of grammar. In particular, Zukowski (2001, 2004, 2009) tested the production of relative clauses and negative questions. Her results strongly suggest that children with WS follow the typical path of language development. First, they showed the typical pattern of performance on the production of relative clauses, that is, better performance on subject than on object relatives; second, children with WS and younger TD children produced negative question errors that cannot be found in the (linguistic) input. Therefore, Zukowski (2001 , 2004 , 2009) suggested that, despite delays in language development, grammatical abilities in individuals with WS develop normally; consequently, the mechanism of grammar acquisition is normal in WS.

A similar claim concerning language development in WS was made by Perovic and Wexler (2007). They suggested that, whereas language develops normally in WS, some particular aspects of language mature very late in individuals with WS. This selective developmental delay concerns those linguistic phenomena acquired late by TD children. The claims by Perovic and Wexler (2007) are supported by experimental evidence showing normal performance for the acquisition of binding (cf. Ring & Clahsen 2005) but significant difficulties in the acquisition of raising structures (e.g., John seems to Maria to be reading a book). On the assumption that some grammatical abilities never mature in WS, Perovic and Wexler (2007) argued in favor of a specific grammatical impairment in WS. In this respect, their proposal is different from the one put forth by Zukowski (2001, 2004, 2009).

In addition, Joffe and Varlokosta (2007) provided further evidence for significant grammatical difficulties in WS. Specifically, they reported lower performance by participants with WS than MA-matched TD controls on the comprehension of passives and the production, comprehension, and repetition of wh-questions.

Overall, the research findings appear to be quite conflicting (see Brock, 2007, for a current review of the literature on language in WS). Possible reasons for the attested discrepancy between different studies can be traced to the following factors, which are discussed below: (1) small samples, (2) selection criteria for controls, and (3) properties of language tests employed in the WS studies.

First, in many studies small samples of individuals with WS participated; thus, it is questionable whether the conclusions based on those studies can be generalized to the whole WS population (Brock, 2007). Second, selection criteria for the control groups seem to significantly affect the conclusions. Having mental retardation, the individuals with WS are expected to perform below their CA peers at least in some of the language tasks, as already shown by studies in the field (e.g., Karmiloff-Smith *et al.*, 1998). Thus, comparing the performance of individuals with WS and that of their CA peers can only show whether the WS participants are behind their CA controls and cannot elucidate the developmental processes for language acquisition in WS. A better way of investigating whether there are any similarities and/or differences in language acquisition by WS and TD children is to compare individuals with WS to MA-matched controls (see Temple *et al.*, 2002, for discussion; and Brock, 2007, for a different view). By keeping MA constant, direct comparisons concerning the development of specific cognitive abilities per se become possible; hence, better understanding of the developmental processes in WS and typical development can be achieved (see Chapter 8).

Another reason for the conflicting findings is related to the language tests employed in the WS studies and in particular to the aspects of language that those tests measure. For example, the TROG has been used as a measure of grammatical abilities in WS (Mervis *et al.*, 2004; Voltera *et al.*, 1996), despite the fact that it is not a pure test of grammar (phonology, morphology, syntax). It also assesses lexical/semantic abilities (e.g., meaning of verbs and prepositions) (Clahsen & Almazan, 1998). As a result, the reliance on language tests that simultaneously measure different linguistic abilities (lexical/semantic and syntactic) cannot constitute a reliable measure or accurate assessment of grammatical abilities. More sophisticated language measures should be designed and employed for research purposes.

It is, therefore, evident that more studies on WS should be carried out in order to get a more precise picture of language abilities in this population. In the next sections, a study of receptive syntactic abilities in Greek-speaking individuals with WS is presented.

New data from the Greek language: Sentence comprehension in Greek children with Williams syndrome

Participants

Five Greek children who were independently diagnosed with WS by multi-disciplinary teams in Greek hospitals in Thessaloniki participated in this study. The diagnoses were confirmed using the fluorescent in situ hybridization (FISH) technique (i.e., a specialized chromosome analysis utilizing specially prepared elastin probes). WS children's MA was derived from the verbal and nonverbal IQ scores calculated on the basis of the Greek version of Wechsler Intelligence Scale for Children-III (WISC-III) test (Georgas *et al.*, 1997), which has been standardized for children aged 6;2–16;10 years. The scores obtained by the three younger children on the WISC-III subscales indicated language ages considerably below 6;2. Hence, the exact calculation of MA was not possible. Further testing of TD children younger than 6;2 indicated that only children with a mean CA of 3;4 and 4;2 reached the raw WS scores on the WISC-III; those ages were taken to be the MAs of the WS children. The individual WS profiles are presented in Table 1.

Fifteen control participants whose CAs corresponded to the MAs of the WS children (+/− 3 months) participated in the experiment; specifically, each WS child was matched to three control children on the basis of his/her MA. The control children constitute the MA control group. Furthermore, another control group of 16 younger typically developing children (YTD) aged 3;6–5;6 years participated in the experiment in order to get a more accurate picture of the typical language development process with respect to the tested structures. In Table 2, the CA and MA of the children with WS as well as the CA of the control groups are presented.

Table 1. Children with Williams syndrome (WS): Chronological age (CA) and mental age (MA)

	CA	MA
WS1	7;9	<6;2 (3;4)
WS2	7;9	<6;2(3;4)
WS3	9;2	<6;2(4;2)
WS4	15	6;9
WS5	10;5	7;2

Table 2. CA and/or MA of children with WS, MA-matched controls, and YTD controls

	CA Mean Range (SD)	MA Mean Range (SD)
WS group	10.1	5
N = 5	7;9–15 (2.94)	3;4–7;2 (1.88)
MA-matched group	5	
N = 15	3;3–7;4 (1.7)	
YTD group	4.4	
N = 16	3;6–5;6 (0.73)	

Experimental materials and procedure

Design and materials

The test sentences consisted of six sentence types with different syntactic properties. In particular, the experimental materials included simple transitive structures with SVO (subject–verb–object) word order as well as structures formed by A-bar movement (e.g., subject and object wh-questions, subject and object clefts), and A-movement (e.g., passive sentences).

Examples of the sentence types are presented below:

Simple transitive sentences with SVO word order
(1) O elefantas   kiniga   ton   pithiko
    the elephant-nom chases   the   monkey-acc
    "The elephant is chasing the monkey"

Subject clefts
(2) O skilos   ine   pu   kinighai   tin katsika
    the dog-nom   is   that chases   the goat-acc
    "It is the dog that is chasing the goat"

Object clefts
(3) O pithikos   ine   pu   htipai   o elefantas
    the monkey-nom is   that hits the   elephant-nom
    "It is the monkey that the elephant is hitting"

Who-subject questions
(4) Pjos   kinijise   ton elefanta?
    who-nom   chased   the elephant-acc
    "Who chased the elephant?"

Who-object questions
(5) Pjon   klotsise   i katsika?
    who-acc   kicked   the goat-nom
    "Who did the goat kick?"

Table 3. Classification of the tested structure

	A- or A-bar movement	Word order	Case/theta-role conflict
Simple transitive sentences (SVO)		SVO	
Subject wh-questions	Yes (A-bar movement)	SVO	
Object wh-questions	Yes (A-bar movement)	OVS	
Subject clefts	Yes (A-bar movement)	SVO	
Object clefts	Yes (A-bar movement)	OVS	Yes
Passives	Yes (A-movement)	SV-by phrase	Yes

Passive sentences

(6) O pithikos   sproxnete   apo   tin tigri
     the monkey-nom   push-3s-passive by   the tiger
     "The monkey is pushed by the tiger"

The above structures differ with respect to the following parameters: (1) presence (or absence) of A- or A-bar movement; (2) word order: SVO or OVS; (3) existence (or not) of conflict between case marking and theta-role: Such a conflict reveals when nominative case is associated with patient theta-role, as is the case with object clefts and passives.

The experimental sentences of this study have been classified in terms of the above parameters. This classification is presented in Table 3.

It was hypothesized that combinations of the above factors should result in a differential degree of acquisition/processing difficulty. In particular, Stavrakaki expected syntactic parsing to be facilitated (1) when morphological contrast cues are activated by associating nominative case with agent theta-role and accusative case with patient theta-role but not the reverse (nominative case with patient theta-role), and (2) when syntactic cues are activated by associating the first preverbal NP with the agent theta-role and the second postverbal NP with the patient theta-role (hence, preference for the SVO word order) (Stavrakaki, 2002). Therefore, it was predicted that co-occurrence of syntactic movement (A-bar movement) with (1) OVS word order and (2) conflict between case marking and theta-role (as is the case with object clefts) makes sentence comprehension extremely difficult. By contrast, it was predicted that co-occurrence of syntactic (A-bar) movement with

(1) SVO word order and (2) absence of conflict between case marking and theta-role (as is the case with subject clefts) facilitates the sentence comprehension process due to available syntactic (SVO word order) and morphological (nominative case marking corresponds to the agent theta-role) cues.

For each sentence type presented above, there were 14 exemplars except for the wh-questions. Concerning wh-questions, eight stories for each question type were used when the children with WS and MA controls were tested, whereas four stories for each question type were used when YTD children were tested.

Procedure

An acting-out task was employed for all sentences except for wh-questions. This task requires the subject to manipulate toy animals in such a way so as to demonstrate the thematic roles of nouns in verbally presented sentences. Before beginning the task, the children were asked to identify all animals by pointing to them in turn when the experimenter named them. They were also encouraged to play with the toys in order to be familiar with them. Finally, the children were instructed to do what the experimenter asked of them.

A somewhat different method, which is nevertheless based on a toy manipulation task, was used for who-questions (Crain & Thornton, 1998). The children were told that they should help the puppet understand what was going on in the story by telling the puppet the answer. Three figurines were placed on the table; for example, one dog, one elephant, and one fox. The experimenter told the child a story in which the fox was chasing the dog and after that the dog was chasing the elephant. At the same time, the experimenter showed that the fox was chasing the dog and the dog was chasing the elephant. At the end, the child should help the puppet answer the following question: "Who chased the dog?"

Results

The correct performance of all groups on the test sentences is presented in Table 4.

Table 4 indicates that all TD children (MA and YTD controls) showed ceiling performance on all structures with SVO word order (simple transitive sentences with SVO word order, subject clefts, and subject wh-questions). Although they showed near-ceiling performance on who-object questions, they had significant problems with object clefts and passive sentences. The individuals with WS showed a similar pattern. In particular, they showed ceiling and near-ceiling performance on all structures with SVO word order and near-ceiling performance on who-object questions. The performance of the WS group on object vs. subject questions did not reach significance (Wilcoxon test $Z = 0.447$, $p = 0.655$). In addition, the WS children performed like TD children and showed low level of performance on

Table 4. Correct performance (%) of all groups on the tested structures

	Transitive sentences (SVO) Mean Range (SD)	Who-subject questions Mean Range (SD)	Subject clefts Mean Range (SD)	Who-object questions Mean Range (SD)	Object clefts Mean Range (SD)	Passive sentences Mean Range (SD)
YTD	100 (224/224) 100–100 (.0)	100 (64/64) 100–100 (.0)	100 (224/224) 100–100 (.0)	87.5 (56/64) 75–100 (12.9)	36.6 (82/224) 0–100 (32.1)	57.6 (129/224) 14.3–100 (34.5)
WS group	100 (70/70) 100–100 (.0)	90 (36/40) 75–100 (13.69)	100 (70/70) 100–100 (.0)	92.5 (37/40) 75–100 (11.18)	55.7 (39/70) 0–100 (51.6)	65.7 (46/70) 0–100 (42)
MA-matched Group	100 (210/210) 100–100 (.0)	100 (120/120) 100–100 (.0)	100 (210/210) 100–100 (.0)	97.5 (117/120) 75–100 (7)	48.09 (101/210) 0–100 (36.6)	53.8 (113/210) 0–100 (35.8)

object clefts and passive sentences. In sum, all groups showed the same pattern of performance with low correctness scores for object clefts and passive sentences and high correctness scores for all sentences with SVO word order and object wh-questions. Therefore, the same structures were difficult for all groups. Statistics confirmed the above observations. A 3×6 analysis of variance with the variables Group $\times$ Sentence Type was carried out to investigate the data. The main effect of Sentence Type was significant [$F(5, 165) = 35.313, p < 0.001$], but neither the main effect of Group [$F(2, 33) = 1658,119, p = 0.674$] nor the interaction of Subject Group $\times$ Sentence Type were significant [$F(10, 165) = 0.711, p = 0.713$]. These findings reflect the fact that all groups showed similar performance on the test structures.

Further analysis of the individual WS children's performance indicated significant within group variation. In Table 5 , the performance of each child with WS on all sentences for which no ceiling performance was found is presented.

While the two older children with WS performed at ceiling, as predicted by their MA (6;9 and 7;2, respectively), the younger children with WS whose MA ranged from 3.4 to 4.2 showed heterogeneous performance. Despite being heterogeneous, the performance of these children with WS is within the normal range as shown by comparing performance in the three youngest children with WS (YWS) to 9 controls on object clefts and passives in Table 6.

Table 5. Performance (%) on subject and object questions, object clefts, and passive sentences for children with WS

	MA	Subject questions	Object questions	Object clefts	Passives
WS1	3;4	75	75	0	78.5
		(6/8)	(6/8)	(0/14)	(11/14)
WS2	3;4	75	100	78.5	0
		(6/8)	(8/8)	(11/14)	(0/14)
WS3	4;2	100	87.5	0	50
		(8/8)	(7/8)	(0/14)	(7/14)
WS4	6;9	100	100	100	100
		(8/8)	(8/8)	(14/14)	(14/14)
WS5	7;2	100	100	100	100
		(8/8)	(8/8)	(14/14)	(14/14)

Table 6. Correct performance (%) of the YWS children (N = 3) compared to that of their MA-matched controls (N = 9)

	Transitive sentences (SVO) Mean Range (SD)	Who-subject questions Mean Range (SD)	Subject clefts Mean Range (SD)	Who-object questions Mean Range (SD)	Object clefts Mean Range (SD)	Passive sentences Mean Range (SD)
YWS group	100	83.33	100	87.5	26.2	42.83
N = 3	(42/42)	(20/24)	(42/42)	(21/24)	(11/42)	(18/42)
	100–10	75–100	100–100	75–100	0–78.5	0–78.5
	(.0)	(14.43)	(.0)	(12.5)	(45.32)	(39.73)
MA group	100	100	100	95.83	28.5	28.5
N = 9	(126/126)	(72/72)	(126/126)	(69/72)	(36/126)	(36/126)
	100–100	100–100	100–100	75–100	0–100	0–50
	(.0)	(.0)	(.0)	(8.83)	(31.13)	(20.82)

Further comparisons did not show any significant differences between the performance of the YWS participants and their corresponding MA-matched control group, except for the case of subject wh-questions (Mann-Whitney U test, $U = 4.5$; $p = 0.010$]. The YWS children performed better on object than subject wh-questions. This pattern of performance was not shown by TD children matched for MA.

Table 7. TDC and children with WS: The proportion (%) of error types out of the total number (N) of errors produced

	Object questions		Object clefts		Passive sentences	
	TDC N = 11	WS N = 3	TDC N = 251	WS n = 31	TDC N = 192	WS N = 24
Reversal of theta-roles	72.7	33.33	100	100	92.2	95.83
Reciprocal interpretation					7.8	4.16
Case error	27.3	33.33				
Gender error		33.33				

Error analysis indicated that TD children and children with WS showed a similar pattern of performance. Table 7 presents the error types produced by all TD children (MA-matched and YTD controls) and participants with WS.

Both groups produced reversal of theta-role errors and case errors while interpreting object-questions. Whereas the former is a receptive error, the latter is a production error and, thus, not related to the receptive abilities of the participants. Case errors were only included in the error types because they do not constitute adult responses. Recall that children were required to tell the puppet the answer in the wh-question comprehension task. Some children produced correct determiner phrase (DP) marked for incorrect case, that is, nominative instead of accusative. One child with WS made a gender error and produced the correct DP marked for incorrect gender. Again this is a production and not a comprehension error. It was included in error types because it does not constitute an adult response.

Although the younger of the WS participants produced a few reversal of theta-role errors in the comprehension of subject wh-questions, the TD children did not. By contrast, both TD (MA-matched controls and YTD children) and WS children produced the same types of errors in the interpretation of passive sentences. Specifically, they produced reversal of theta-role errors and reciprocal interpretation errors. The latter are allowed in Greek due to the fact that both passive and reciprocal verb forms share the same suffix -*me*. In addition, children with WS and TD children made theta-role errors in the interpretation of object clefts; hence, they misinterpreted object clefts as subject clefts.

Discussion

This study investigated the receptive linguistic abilities of Greek children with WS compared to children with typical development to provide a characterization of the language abilities of the WS participants as impaired, normal, or delayed. The main findings are as follows.

The results concerning TD children indicate that they performed at ceiling on structures with SVO word order and showed a high level of correct performance on object wh-questions. Therefore, they exhibited knowledge of syntactic operations required for wh-question formation. However, they demonstrated low performance on the interpretation of object clefts and passive sentences. Their low performance on object clefts can be attributed to the linking status of relative operators in object clefts (cf. Wexler, 1991; Guasti & Shlonsky, 1995). In particular, whereas the formation of wh-questions in Greek requires overt raising of a wh-operator to the clause initial position, thus creating an A-bar chain with the wh-operator in Spec-CP binding a variable in the base position (Browing, 1987; Chomsky, 1986), the formation of clefts requires a relative operator moved to an A-bar position, which needs to be co-indexed with its variable and with the head NP, hence, the linking status of the relative operator. (Note: Spec-CP indicates "the specifier position within CP" [Radford, 1997, p. 528]. CP is the complementizer phrase "headed by a complementizer" [Radford, 1997, p. 499]). Therefore, the observed difficulties with object clefts are highly related to the linking status of the relative operator (Guasti and Shlonsky, 1995; Wexler, 1991). In addition to demanding syntactic processes taking place in object clefts, the association of the patient theta-role with nominative case makes these structures even more difficult. Due to misleading surface morphological cues (nominative case is associated with patient theta-role instead of agent theta-role), children have to rely on syntactic operations and overcome "misleading" directions from linguistic input.

Similar constraints may hold for the acquisition of A-movement as TD children showed a low level of correct performance on passives. Borer and Wexler (1987, 1992) claimed that specific maturational constraints are required for the acquisition of passive sentences. Evidence for late acquisition of verbal passives of action verbs by Greek children comes from a study by Terzi and Wexler (2002). Based on comprehension data, Terzi and Wexler (2002) have claimed that children's low performance on passives can be interpreted in terms of the A-Chain Deficit Hypothesis, according to which the acquisition of A-chains is only possible after a particular point of age maturation (Borer & Wexler, 1992). Stavrakaki suggests that, due to unavailable surface cues for the interpretation of passives (surface word order cues or morphological cues, i.e., association of morphological case with theta-role, see the Design and materials section), children should only rely on syntactic knowledge, which is, nevertheless, late acquired (Terzi & Wexler, 2002). This study revealed many similarities between the WS and TD participants. First, the participants with WS showed a very high level of performance on the structures with SVO word order and who-object questions. With the exception of the YWS participants' lower performance on the who-subject compared to that shown by the YTD group, analyses revealed the same level of performance on all tested structures by WS participants and their correspondent MA-matched controls. One possible interpretation for the lower performance of the YWS participants on subject wh-questions compared to that of the YTD group is the ceiling level of performance on subject wh-questions shown by the YTD group. Another interpretation concerns a possible developmental strategy employed by the WS individuals. Noticeably, two of the YWS participants performed better on object than subject wh-questions, a pattern not found in typical development. This peculiar pattern of the WS children's performance, that is, better accuracy performance scores for object than subject wh-questions, was also reported in a recent study on the production of wh-questions by Greek children with WS (Stavrakaki, 2004). In particular, one child with WS in that study performed better on the production of who-object than who-subject questions. This performance was interpreted as showing a preference for grammatical processes and rules, in particular wh-operator movement (required for object wh-questions) over simple heuristic strategies, in particular, use of the SVO word order strategy (sufficient for successful subject wh-question production).

The proposed interpretation of the present data is along the same lines: Individuals with WS show a strong preference for overusing wh-movement, hence, their better performance on object than subject wh-questions. These findings are compatible with the profile of children with WS described in the literature. Specifically, Clahsen and Almazan (1998) proposed that these children overuse grammatical rules of past tense formation in English as shown by the overgeneralization of the regular suffix both to existing regular forms and to novel words rhyming with existing irregulars. Apart from the stronger than usual reliance on grammatical rules, the children with WS in this study did not show any differences from TD children. They performed similarly low on object clefts and passive sentences as controls. In addition, error analysis indicated the same error types for WS and TD participants. Therefore, the performance of children with WS did not differ from that of TD children in both quantitative and qualitative terms as shown by accuracy scores and error analysis. Consequently, the performance of children with WS cannot be characterized as impaired or even delayed when compared to the performance of TD children.

In sum, TD children and children with WS indicated knowledge of complex syntactic structures. The low performance on object clefts and passives is related to the specific acquisition requirements for these structures, which holds true for both TD children and individuals with WS. In this respect, the results of the present study are taken to support the view that, as far as the reception of syntax is concerned, children with WS show normal abilities consistent with their mental age (cf. Clahsen *et al.*, 2004).

REFERENCES

Bartke, S. (2004). Passives in German children with Williams syndrome. In S. Bartke & J. Siegmuller (Eds.), *Williams Syndrome Across Languages*. Amsterdam/Philadelphia: John Benjamins.

Bellugi, U., Marks, S., Bihrle, A., & Sabo, H. (1988). Dissociation between language and cognitive functions in Williams syndrome. In D. Bishop & K. Mogford (Eds.). *Language Development in Exceptional Circumstances*. London: Churchill Livingstone.

Bishop, D. (1989). *Test for the Reception of Grammar*, 2nd edn. Manchester, UK: Chapel Press.

Borer, H. & Wexler, K. (1987). The maturation of syntax, In T. Rooper & E. Williams (Eds.), *Parameter Setting*. Dordrecht: Reiedel Publishing Company.

Borer, H. & Wexler, K. (1992). Bi-unique relations and the maturation of grammatical principles. *Natural Language and Linguistic Theory*, **10**, 147–89.

Brock, J. (2007). Language abilities in Williams syndrome: A critical review. *Development and Psychopathology*, **19**, 97–127.

Browing, M. (1987). Null operator constructions. Unpublished Doctoral Dissertation, Massachusetts Institute of Technology, Cambridge.

Chomsky, N. (1981). *Lectures on Government and Binding*. Dordecht: Foris.

Chomsky, N. (1986). *Knowledge of Language: Its Nature, Origin and Use*. New York: Praeger.

Clahsen, H. & Almazan, A. (1998). Syntax and morphology in children with Williams syndrome. *Cognition*, **68**, 167–98.

Clahsen, H., Ring, M., & Temple, C. (2004). Lexical and morphological skills in English-speaking children with Williams syndrome. In S. Bartke & J. Siegmuller (Eds.), *Williams Syndrome Across Languages*. Amsterdam/Philadelphia: John Benjamins.

Clahsen, H. & Temple, C. (2003). Words and rules in Williams syndrome. In Y. Levy & J. Schaeffer (Eds.), *Language Competence Across Populations*. Hillsdale, NJ: Erlbaum.

Crain, S. & Thornton, R. (1998). *Investigations in Universal Grammar*. Cambridge MA: MIT Press.

Doll, A. & Grzeschik, K. H. (2001). Characterization of two novel genes, WBSCR20 and WBSCR22 deleted in Williams-Beuren syndrome. *Cytogenesis and Cell Genetics*, **95**, 20–7.

Ewart, A. K., Morris, C. A., Atkinson, D., *et al.* (1993). Hemizygosity at the elastin locus in a developmental disorder, Williams syndrome. *Nature Genetics*, **5**, 11–6.

Georgas, D., Paraskevopoulos, I., Bezevengis, I., & Giannitsas, N. (1997). *Guidelines for the Greek WISC III*. Athens: Ellinika Grammata.

Gleitman, L. R. (1990). The structural sources of verb meanings. *Language Acquisition*, **1**, 3–55.

Guasti, M. T. & Shlonsky, R. (1995). The acquisition of French relatives reconsidered. *Language Acquisition*, **4**, 257–76.

Joffe, V. L. & Varlokosta, S. (2007). Patterns of syntactic development in children with Williams syndrome and Down's syndrome: Evidence from passives and Wh-questions. *Clinical Linguistics and Phonetics*, **21**(9), 705–27.

Jordan, H., Reiss, J. E., Hoffman, J. E., & Landau, B. (2002). Intact perception of biological motion in the face of profound spatial deficits: Williams syndrome. *Psychological Science*, **13**(2), 162–7.

Karmiloff-Smith, A. (1998). Development itself is the key to understand developmental disorders. *Trends in Cognitive Sciences*, **2**, 389–398.

Karmiloff-Smith, A., Klima, E., Bellugi, U., Grant, G., & Baron-Cohen, S. (1997). Is there a social module? Language, face processing and theory of mind in individuals with Williams syndrome. *Journal of Cognitive Neuroscience*, **7**, 196–208.

Karmiloff-Smith, A., Tyler, L., Voice, K., *et al.* (1998). Linguistic dissociations in WS: Evaluating receptive syntax in on-line and off-line tasks. *Neuropsychologia*, **36**, 343–51.

Korenberg, J. R., Chen, X.-N., Hirota, H., *et al.* (2000). Genome structure and cognitive map of Williams syndrome. *Journal of Cognitive Neuroscience*, **12**, S89-S107.

Mervis, C. B., Robinson, B. E., Bertand, J., Morris, C. A., Klein-Tasman, B. P., & Armstrong, S. C. (2000). The Williams syndrome cognitive profile. *Brain and Cognition*, **44**, 604–28.

Mervis, C. B., Robinson, B. E., Rowe, M., Becerra, A., & Klein-Tasman, B. P (2004). Relations between language and cognition in Williams syndrome. In S. Bartke & J. Siegmuller (Eds.), *Williams Syndrome Across Languages*. Amsterdam/Philadelphia: John Benjamins.

Perovic, A. & Wexler, K. (2007). Complex grammar in Williams Syndrome. *Journal of Clinical Linguistics and Phonetics*, **21**, 729–45.

Pinker, S. (1999). *Words and Rules*. London: Weidenfeld Nicolson.

Radford, A. (1997). *Syntactic Theory and the Structure of English. A Minimalist Approach.* Cambridge: Cambridge University Press.

Ring, M. & Clahsen, H. (2005). Distinct patterns of language impairment in Down's syndrome, Williams syndrome, and SLI: The case of syntactic chains. *Journal of Neurolinguistics*, **18**, 479–501.

Stavrakaki, S. (2002). Sentence comprehension in Greek SLI children. In N. Hewlett, L. Kelly, & F. Windsor (Eds.), *Investigations in Clinical Phonetics and Linguistics*. Hillsdale, NJ: Erlbaum.

Stavrakaki, S. (2004). Wh-questions in Greek children with Williams syndrome: A comparison with SLI and normal development. In S. Bartke & J. Siegmuller (Eds.), *Williams Syndrome Across Languages*. Amsterdam/Philadelphia: John Benjamins.

Tager-Flusberg, H., Plesa-Skwerer, D., Faja, S., & Joseph, M. (2003). People with Williams syndrome process faces holistically. *Cognition*, **88**(1), 11–24.

Tager-Flusberg, H. & Sullivan K. (2000). A componential view of theory of mind: Evidence from Williams syndrome. *Cognition*, **76**(1), 59–90.

Temple, C., Almazan, M., & Sherwood, S. (2002). Lexical skills in Williams syndrome: A cognitive neuropsychological analysis. *Journal of Neurolinguistics*, **15**, 463–95.

Terzi, A. & Wexler, K. (2002). A-chains and S-homophones in children's grammar: Evidence from Greek passives. *Proc NELS*, **32**, 519–39.

Thomas, M., Grant, J., Barham, Z., *et al.* (2001). Past tense formation in Williams syndrome. *Language and Cognitive Processes*, **16**, 143–76.

Thomas, M. & Karmiloff-Smith, A. (2002). Are developmental disorders like cases of adult brain damage: Implications from connectionist modeling. *Behavioral and Brain Sciences*, **25**(6), 727–88.

Volterra, V., Capirci, O., & Caselli, C. (2001). What atypical populations can reveal about language development: The contrast between deafness and Williams syndrome. *Language and Cognitive Processes*, **16**, 219–39.

Volterra, V., Capirci, O., Pezzini, G., Sabbadini, L., & Vicari, S. (1996). Linguistic abilities in Italian children with Williams syndrome. *Cortex*, **32**, 663–77.

Wexler, K. (1991). Some issues in the growth of control. *MIT Occasional Papers in Linguistics* (No 44). Department of Brain and Cognitive Science, Massachusetts Institute of Technology, Cambridge.

Zukowski, A. (2001). Uncovering grammatical competence in children with Williams syndrome. *Unpublished Doctoral Dissertation*, Boston University.

Zukowski, A. (2004). Investigating knowledge of complex syntax: Insights from experimental studies of Williams Syndrome. In M. Rice & S. Warren (Eds.), *Developmental Language Disorders: From Phenotypes to Etiologies*. Mahwah, NJ: Lawrence Erlbaum Associates.

Zukowski, A. (2009). Elicited production of relative clauses reflects intact grammatical knowledge in Williams syndrome. *Language and Cognitive Processes*, **24**, 1–43.

6

Language in Down syndrome: A life-span perspective

Jean A. Rondal

Down syndrome (DS), or trisomy 21, is divided according to three etiological subcategories: (1) standard trisomy, (2) mosaicism, and (3) translocation. In 97% of all cases (the standard trisomy 21 subcategory), the genetic error takes place in the ovula or the spermatozoid before syngamy or during the first cell division. All the living cells of the embryo receive three chromosome 21s. In 1% of all cases (Hamerton *et al.*, 1965; 2% according to Richards, 1969; the mosaicism subcatregory), the genetic error takes place during the second or the third cell division. In those cases, the embryo develops with a mosaic of normal cells containing the regular number of 46 chromosomes and cells with three chromosome 21s. In the remaining 2% (1%, according to Richards) of all cases (the translocation subcategory), the additional chromosomic material is not a triplicate of chromosome 21 but a part or the totality of another chromosome (often chromosome 14 or 22). In about 66% of the translocation cases, the genetic error takes place during the formation of the ovula or the spermatozoid, or during the first division of the embryo cell. In 34% of the cases, one of the parents, although phenotypically normal in all respects, carries the translocation in his/her genotype.

A natural question is "Does the difference in karyotype make a difference through its variations in the psychological outcomes of Down syndrome?" This question was first raised by Clarke *et al.* (1961), who described a case of trisomy mosaicism in a girl of average intelligence presenting some features of the syndrome. Since then, other reports have explored frequency of aberrant cells and level of intelligence. Overall, findings (see Gibson, 1981, for a review of the literature) suggest that (1) mosaic DS subjects have less severe retardation than translocation or standard trisomy DS subjects and (2) translocation DS subjects display less intellectual deficit than standard trisomy DS subjects. But the extent of agreement between the studies is far from perfect.

Few specific data exist on the same problem regarding language capacities. Fishler and Koch (1991) have reported a mean IQ difference of 12 points (on

Wechsler's scales) between a group of 30 individuals with standard trisomy 21 (mean IQ 52, SD 14.6) and a group of mosaic DS subjects (mean IQ 64, SD 13.8). The two groups were matched for CA (between 2 and 18 years), sex, and parental socio-economic background. As indicated by the authors, many subjects with mosaicism (but none of the regular DS subjects) showed better verbal abilities (actually receptive lexical ability, as assessed by the Peabody Picture Vocabulary Test), and some demonstrated normal or normal-like visuo-perceptual skills on paper-and-pencil tasks.

As the most common chromosomal cause of intellectual disabilities (ID), DS affects about 1 in 800 births, and increased risks of trisomy 21 are seen among women with advanced maternal age. DS enjoys more behavioral research than all other ID syndromes combined.

Benda's classical curve of mental growth for DS individuals (Benda, 1949) culminates around 40 months MA reached between 10 and 15 years CA. Modal IQ in standard trisomy 21 is between 45 and 50 points (Gibson, 1981). The literature on psychological development sees mental evolution in DS in three "stages" (Gibson, 1981). Mental growth is steady during the first 18 months MA, developed over 4 or 5 years CA. This phase witnesses the DS child's evolution through the stages of Piaget's sensori-motor intellectual subcategories. The beginning of conceptual–symbolic development is also evident. The second and third periods of mental growth occur between 5 and approximately 15 years CA. They cover the MA range from 2 to 5 years. Five years MA seems to be the realistic upper limit of mental growth for most DS subjects, which they reach between 12 and 15 years CA. It is known, however, that mental development may continue beyond this level into the third decade of life for a number of DS persons, albeit more slowly (Berry *et al.*, 1984).

Speech and language development

Detailed reviews of the literature on the development of speech, language, and communication skills in persons with DS and other mental handicaps are readily available (e.g., Barrett & Diniz, 1989; Chapman, 2003; Rondal, 1975, 1984; Rondal & Edwards, 1997). The following presentation will only summarize major data.

Prelinguistic development

Prelinguistic development covers the first 18 months in TD infants. It may be quite extended in DS, and there is large inter-individual variability. Delays tend to be reduced nowadays as a result of better care and early stimulation and intervention procedures.

Neurological examinations show hypotonia and abnormalities in the early reflexes and automatisms in DS neonates (including palmar and plantar reflexes; Landau reaction, i.e., ventral suspension; Moro response; and automatic stepping). Early motor development is usually delayed, largely due to congenital hypotonia.

It is known that TD neonates can recognize (i.e., discriminate from other corresponding language material) their mother's speech and tongue, providing that it is normally intonated. TD infants a few days and weeks old can discriminate all the sounds occurring in natural languages, on the basis of place of articulation (e.g., p, t, k), mode of articulation (d, n), oral and nasal vowels (a, i, u, an, in; the latter in French, for example), and so on. The neonates' overall discriminative ability for speech sounds decreases over the first year of life, except for the phoneme sounds characteristic of the community language. For instance, Japanese babies are able to distinguish r and l sounds, whereas older Japanese children and adults no longer can, as these phonemes do not exist in Japanese. This loss of sensitivity is cognitive or attentional but not neurosensorial. Research shows that only those sounds that share one or several dimensions with maternal phonemes are distinguished, i.e., sounds that are potential competitors for the maternal ones are "faded away" (on a statistical basis). Less frequent sounds are not primed and disappear from the activated attentional/memory register.

Unfortunately, we know almost nothing about these key aspects of early language sensitization in DS babies. Frequently reported hearing loss and attentional difficulties may hinder early sound discrimination and familiarization with maternal language early on in DS development.

As for babbling, four major periods can be identified: Stage 1 (0–2 months in TD babies) involves reflex or quasi-reflex vocalizations (crying and vegetative sounds); Stage 2 (2–4 months) is characterized by cooing sounds tied to smiles and prevocalic sounds; Stage 3 (4–8 months) involves quasi-vowels, clicks, palatalized or pharyngealized consonants, affricates, etc.; and Stage 4 (8–10 months) is characterized by canonical babbling (production of well formed syllables; e.g., ba, pa, da, ta, ga, ka), often reduplicated (e.g., bababa, mamama, tatata, etc), then variegated (consisting of consonants and vowels that differ).

Before approximately 6 months of age, infants' babbling appears to be only minimally influenced by the community language. Sounds that do not belong to the maternal tongue are readily produced. Between 6 and 12 months, a clear influence of the linguistic environment can be demonstrated. In some way, the older infant babbles in his/her mother tongue.

Insufficient data are available on babbling development in DS. The research on this should be enlarged, as well as the one on sound perception and discrimination, if one wants to be able to carry out an efficient prelinguistic intervention designed to foster more rapid language development in these children. Babbling sounds are mostly similar in types and tokens in TD and DS children (Smith & Oller, 1981). However, there is a 3-month delay on average regarding the onset of reduplicated babbling in the latter infants.

Reduplicated babbling is a distinct precursor to meaningful speech. Significant positive correlations have been found for the age of onset of reduplicated babbling in infants with DS and their scores at 27 months on the early Social-Communication Scales (Mundy *et al.*, 1984), which have predictive value with respect to subsequent development of verbal communication.

Another aspect of babbling (*interactive babbling*) has been studied and has been described as "prelinguistic phrasing" or intermittent babbling, approximately 3 seconds long, characterized by the prosody and structure that later underlie speech (for example, phrase-ending syllables last longer than other syllables, which may be a signal prefiguring turn-taking organization). Babies with DS display the same prosodic organization in prelinguistic phrases as TD infants (but they are delayed by several months) and when they do, they take longer to finish a phrase (an average of more than 5 seconds). This probably explains why mothers and their babies with DS are found to vocalize simultaneously more often than mothers and TD babies of the same CAs.

Speech

Articulatory Problems

Between 70% and 90% of individuals with moderate or severe ID (including those with DS) have serious articulatory difficulties. Individuals with DS are particularly prone to slow articulatory development and persisting (sometimes lifelong) difficulties.

Responsible factors include the following: (1) Peripheral anatomical factors: buccal cavity too small for tongue affecting sound resonance; protruding tongue; cleft or short hard palate; deformities resulting in defective dental occlusion; larynx located high in the neck; and hypotonia of speech muscles involving tongue, lips, soft palate, and breathing muscles (Spitzer *et al.*, 1961). (2) Auditory defects (60% or more of the DS samples), mainly 25 to 55 decibel losses over the frequencies 500, 1000, and 2000 Hertz; impairment being roughly half conductive and half sensorineural or mixed. (3) Deficits in motor coordination and timing (Rosin *et al.*, 1987). (4) Voice problems, including hoarseness; higher or lower fundamental frequencies than normal (Montague & Hollien, 1973).

Phonological development

Articulatory development (i.e., the setting up of phonological contrasts in production) is slow and difficult in many children with DS for a number of reasons, including the delays and uncertainties of lexical development, but the overall progression appears to parallel development in TD children (e.g., Menn, 1983; Smith & Oller, 1981; Stoel-Gammon, 2001). Vowels, semivowels, and nasal and stop consonants are produced first. The fricatives [f],[θ],[s],[ʃ], [v], [z],[δ], and [z] are more difficult to articulate. They take longer to be mastered (when they are). Intelligibility of speech remains low in most individuals with DS (Rondal, 1978; Ryan, 1975). The articulatory simplifications are of the same type, albeit more inconsistent and more variable from trial to trial in the same subjects and from subject to subject, even at comparable IQ and MA levels, as those observed in the speech of TD children (mainly feature changes, cluster reductions, and assimilations) (Dodd, 1976; Dodd & Leahy, 1989; Rosin *et al.*, 1988; Van Borsel, 1993). Most adolescents and adults with DS exhibit a pattern of phonological performance similar to that of older children with DS (Rondal & Lambert, 1983; Van Borsel, 1988).

As for nonsegmental phonology (prosody), systematic studies in children with DS are nonexistent. Anecdotal observations suggest that the prosody of these children may be slightly more advanced than other linguistic skills (Rondal & Edwards, 1997). However, in the absence of quantitative data, no firm conclusion is possible. Contrastive intonational patterns are used to support the emerging conversational skills but with some inconsistency.

Lexical Development

From comparative studies in DS and typical individuals, it appears that MA is a good predictor of receptive lexical developmental level. Word understanding begins at the same MA in DS and TD infants, and there are many similarities in the progressions (Cunnigham & Sloper, 1984). Lexical development proceeds with growth in MA, which follows CA with increasing delays in individuals with DS (Rondal, 1985).

The relationship between MA and expressive lexical development (not to be confounded with lexical definitions, i.e., a metalinguistic task at which ID persons have little aptitude for cognitive reasons) is more variable, because additional variables come into play (prominently the problems associated with articulatory development and motor programming), hence, the dissociations observed between lexical understanding and expression in these individuals. The onset of expressive language is typically markedly delayed in DS. In some studies, cohorts of CA 4-year-olds have expressive vocabularies of 50 words on average, which is about the median value of 16- to 18-month-old TD infants (Smith & Stoel-Gammon, 1983).

Lexical learning may look simple. It is actually a complex task involving segmenting the input speech flow into candidate lexical units; establishing relevant (i.e., conventional) associations between forms, meaning, and categories of referents; maintaining the information in short-term memory (STM) for the time needed to allow registration in longer term stores; and organizing the lexical units in semantic memory (long-term memory, LTM) to ensure permanent storage and efficient retrieval.

Segmenting

Except for the fact that, globally, the language input to children with DS is comparable to that of TD children at similar levels of language development, relatively little is known about the way infants with DS learn to segment the input speech to which they are exposed into relevant lexical units (see Chapter 8).

Constraints on Lexical Learning

Several strategies, hypotheses, or constraints bearing on the acquisition of the early lexical repertoires, particularly the nouns at the basic level, have been proposed for TD children (Mervis, 1987). They are meant to help meet the challenge created by the large number of logically plausible alternatives regarding the relationship between a lexical form and its possible meaning(s)–referent(s). Lexical strategies consist of the following: (1) Whole objects (a new name refers to a whole referent and not to one of its properties, qualities, parts, substance, etc.); (2) Mutual exclusivity (each object corresponds to a different name); (3) Taxonomy (lexical categories are constituted of similar objects and not, for example, of objects that can be associated thematically); (4) Form; (5) Function; (6) Contrast (every formal difference codes for a difference in meaning and/or normal class status, e.g., noun–verb, object–attribute, etc.); (7) Conventionality (words have conventional meaning that are stable over time); (8) Reference; (9) Extensionality (words come to refer to more than their initial referents; formal and functional similarities and associations control the extension); and (10) New name–category without a name (new words usually refer to categories for which one does not have a name yet, probably involved in the so-called fast mapping ability).

Research with ID and TD children suggests that children with DS between CA 5–8 years exhibit similar fast mapping ability as MA-matched TD children. The strategy "New name–category without a name" is not available at the beginning of lexical development (CA 2–3 years) in children with DS (that is also the case for TD infants earlier in development). Children with DS who subsequently have access to this principle proceed more rapidly in their lexical acquisitions (Mervis & Becerra, 2003; Mervis & Bertrand, 1994 , 1995).

Short-Term Memory

It has been suggested that auditory–vocal short-term memory (AV-STM) plays an important role in lexical learning (Baddeley, 1980). A mechanism that may account for the relationship between AV-STM and lexical development is that the longer a new word is kept in STM, the better the odds that it will be learned (i.e., passed onto LTM) (Gathercole & Baddeley, 1993). Individuals with DS typically have shorter and more unstable AV-STM (and slightly better visuo-spatial STM; Marcell & Armstrong, 1982, Marcell & Weeks, 1988), which may account, at least partially, for the slowness and limitations of their lexical learning (Jarrold & Baddeley, 1997; Jarrold *et al.*, 1999; MacKenzie & Hulme, 1987).

Lexical Organization in LTM

Fast and reliable retrieval is needed to produce and understand a linguistic utterance in real time (i.e., several words are produced per second during every-day conversations). Such ability also depends on the quality of the organization in LTM. Although this aspect of lexical functioning is still far from satisfactorily explained in typical individuals, a few organizing principles and dimensions have been studied, for example, lexical prototypicality and the hierarchical dimensions of semantic fields.

Prototypicality (or "best category example") means that, in a number of lexical categories, one can readily identify individual referents presenting at the same time most if not all of the definitional characteristics of the category and few or none of the characteristics of neighboring classes (e.g., among birds, eagle, sparrows, and crows are most often considered prototypes of the general category, whereas ducks, swans, and hens are not) (Rosch, 1978). By hierarchical dimension, one means a structure based on two types of relations, i.e., a hierarchy of subsets and a series of attributions. Consider, for instance, the three-level hierarchy composed of superordinate, basic, and subordinate levels, holding in the case of the categories animal, dog, German Shepherd (Rosch, 1978).

Studies show that subjects with DS tend to represent the meaning of a number of noun categories by relying on lexical prototypes (see Barrett & Diniz, 1989, for review). They gradually extend their lexical categories to include other items on the basis of similarity to the prototypes. The closer the new item to the prototype, the faster it is identified as belonging to the same category (Tager-Flusberg, 1986). Individuals with DS acquire the notions of superordinate and subordinate relationships, although with significant delays (Barrett & Diniz, 1989). The basic level is dominant. Items at this level are learned, memorized, recognized, and recalled more reliably and more rapidly. Their knowledge of items at nonbasic levels is less advanced and remains unstable (Tager-Flusberg, 1986).

Grammar

Semantic Structural Development

Semantic structural development may be considered the building blocks for grammatical development. Individuals with DS are delayed in semantic development in proportion to their cognitive deficit. When they start to combine two and three words within the same utterance, children with DS appear to understand and to express the same range of relational meanings or thematic roles and relations as reported in typical combinatorial language (Coggins, 1979; Duchan & Erickson, 1976; Layton & Sharifi, 1979; Rondal, 1978). Examples of early thematic relations are notice or existence; denial or disappearance; recurrence, attribution (qualitative or quantitative); possession; location; agent; patient; instrument; source; agent–action; action–patient; agent–action–patient.

Therefore, despite noticeable CA delays, children with DS do develop the regular semantic basis for combinatorial language functioning.

Morphosyntactic Development

Further delays in grammatical development are due to particular difficulties with a number of morphosyntactical dimensions of language. Some find their source in the cognitive limitations of these persons, others in problems relative to the linguistic organization itself. Morphosyntactic development is rarely complete in DS subjects. Some progress is obvious, however, with increased CA (Lenneberg *et al.*, 1964). It is reflected in the progressive lengthening of the utterances as captured by mean length of utterance (MLU; Brown, 1973). Table 1 summarizes MLU data obtained by Rondal and colleagues (Rondal, 1978; Rondal & Lambert, 1983; Rondal *et al.*, 1980) through spontaneous speech analyses in free-play and free-conversation conditions. The adult MLU data exhibit larger interindividual variability to the extent that the mean reported may be partially misleading as a summary index for this group of subjects.

The slowness and limitation of MLU development in children with DS corresponds to important shortcomings in morphosyntax. However, word order in those languages that rely on sequential devices to express thematic relations is usually correct. The production of grammatical words (functors, i.e., articles, prepositions, pronouns, modals, auxiliaries, copula, conjunctions) is reduced in younger DS children, and often remains unstable in older subjects. Children and adolescents with DS produce proportions of grammatical (inflexional) morphemes similar to MLU-matched TD children. Often, however, children with DS are more variable in their production, but there is no evidence of deviance in their development.

Children and adolescents with DS have serious limitations in the comprehension of morphosyntactic structures, and they lag behind MA-matched TD

Table 1. MLU and standard deviations (SD) in DS subjects

Study	Chronological age[a]		MLU[b]	
	Group mean	SD[c]	Group mean	SD
Rondal (1978)[d]				
Group 1	4.01	0.09	1.26	0.23
Group 2	6.06	2.01	1.94	0.19
Group 3	9.06	1.09	2.87	0.14
Rondal, Lambert, & Sohier (1980)[e]	11.06	1.08	3.40	0.95
Rondal & Lambert (1983)[d]	26.00	1.07	5.98	2.62

[a] In years and months.
[b] Computed in number of words plus grammatical morphemes after Brown's rules (1973).
[c] Standard deviation.
[d] Study conducted with American English-speaking subjects.
[e] Study conducted with Belgian French-speaking subjects.

controls in this respect as well. Passive voice understanding is problematic. Younger TD children tend to decode reversible passive sentences as if they were corresponding actives (The blue car is followed by the red car). The same trend is found in children and adolescents with DS, and there is no clear indication that this situation changes with development (Rondal, 1995). Actional passives (i.e., sentences constructed around action verbs, e.g., push, carry) as opposed to mental or experience verbs (e.g., imagine, like, see) are facilitative in TD children (Rondal *et al.*, 1990), but have no such effect in children with DS for whom it may be supposed that the formal complexity blocks the otherwise facilitating semantic effect.

Pragmatics

Although formally reduced, the language of individuals with DS is not devoid of communicative value. Conversational topics are dealt with in such a way as to allow for the necessary continuity in the exchange between interlocutors. Language content is informative and new information is exchanged. Major illocutionary types of sentences are used. Other research (e.g., Owings *et al.*, 1981) demonstrates the capacity of moderately and severely ID adults (including individuals with DS) to take part efficiently in conversation with TD persons or other ID people at least in simplified contexts (i.e., dyadic or triadic ordinary conversation in familiar settings). In experimental settings, young adults with mild to moderate ID are able to judge topic maintenance correctly. ID adults exhibit similar types of conversational controls as typical adults. Rosenberg and colleagues (Abbeduto & Rosenberg, 1980; Rosenberg & Abbeduto, 1993) have examined the communicative competence of moderately to mildly ID adults engaged in triadic conversation with peers with mental retardation. The conversational turn-taking organization functions well in these individuals. They are able to recognize those illocutionary acts requiring a response on the interlocutor's part from those that do not. The exchange of information is active and correctly controlled. However, limitations do exist. ID subjects express fewer indirect speech acts (Abbeduto & Rosenberg, 1980), and they formulate few clarification requests in uninformative extralinguistic contexts in comparison with MA-matched TD subjects (Abbeduto *et al.*, 1991).

Younger subjects with DS already make use of a variety of illocutionary devices in relating verbally to the interlocutor, as shown in the data gathered by Rondal (1978). Those data were obtained in free-play interactions at home with the mothers. In such situations, mothers (of ID as well as of TD children) are known to lead the interaction, asking questions and giving orders more frequently than the children. Correspondingly, studies by Leifer and Lewis (1984) and Scherer and Owings (1984) demonstrate nontrivial conversational capacities and an ability to respond correctly to simple verbal requests in children with DS around 5 years CA.

Discourse

Reilly *et al.* (1991) compared cognitively matched adolescents with Williams syndrome (WS) and DS in a story-telling task. The subjects were introduced to a wordless picture book (Frog, where are you?) and asked to construct a story from the pictures as they progressed page by page through the book. In contrast to subjects with DS, the adolescents with WS told coherent and complex narratives making extensive use of affective prosody. The participants with WS, but not those with DS, enriched the referential contents of their stories with narrative, and affective and social cognitive devices. For example, subjects with WS used more features such as affective and mental verbs, emphatic and intensifier forms, negative markers, causal connectors, as well as onomatopoeic forms.

A study by Chapman *et al.* (1991) indirectly confirms the particular difficulty of children and adolescents with DS in online story processing. In such contexts, these subjects no longer demonstrate the fast-mapping ability with novel words that they exhibit in simpler event contexts. In story contexts, subjects with DS encounter additional difficulties in processing the narrative structure and in memory for story gist generally. These difficulties interfere with inferring the likely referent of the novel words, preventing the fast-mapping production forms observed in event contexts from occurring.

More generally, however, Chapman *et al.* (1992) report significant increases in the narratives of older adolescents with DS (CAs between 16 and 20 years) in comparison with children and younger adolescents with DS aged 5 to 16 years. Chapman (1995) suggests that these data contradict the hypothesis of a critical period (CP) in language development of children with mental retardation, which would terminate before or around puberty. As discussed below, contemporary views of the CP hypothesis are modular and tend to restrict temporal constraints to the computational aspects of language development. The discursive dimension is not specifically concerned with the grammatical, thematic semantic, or information structure of language (Halliday, 1985). It relates to the network of relationships between clauses and/or paragraphs allowing for textual cohesion. It may be expected that at least some adolescents and adults with DS can continue to progress in this aspect as well as in other cognitive aspects of the language system given adequate opportunities and stimulation.

The Critical Period Problem

The question of whether there exists a critical period for first language acquisition has practical relevance for ID and DS children, given that they usually fail to complete the developmental course by the end of childhood. The notion of a CP for language development was first proposed by Lenneberg (1967). Outside the field of ID, a series of data (e.g., Curtiss, 1989; Mayberry *et al.*, 1983; Newport, 1992; Ploog, 1984) support a milder and slightly diverse form of a CP hypothesis. It is limited to two (major) language components, phonology and morphosyntax, with different developmental time windows (the phonological CP is shorter than the morphosyntactic one). The CPs relate to a native brain ability to implicitly extract regularities regarding distributional features of language.

Lenneberg *et al.* (1964) reported data supporting the hypothesis of a "freeze" in language acquisition in individuals with DS after roughly 14 years of age. Sixty-one individuals with DS aged CA 3–22 years at the beginning of the study were followed over a 3-year period. Those who had reached puberty failed to make further progress in language structures. This was in contrast to younger subjects for whom some growth was observed. However, judging from the unclear report of Lenneberg *et al.* (1964) on this point, it seems that only 4 subjects were beyond CA 14 years when tested, which is too limited a subsample to allow for generalization.

We have recorded the spontaneous speech of 24 French-speaking adolescents with moderate ID, of mixed etiologies, in dyadic conversational interaction with a typical adult (Rondal *et al.*, 1980). Mean MLU for the 16 subjects whose ages were between 14 and 18 years was 5.52. Mean MLU for the ID subjects aged 12–14 years was 5.15, which is not significantly different from that of the older group. None of the other language measures yielded a significant difference between younger and older subjects (type–token ratio, proportion of correct articles, proportion of correct verbal inflections, proportion of sentence complexity, proportion of information, or proportion of new information).

Fowler (1988) has supplied conversational MLU data from a group of adolescents with DS (aged 12–19 years). She split her group into lower IQ (Stanford-Binet score, 38–48) and higher IQ (55–64) subjects. Mean MLU in words plus grammatical morphemes reached 3.58 in the lower IQ group and 3.78 in the higher IQ group (with noticeable intersubject differences in the two groups). These MLU figures may be compared to the middle age DS group (7–12 years) also studied by Fowler (1988). Corresponding MLU data for this group were 2.56 in the lower IQ group and 4.03 in the higher group. Corresponding results were obtained by Fowler (1988) with a second measure, the Index of Productive Syntax, which awards points for the occurrence of 56 kinds of morphological and syntactic forms in the speech sample. In another study, Fowler *et al.* (1994) reported no further modification in MLU over a 2½- to 4-year period following initial measurement in four adolescents with DS (mean CA 12 years and 7 months at the beginning of the study), as MLU remained in the range 3–3.50.

Regarding speech, Buckley and Sacks (1987) report that the speech of over half of the adolescent girls and about 80% of the adolescent boys in their survey were rated by parents as unintelligible to strangers. Intelligibility of speech in adolescents with DS does not seem to undergo much change, as indicated by the reports of Lenneberg (1967), Ryan (1975), and Rondal (1978). Bray and Woolnough (1988) confirm that intelligibility of speech is a serious problem in many children and adolescents with DS (12–16 years), even for those displaying more advanced syntax.

Van Borsel (1988) has reported a comprehensive analysis of the elicited speech of five Dutch-speaking girls with DS (CAs: 16 to 20 years). The work included a phonetic, substitution, and phonological process analysis. All Dutch phonemes occurred in the corpus of each subject, except the low-frequency loan-phonemes /ß/ and /Ω/. Results indicate that the speech errors of the adolescents with DS are for the most part identical to the error patterns observed in young TD children.

Observations regarding several aspects of the language of French-speaking children, adolescents, and adults with DS can be found in the doctoral work of Annick Comblain (1995) at the Laboratory for Psycholinguistics of the University of Liège. Comblain (1995; see also Rondal & Comblain, 1996) conducted a series of language tasks on 11 children with DS (8 girls and 3 boys), aged 7 to 13 years; 16 adolescents with DS (9 girls and 7 boys), aged 14 to 21 years;

and 15 adults with DS (9 females and 6 males), aged 24 to 42 years. All subjects had standard trisomy 21. The MLU values reported for the child and adolescent groups are globally consistent with those of Rondal *et al.* (1980), Fowler (1988), and Fowler *et al.* (1994), suggesting no change in productive morphosyntactic ability from late adolescence to adulthood.

Chapman *et al.* (1998) have reported contradictory results from cohorts of individuals with DS aged between 5 and 20 years. MLU increased with CA throughout the age range in both conversational and narrative language samples. MLU increases were larger in narrative than in conversational context, most notably after age 16, although individual variability was also greater at this point. The data of Chapman *et al.* may not be representative of the DS population as the 12- to 16-year-old age group scored relatively low compared to the younger age group (as well as to comparable age-group samples in Fowler's 1988 study, mentioned before, and even with regard to the MLU data reported by Rondal, 1978, for his English-speaking children around 12 years of age), and this discrepancy appears to be, in large part, responsible for the MLU difference observed between the older group (16–20 years) and the younger group. Thordadottir *et al.* (2002) also claim that syntactic development in individuals with DS continues in late adolescence. They document that, in narrative languages samples, both older children and adolescents with DS and a group of TD children matched on MLU, used conjoined and subordinate sentence forms (10% of the time). It is interesting to observe that some subjects with DS sometimes do use complex syntactic forms to a limited extent. However, it is hard to see why the authors have interpreted their data as contradicting previous conclusions regarding the CP question given that these data concern solely the adolescent years.

In conclusion, there is no clear indication of continued development of phonological and morphosyntactic aspects of language beyond mid-adolescence (earlier for the phonological aspects) in individuals with DS. There may be some continued progress, at least in some individuals, regarding other aspects of language, for example, lexical, pragmatical, and communicative abilities (Abbeduto *et al.*, 1988; Berry *et al.*, 1984; Owings *et al.*, 1981; Zetlin & Sabsay, 1980), which have yet to be investigated more thoroughly.

Interindividual variability

Many, but not all, individuals with a given syndrome will show the syndrome's characteristic behaviors. However, each individual will not show the behavior to the same extent. Some within-syndrome variability exists in every ID genetic syndrome (Hodapp & Dykens, 2004). Regarding physical outcomes, for example, although many professionals consider epicanthal folds as the hallmark facial characteristic of individuals with DS, at least during infancy, only around

60% of DS infants show this characteristic (Pueschel, 1995). The same is true for the various domains of behavior and development.

The reasons for within-syndrome variability, an issue still insufficiently researched as of today, are undoubtedly complex. Some have to do with the ways in which genetic effects are probabilistic. Genetics is better conceptualized as predisposing a person to have one or another etiology-related neurobehavioral trait expressed to a certain extent in his/her phenotype. Essentially, genes provide the starting point in complex multidirectional epigenetic pathways. The interactions between genotype and environmental events from the time of conception on determine the spans of individual variation. The behavioral phenotypes may also change at different CAs, often with relative strengths becoming stronger with age and weaknesses becoming weaker. Cascade effects may be operating in such ways that early propensities lead to greater personal interest as well as other people's interest, and this greater interest and increased time spent performing these activities, in turn, leads to increased skills. In this perspective, family background variables have not been studied sufficiently, although they are considered customarily to have a role in the individual differences between individuals with DS and other ID syndromes.

Some individual differences in language development may be particularly striking. Studies have appeared of individuals with DS who have atypical language abilities, that is, language characteristics that are not currently observed in the syndrome (cf. Rondal, 1995; Rondal & Edwards, 1997). As discussed in Rondal (2003), the major determinants of morphosyntactic and phonological differences between atypical and typical individuals with DS may operate at the level of the brain. There may exist significant within-syndrome variability in some brain areas of persons with DS devoted to language, consequent upon genetic variations. Of importance, is the observation that language-exceptional individuals with DS are atypical only with respect to the phonological and morphosyntactic aspects of language, which is consistent with a modular conception of basic language organization.

Language aging

It would seem that physically and biochemically some earlier aging process is at work in DS already objectifiable in the forties and even before (Van Buggenhout et al., 2001); this is independent of the susceptibility to develop an Alzheimer-like degenerative brain pathology seen in 15% to 20% of individuals with DS (Rondal et al., 2003). Cognitively and linguistically, however, things are less clear. Fenner et al. (1987) reported a decline in mental age in less than one-third of their total sample (n = 39) of persons with DS between 20 and 49 years and in just over one-third of the subjects older than 35 years. Ribes and Sanny (2000) have documented a decline of short-term and longer-term memory, vocabulary use, and expressive as well as receptive language abilities, in adults with DS. According to their data, the cognitive and language abilities evaluated showed a slight decline between the ages of 20 and 40 years. However, a more marked decline takes place beyond 40 years. Along similar lines, Moss *et al.* (2000) have reported a significant inverse relation between increasing age and several aspects of auditory linguistic comprehension in a cohort of participants with DS aged between 32 and 65 years. Correspondingly, Prasher (1996) has documented an age-associated decline in short-term memory, speech, practical skills, and general level of activity and interest, in approximatively 20% of persons with DS aged 50 to 71 years.

Other research reports are less definitive. Little to no change in nonverbal reasoning, memory, language (receptive and expressive vocabulary), planning and attention, perceptual–motor, and adaptive skills, until close to 60 years, is suggested in a study by Das *et al.* (1995). The same authors remark, however, that their older DS participants (those over 60 years) showed poorer performance than those in younger groups, on tasks requiring attention and planning. George *et al.* (2001) conducted a 4-year longitudinal study of 12 participants with DS (6 women and 6 men), aged 36 to 48 years at the beginning of the study. The language functions (receptive as well as productive; with tasks concerning the lexical, morphosyntactic, and discursive aspects of language) were assessed at 1-year intervals, as well as a number of nonverbal cognitive abilities. Short-term memory, auditory–verbal as well as visuo-spatial, and episodic memory (using an adaptation of the child Rivermead Behavioral Memory Test, Wilson *et al.*, 1991), visual perception, visuo-spatial functions, executive functions, and reasoning (evaluated with the K-ABC, Kaufman & Kaufman, 1993), and attention were also studied. None of the analyses yielded significant results, failing to corroborate the null hypothesis of a language change and/or a change in nonverbal cognitive functions over the 4 years of the study. Comparing the language data obtained from the receptive subtests of the Batterie pour l'Evaluation de la Morpho-Syntaxe (Comblain, 1995) with the corresponding data reported by Comblain (1994, 1996) from her study of adolescents (mean CA, 16 years and 7 months) and younger adults (mean CA 26 years and 9 months) (the three cohorts having comparable mental age (4 years and 4 months, standard deviation 8 months, for the adolescents; 4 years and 7 months, standard deviation 9 months, for the younger adults; 4 years and 4 months, standard deviation 6 months, for the older adults), Rondal and Comblain (2002) argue that no marked change takes place in the receptive morphosyntactic abilities of persons with DS in the interval of time between late adolescence and roughly 50 years of age.

Other longitudinal studies have reported similar observations. Devenny *et al.* (1992), and Burt *et al.* (1995) did not observe significant changes in the cognitive functioning of individuals with DS aged between 27 and 55 years, and 22 and 56 years, in two studies respectively, over 3- to 5-year time intervals. Devenny *et al.* (1996) report only four cases of cognitive involution in 91 subjects with DS followed for several years beyond the age of 50 years.

Conclusions

Thanks to the extensive research that has been conducted for the past 50 years or so, we now have at our disposal a rich data base of information on the language of individuals with DS across the life span. Systematic information, however, is still needed regarding prelinguistic development, particularly in the first weeks and months of life, even if only to determine whether or not the sensitivity toward the prosodic and distributional aspects of language input seen in TD babies can also be found in DS infants. The data on language in the later adult and elderly years is incomplete and insufficient. However, when analyzed in sufficient detail, the language of persons with DS demonstrates quantitative differences, significant delays, and incompleteness, particularly regarding more complex aspects of language, but not qualitative differences; that is, there is no evidence of aberrant developmental patterns or deviant processes or mechanisms.

REFERENCES

Abbeduto, L., & Rosenberg, S. (1980). The communicative competence of mildly retarded adults. *Applied Psycholinguistics*, **1**, 405–26.

Abbeduto, L., Davies, B., & Furman, L. (1988). The development of speech act comprehension in mentally retarded individuals and nonretarded children. *Child Development*, **59**, 1460–72.

Abbeduto, L., Davies, B., Solesby, S., & Furman, L. (1991). Identifying the referents of spoken messages: Use of context and clarification request by children with and without mental retardation. *American Journal of Mental Retardation*, **95**, 551–62.

Baddeley, A. (1980). *Human Memory*. Hillsdale, NJ: Erlbaum.

Barrett, M. & Diniz, F. (1989). Lexical development in mentally handicapped children. In M. Beveridge, G. Conti-Ramsden, & I. Leudar (Eds.), *Language and Communication in Mentally Handicapped People* (pp. 3–32). London: Chapman and Hall.

Benda, C. (1949). *Mongolism and Cretinism*. New York: Grune & Startton.

Berry, P., Groenweg, G., Gibson, D., & Brown, R. (1984). Mental development of adults with Down's syndrome. *American Journal of Mental Deficiency*, **89**, 252–6.

Bray, M. & Woolnough, L. (1988). The language of children with Down's syndrome aged 12 to 16 years. *Child Language Teaching and Therapy*, **4**, 311–21.

Brown, R. (1973). *A First Language*. Cambridge, MA: Harvard University Press.

Buckley, S. & Sacks, B. (1987). *The adolescent with Down's syndrome –Life for the teenager teaching and the family*. Portsmouth, UK: Portsmouth Down's syndrome Trust.

Burt, D., Loveland, K., Chen, Y.-W., Chuang, A., Lewis, K., & Cherry, L. (1995). Ageing in adults with Down syndrome: Report from a longitudinal study. *American Journal of Mental Retardation*, **100**, 262–70.

Chapman, R. (1995). Language development in children and adolescents with Down's syndrome. In P. Fletcher & B. McWhinney (Eds.), *The Handbook of Child Language* (pp. 641–63). Oxford: Blackwell.

Chapman, R. (2003). Language and communication in individuals with Down syndrome. In L. Abbeduto (Ed.), *Language and Communication in Mental Retardation* (pp. 1–34). New York: Academic Press.

Chapman, R., Schwartz, S., & Kay-Raining Bird, E. (1991). Language skills of children and adolescents with Down's syndrome: I. Comprehension. *Journal Speech and Hearing Research*, **34**, 1106–20.

Chapman, R., Schwartz, S., & Kay-Raining Bird, E. (1992, August). *Language production of children and adolescents with Down's syndrome*. Paper presented at the 9th World Congress of the International Association for the Scientific Study of Mental Deficiency. Gold Coast: Australia.

Chapman, R., Seung, H., Schwartz, S., & Kay-Raining Bird, E. (1998). Language skills of children and adolescents with Down syndrome: Production deficits. *Journal of Speech and Hearing Research*, **41**, 861–73.

Clarke, C. M., Edwards, J. H., & Smallpeice, V. (1961). Trisomy 21 normal mosaicism in an intelligent child with some mongoloid characters. *Lancet*, 1028–30.

Coggins, T. (1979). Relational meaning encoded in two-word utterance of stage 1 in Down's syndrome children. *Journal of Speech and Hearing Research*, **22**, 166–78.

Comblain, A. (1994). Working memory in Down's syndrome: Training rehearsal strategy. *Down Syndrome Research and Practice*, **2**, 123–6.

Comblain, A. (1995). *Batterie pour l'évaluation de la morpho-syntaxe*. Unpublished manuscript, University of Liège, Belgium.

Comblain, A. (1996). *Mémoire de travail et langage dans le syndrome de Down*. Unpublished doctoral dissertation (Logopedics), University of Liège, Belgium.

Cunningham, C. & Sloper, P. (1984). The relationship between maternal ratings of first word vocabulary and Reynell language scores. *British Journal of Educational Psychology*, **54**, 160–7.

Curtiss, S. (1989). Abnormal language acquisition and the modularity of language. In F. Newmeyer, (Ed.), *Linguistics: The Cambridge Survey* (Vol. 2, pp. 96–116). Cambridge, UK: Cambridge University Press.

Das, J. P., Divis, B., Alexander, J., Parrila, R., & Naglieri, J. (1995). Cognitive decline due to aging among persons with Down syndrome. *Research in Developmental Disabilities*, **16**, 461–78.

Devenny, D., Hill, A., Patxot, D., Silverman, W., & Wisniewsky, H. (1992). Ageing in higher functioning adults with Down's syndrome: A longitudinal study. *Journal of Intellectual Disability Research*, **36**, 241–50.

Devenny, D., Silverman, W., Hill, A., Jenkins, E., Sersen, E., & Wisniewski, H. (1996). Normal ageing in adult with Down's syndrome: A longitudinal study. *Journal of Intellectual Disability Research*, **40**, 208–21.

Dodd, B. (1976). A comparison of the phonological systems of mental-age-matched severely subnormal and Down's syndrome children. *British Journal of Disorders of Communication*, **11**, 27–42.

Dodd, B. & Leahy, Y. (1989). Phonological disorders and mental handicap. In M. Beveridge, G. Conti-Ramsden, & Y. Leudar (Eds.), *Language and Communication in Mentally Handicapped People* (pp. 33–56). London: Chapman & Hall.

Duchan, J. F. & Erickson, J. G. (1976). Normal and nonretarded children's understanding of semantic relations in different verbals contexts. *Journal of Speech and Hearing Research*, **19**, 767–76.

Fenner, M., Hewitt, K., & Torpy, D. (1987). Down's syndrome: Intellectual and behavioural functioning during adulthood. *Journal of Mental Deficiency Research*, **31**, 241–9.

Fishler, K. & Koch, R. (1991). Mental development in Down's syndrome mosaicism. *American Journal on Mental Retardation*, **96**, 345–51.

Fowler, A. (1988). Determinants of rate of language growth in children with Down's syndrome. In L. Nadel (Ed.), *The Psychobiology of Down's Syndrome* (pp. 217–45). Cambridge, MA: MIT Press.

Fowler, A., Gelman, R., & Gleitman, L. (1994). The course of language learning in children with Down's syndrome. In H. Tager-Flusberg (Ed.), *Constraints on Language Acquisition. Studies of Atypical Children* (pp. 91–140). Hillsdale, NJ: Erlbaum.

Gathercole, S. & Baddeley, A. (1993). *Working Memory and Language*. Hillsdale, NJ: Erlbaum.

George, M., Thewis, B., Van der Linden, M., Salmon, E., & Rondal, J. A. (2001). Elaboration d'une batterie d'évaluation des fonctions cognitives de sujets âgés porteurs d'un syndrome de Down. *Revue de Neuropsychologie*, **11**(4), 549–79.

Gibson, D. (1981). Down's syndrome: *The Psychology of Mongolism*. Cambridge, UK: Cambridge University Press.

Halliday, M. (1985). *An Introduction to Functional Grammar*. London: Arnold.

Hamerton, J., Giannelli, F., & Polani, P. (1965). Cytogenetics of Down's syndrome (mongolism) I. Data on consecutive series of patients referred for genetic counselling and diagnosis. *Cytogenetics*, **4**, 171–85.

Hodapp, R. & Dykens, E. (2004). Genetic and behavioural aspects: Application to maladaptive behaviour and cognition. In J. A. Rondal, R. Hodapp, S. Soresi, E. Dykens, & L. Nota, *Intellectual Disabilities. Genetics, Behaviour and Inclusion* (pp. 13–48). London: Whurr.

Jarrold, C. & Baddeley, A. (1997). Short-term memory for verbal and visuospatial information in Down's syndrome. *Cognitive Neuropsychiatry*, **2**, 101–22.

Jarrold, C., Baddeley, A., & Phillips, C. (1999). Down syndrome and the phonological loop: The evidence for an important verbal short-term memory deficit. *Down Syndrom Research and Practice*, **6**, 61–75.

Kaufman, A. & Kaufman, N. (1993). *Batterie pour l'Examen Psychologique de l'Enfant*. Paris: Editions du Centre de Psychologie Appliquée.

Layton, T. & Sharifi, H. (1979). Meaning and structure of Down's syndrome and nonretarded children spontaneous speech. *American Journal of Mental Deficiency*, **83**, 439–445.

Leifer, J. & Lewis (1984). Acquisition of conversational response skills by young Down syndrome and nonretarded young children. *American Journal of Mental Deficiency*, **88**, 610–8.

Lenneberg, E. (1967). *Biological Foundations of Language*. New York: Wiley.

Lenneberg, E., Nichols, L., & Rosenberger, E. (1964). Primitive stages of development in mongolism. In D. McRioch & A. Weinstein (Eds.), *Disorders of Communication* (pp. 119–137). Baltimore: Williams & Wilkins.

Mackenzie, S. & Hulme, C. (1987). Memory span development in Down'syndrome, severely subnormal and normal subjects. *Cognitive Neurospsychology*, **4**, 303–19.

Marcell, M. & Armstrong, V. (1982). Auditory and visual sequential memory of Down syndrome and nonretarded children. *American Journal of Mental Deficiency*, **87**, 86–95.

Marcell, M. & Weeks, S. (1988). Short-term memory difficulties and Down's syndrome. *Journal of Mental Deficiency Research*, **32**, 153–62.

Mayberry, R., Fisher, S., & Hatfield, N. (1983). Sentence repetition in American Sign Language. In J. Kyle & B. Woll (Eds.), *Language in Sign: International Perspective on Sign Language* (pp. 206–214). London: Croom Helm.

Menn, L. (1983). Development of articulatory, phonetic, and phonological capabilities. In B. Butterworth (Ed.), *Language Production* (Vol. 2, pp. 3–50). New York: Academic Press.

Mervis, C. (1987). Child-basic object categories and early lexical development. In U. Neisser (Ed.), *Concepts and Conceptual Development: Ecological and Intellectual Factors in Categorization* (pp. 201–33). Cambridge, UK: Cambridge University Press.

Mervis, C. & Becerra, A. (2003). Lexical development and intervention. In J. A. Rondal & S. Buckley (Eds.), *Speech and Language Intervention in Down Syndrome* (pp. 63–85). London: Whurr.

Mervis, C. & Bertrand, J. (1994). Acquisition of the novel name-nameless category principle. *Child Development*, **65**, 1646–62.

Mervis, C. & Bertrand, J. (1995). Acquisition of the novel name-nameless category principle by young children who have Down syndrome. *American Journal of Mental Retardation*, **100**, 231–43.

Montague, J., & Hollien, H. (1973). Perceived voice quality disorders in Down's syndrome children. Journal of Human Communication Disorders, **6**, 76–87.

Moss, S., Tomoeda, C., & Bayles, K. (2000). Comparison of the cognitive linguistic profiles of Down syndrome adults with and without dementia to individuals with Alzeimer's desease. *Journal of Medical Speech Language Pathology*, **8**, 69–81.

Mundy, P., Seibert, J., & Hogan, A. (1984). Relationship between sensorimotor and early communication abilities in developmentally delayed children. *Merill-Palmer Quarterly*, **30**, 33–48.

Newport, E. (1992). Contrasting conception of the critical period for language. In S. Carey & R. Gelman (Eds.), *The Epigenesis of Mind: Essays on Biology and Cognition* (pp. 11–130). Hillsdale, NJ: Erlbaum.

Owings, N., McManus, M., & Scherer, N. (1981). A deinstitutionalized retarded adult's use of communication functions in a natural setting, *British Journal of Disorders of Communication*, **16**, 119–23.

Ploog, D. (1984). Comment on J. Leiber's paper. In R. Harre & V. Reynolds (Eds.), *The Meaning of Primate Signals* (pp. 88). Cambridge, UK: Cambridge University Press.

Prasher, V. (1996). Age-associated functional decline in adults with Down's syndrome. *European Journal of Psychiatry*, **10**, 129–35.

Pueschel, S. (1995). Caracteristicas fisicas de las personas con syndrome de Down. In J. Perera (Ed.), *Especificidad en el sindrome de Down* (pp. 53–63). Barcelona: Masson.

Reilly, J., Klima, E., & Bellugi, U. (1991). Once more with feeling: Affect and language in atypical populations. *Development Psychopathology*, **2**, 367–91.

Ribes, R. & Sanny, J. (2000). Declive cognitivo en memoria y lenguaje: Indicadores del proceso de envejecimiento psicologico en la persona con sindrome de Down. *Revista Sindrome de Down*, **17**, 54–9.

Richards, B. W. (1969). Mosaic mongolism. *Journal of Intellectual Disability Research*, **13**, 66–83.

Rondal, J. A. (1975). Développement du langage et retard mental: Une revue critique de la littérature en langue anglaise. *L'Année Psychologique*, **75**, 513–47.

Rondal, J. A. (1978). Maternal speech to normal and Down's syndrome children matched for mean length of utterance. In E. Meyers (Ed.), *Quality of Life in Severely and Profoundly Mentally Retarded People: Research Foundations for Improvement* (pp. 193–265). Monograph Series n°3. Washington, DC: American Association on Mental Deficiency.

Rondal, J. A. (1984). Linguistic development in metal retardation. In J. Dobbing, A. D. B. Clarke, J. Corbett, J. Hog, & R. Robinson (Eds.), *Scientific Studies in Mental Retardation* (pp. 323–345). London: The Royal Society of Medicine and Macmillan.

Rondal, J. A. (1985). Adult-Child Interactions and the Process of Language Acquisition. New York: Praeger.

Rondal, J. A. (1995). *Exceptional Language Development in Down Syndrome*. New York: Cambridge University Press.

Rondal, J. A. (2003). Atypical language development in individual with mental retardation: Theoretical implications. In L. Abbeduto (Ed.), *Language and Communication in Mental Retardation. International Review of Research in Mental Retardation* (Vol. 27, pp. 281–308). New York: Academic Press.

Rondal, J. A. & Comblain, A. (1996). Language in adults with Down syndrome. *Down Syndrome Research and Practice*, **4**, 3–14.

Rondal, J. A. & Comblain, A. (2002). Language in ageing persons with Down syndrome. *Down Syndrome Research and Practice*, **8**(1), 1–19.

Rondal, J. A. & Edwards, S. (1997). *Language in mental retardation*. London: Whurr.

Rondal, J. A., Elbouz, M., Ylieff, M., & Docquier, L. (2003). Françoise, a fifteen-year follow up. *Down Syndrome Research and Practice*, **8**(3), 89–99.

Rondal, J. A. & Lambert, J. L. (1983). The speech of mentally retarded adults in a dyadic communication situation: Some formal and informative aspects. *Psychologica Belgica*, **23**, 49–56.

Rondal, J. A., Lambert, J. L., & Sohier, C. (1980). L'imitation verbale et non verbale chez l'enfant retardé mental mongolien et non mongolien. *Enfance*, **3**, 107–22.

Rondal, J. A., Thibaut, J. P., & Cession, A. (1990). Transitivity effects on children's sentence comprehension. *European Bulletin of Cognitive Psychology*, **10**, 385–400.

Rosch, E. (1978). Human categorization. In N. Warren (Ed.), *Advances in Cross-Cultural Psychology* (Vol. 1, pp. 122–48). Hillsdale, NJ: Erlbaum.

Rosenberg, S. & Abbeduto, L. (1993). *Language and Communication in Mental Retardation. Development, Processes, and Intervention*. Hillsdale, NJ: Erlbaum.

Rosin, M., Swift, E., & Bless, D. (1987, May). *Communication Profiles of People with Down's Syndrome*. Communication presented at the Annual Convention of the American Speech and Hearing Association, New Orleans.

Rosin, M., Swift, E., & Bless, D., & Vetter, D. (1988). Communication profiles of adolescents with Down's syndrome. *Journal of Childhood Communication Disorders*, **12**, 49–64.

Ryan, J. (1975). Mental subnormality and language development. In E. Lenneberg (Ed.), *Foundations of Language Development: A Multidisciplinary Approach* (Vol. 2, pp. 269–77). New York: Wiley.

Scherer, N. & Owings, N. (1984). Learning to be contingent: Retarded children's responses to their mothers' requests. *Language and Speech*, **27**, 255–67.

Smith, B. & Oller, K. (1981). A comparative study of pre-meaningful vocalizations produced by normally developing and Down's syndrome infants. *Journal of Speech and Hearing Disorders*, **46**, 46–51.

Smith, B. & Stoel-Gammon, C. (1983). A longitudinal study of the development of stop consonant production in normal and Down's syndrome children. *Journal of Speech and Hearing Disorders*, **48**, 114–8.

Spitzer, R., Rabinowitch, J., & Wybar, K. (1961). A study of the abnormalities of the skull, teeth and lenses in mongolism. *Canadian Medical Association Journal*, **82**, 567–72.

Stoel-Gammon, C. (2001). Down syndrome phonology: Developmental patterns and intervention strategies. *Down Syndrome Research and Practice*, **7**, 93–100.

Tager-Flusberg, H. (1986). Constraints on the representation of word meaning: Evidence from autistic and mentally retarded children. In S. Kuczaj & M. Barrett (Eds.), *The Development of Word Meaning* (pp. 69–81). New York: Springer.

Thordadottir, E., Chapman, R., & Wagner, L. (2002). Complex sentence production by adolescents with Down syndrome. *Applied Psycholinguistics*, **23**(2), 163–83.

Van Borsel, J. (1988). An analysis of the speech of five Down's syndrome adolescents. *Journal of Communication Disorders*, **21**, 409–22.

Van Borsel, J. (1993). *De articulatie bij adolescenten en volwassenen met het syndroom van Down*. Unpublished doctoral dissertation. Vrije Universiteit Brussels, Brussels.

Van Buggenhout, G., Lukusa, T., Trommelen, J., De Bal, C., Hamel, B., & Fryns, J.-P. (2001). Une étude pluri disciplinaire du syndrome de Down dans une population résidentielle d'arriérés mentaux d'âge avancé: Implications pour le suivi médical. *Journal de la Trisomie* 21(2), 7–13.

Wilson, B., Ivani-Chalian, R., & Aldrich, F. (1991). *The Child Rivermead Behavioural Memory Test*. San Antonio, TX: Thames Valley Test Company.

Zetlin, A. & Sabsay, S. (1980, Match).*Characteristics of verbal interaction among moderately retarded peers*. Paper presented at the Gatlinburg Conference on Research in Mental Retardation, Gatlinburg, TN.

7

Genetic disorders as models of mathematics learning disability: Fragile X and Turner syndromes

Melissa M. Murphy, Michèle M. M. Mazzocco, and Michael McCloskey

Neurodevelopmental disorders and mathematics learning disability

Poor math achievement is well documented in both children and adults with fragile X or Turner syndrome (Bennetto *et al.*, 2001; Brainard *et al.*, 1991; Grigsby *et al.*, 1990; Mazzocco, 1998, 2001; Rovet, 1993; Rovet *et al.*, 1994; Temple & Marriott, 1998). However, there is limited understanding of the cognitive mechanisms that contribute to these poor math outcomes. Specification of these underlying causes is the necessary next step in research on the cognitive phenotypes for these disorders (Mazzocco & McCloskey, 2005). Our efforts to understand the origins of mathematical cognition in fragile X and Turner syndromes are guided by existing knowledge in the field of mathematics learning disability (MLD). This body of research provides a conceptual framework for the contribution of different cognitive systems, such as executive function, visual–spatial, and language skills, to overall competence in mathematics (see Geary, 1993, 1994) as elaborated later in this chapter. Accordingly, the assessment of math ability in persons with fragile X or Turner syndrome is most informative when examined in the context of the overall cognitive phenotype, or the set of cognitive characteristics, associated with each disorder.

Although models of MLD are informative for understanding mathematical functioning in genetic conditions such as fragile X or Turner syndrome, the study of these syndromes may also inform the broader field of MLD research. In this chapter, we propose that fragile X and Turner syndromes provide models of the neurocognitive pathways that lead to MLD because these syndromes are associated with deficits in both math and related skills. For example, deficits in executive function associated with fragile X syndrome may be useful for illustrating the role

Melissa M. Murphy is now at the School of Education at the College of Notre Dame of Maryland, Baltimore, MD. Preparation of this chapter was supported, in part, by grant R01 HD34061 from the National Institute of Child Health and Human Development (NICHD) awarded to Dr. Mazzocco.

of working memory, attention, and inhibition in aspects of poor math performance, such as counting or arithmetic calculations. Similarly, efforts to understand
the link between visual–spatial deficits and poor math performance in Turner
syndrome may inform the extent to which visual–spatial skills contribute to
MLD. As models of pathways to MLD, these syndromes have the potential to
reveal the complexities inherent in attempting to differentiate the relationship
between math and each of the aforementioned cognitive systems. Toward this
end, we describe the profile of math and math-related skills among females with
fragile X or Turner syndrome focusing primarily on the relationship between math
and executive function/working memory, visual–spatial ability, and language skills.

When studying the cognitive features of any phenotype, it is necessary to address
the degree to which phenotype descriptions are specific to the syndrome in question. Recently, attention has been directed toward understanding the relationship
between math and related skills in Williams syndrome, which like fragile X and
Turner syndromes is associated with a specific genetic cause and a distinct cognitive
phenotype. Therefore, in exploring the complexity of the cognitive correlates of
MLD, we also briefly contrast the findings in our review with evidence from studies
of Williams syndrome to further explore individual syndrome models of pathways
to MLD. For the reader unfamiliar with fragile X, Turner, or Williams syndrome,
we provide an overview of each syndrome, below. Note, however, that the emphasis
of this chapter is on the first two of these three syndromes.

Syndrome overview

Fragile X syndrome

The prevalence of fragile X syndrome is approximately 1 in 4,000 to 1 in 9,000 live
births (Crawford *et al.*, 2001). It is caused by a single gene mutation on the long arm
of the X chromosome, which destabilizes the gene, thereby impeding production of
the associated protein called the Fragile X Mental Retardation Protein (FMRP,
Oostra, 1996). The presence of FMRP is integral for the maturation of synapses,
and for neuronal pruning (Greenough *et al.*, 2001) and is, therefore, critical for
optimal neural development.

Fragile X syndrome is associated with a variety of physical and behavioral characteristics, as reviewed elsewhere in detail (Cornish *et al.*, 2007; Chapter 1). Although it
is a leading genetic cause of intellectual disability, only about 50% of females meet
criteria for intellectual disability (Rousseau *et al.*, 1994), compared to almost all males
with the syndrome (Bailey *et al.*, 1998). (Note: This chapter uses the term *intellectual
disability* instead of the term *mental retardation* to reflect changes in nomenclature
within the field of developmental disabilities; see Scholock *et al.*, 2007.) The remaining

half of females with fragile X may present with cognitive impairments, including learning disabilities, or have no noticeable effects of the syndrome (Rousseau *et al.*, 1994). The variability in the degree to which males and females are affected by fragile X is, in part, due to the X-linked nature of the syndrome. In contrast with a male genotype that consists of one X-chromosome, all females have two X-chromosomes present in every cell in the body, only one of which is active (Lyon, 1972). Females with fragile X continue to produce FMRP in cells where the unaffected X remains activated, and so have more of this protein available relative to males, and in turn tend to be less affected than males (Hagerman, 1999).

The variability in cognitive impairments among females with fragile X affords the opportunity to investigate the subtle aspects of the fragile X cognitive phenotype. Toward that end, the work discussed in the present chapter focuses on females with fragile X without intellectual disability. In specific areas of cognitive performance, these females tend to be characterized by relative strengths in verbal memory (Jakala *et al.*, 1997) and limited aspects of visual perception, including the ability to identify missing parts of pictured concrete objects (Bennetto *et al.*, 2001) and to detect shapes in embedded designs (Mazzocco *et al.*, 2006). Areas of relative weaknesses include several aspects of executive function skills (e.g., Bennetto *et al.*, 2001; Mazzocco *et al.*, 1993), which are a set of deliberate, goal-oriented cognitive abilities, including working memory (Kwon *et al.*, 2001; Mazzocco *et al.*, 1993), inhibition, sustained attention, and controlled switching of attention (Cornish *et al.*, 2004). For additional information on the fragile X syndrome, see Cornish *et al.* (2007), Hagerman (2002), or Chapter 1.

Turner syndrome

The prevalence of Turner syndrome is approximately 1 in 2,000 to 1 in 5,000 live female births (Davenport *et al.*, 2007). It is caused by the partial or complete loss of one of the two X-chromosomes typically present in females. In the absence of two X-chromosomes, the ovaries fail to develop, consequently impairing the production of estrogen, a hormone associated with pubertal maturation.

Turner syndrome is associated with a variety of physical and behavioral characteristics, as reviewed elsewhere in greater detail (Rovet, 2004). Unlike fragile X, intellectual disability is not associated with the Turner syndrome phenotype; however, girls with Turner syndrome are at increased risk for learning disabilities, especially in mathematics (Rovet, 1993). Girls with Turner syndrome tend to have significantly higher verbal than performance IQs, despite having overall full scale IQs (FSIQ) in the low-average to average range (Mazzocco, 2001; Rovet, 1993; Rovet *et al.*, 1994; Tamm *et al.*, 2003; Temple & Carney, 1993; Waber, 1979). Similar to fragile X, there is a great deal of individual variability in the extent to which these physical, behavioral, and cognitive characteristics are present among females with Turner syndrome. For additional information, see Davenport and colleagues (2007).

Williams syndrome

The prevalence estimates for Williams syndrome vary from approximately 1 in 7,500 (Strømme, Bjørnstad, & Ramstad, 2002) to 1 in 20,000 to 1 in 50,000 (Greenough *et al.*, 2001; Martin *et al.*, 1984; Semel & Rosner, 2003) live births. The syndrome is caused by a deletion of genes on chromosome 7 (Ewart *et al.*, 1993) that disrupts the production of multiple genes, including one that codes for a kinase protein believed to play a role in brain development (Frangiskakis *et al.*, 1996; Tassabehji *et al.*, 1996). Williams syndrome is characterized, in part, by relative weakness in visual–spatial skills, and relative strength in language skills, such as expressive and receptive vocabulary (see Chapters 5 and 8). Unlike fragile X and Turner syndromes, Williams syndrome is not an X-chromosome linked syndrome. As a result, the effects of Williams syndrome are comparable across males and females, and typically include cognitive impairments consistent with the criteria for intellectual disability. See Mervis and Morris (2007) for additional information.

Framework for studying MLD

Understanding the causes of MLD is a challenging undertaking given the complexity of mathematics and the multiple pathways that can contribute to poor performance (Geary, 2004). Geary (1993, 2004) proposes a model for conceptualizing MLD that captures the complexity within the field of mathematics development and the possible contributions of cognitive competence. Within this model, mastery of a given mathematical domain is dependent on the conceptual and procedural knowledge required for individual domains, which Geary (2004) refers to as "supporting competencies" (p. 8). Inherent in the supporting competencies are cognitive processes that may influence the representation and manipulation of the information that underlies conceptual and procedural knowledge specific to mathematics (see Geary, 2004, for a review). According to Geary's model, although this conceptual and procedural knowledge itself is specific to mathematics, the supporting cognitive competencies are not themselves mathematical in nature. They represent more domain general abilities, such as working memory or verbal short-term memory. From this perspective, MLD may result from difficulty with a given mathematical domain (or domains) or one of several cognitive processes (e.g., working memory) that support development of that knowledge in that domain (Geary, 2004). For example, difficulty representing or manipulating visual–spatial information may lead to problems in aspects of math that rely on such information, including digit alignment when calculating or representing numbers on a mental number line (Mazzocco *et al.*, 2006). Similarly, computational errors may be related, in part, to difficulty maintaining or manipulating information in working memory (Geary *et al.*, 1991, 2007). Moreover, difficulty with spoken or written language comprehension may influence performance on aspects of math with considerable language components, such as story problems (Fuchs & Fuchs, 2002).

Based on evidence collected from studies of children with MLD in the general population, Geary (1993, 2004) proposes three preliminary subtypes of MLD: procedural, semantic memory, and visuo-spatial. The procedural subtype is characterized by difficulty in the use and application of strategies and procedures, such as reliance on developmentally immature strategies and errors in applying procedures, which may be related to problems maintaining and manipulating information in working memory, conceptual understanding of the procedure, or the ability to execute complex sequences of action. The semantic memory subtype is characterized by difficulty in the storage and retrieval of arithmetic information from memory, manifested in frequent errors and slow response times during math fact retrieval. Although representation and manipulation of linguistic information is implicated in this subtype, aspects of executive function, such as inhibition, are under investigation. For instance, difficulty with inhibition may lead to retrieving a solution that is a "near neighbor" in semantic memory to the target problem (e.g., retrieving $3 + 4 = 8$) or operand errors in multiplication (e.g., $4 \times 5 = 25$). The third subtype, visuo-spatial, addresses the role of visual–spatial deficits in math performance, but is the least explored of the three subtypes.

Studying the sources of poor math performance in fragile X and Turner syndromes can provide a means by which to test hypotheses concerning the pathways to MLD described by Geary (Geary, 1993, 2004). Both of these syndromes have well documented math difficulty and deficits in math-related skills, but also are distinguished from each other on the basis of performance on specific math skills, such as knowledge of counting principles (Murphy *et al.*, 2006) and the types of errors made during math calculations (Mazzocco, 1998). Moreover, differences between the syndromes are evident in areas that support the conceptual and procedural knowledge needed for mathematical competence, such as visual–spatial ability (Cornish *et al.*, 1998; Kwon *et al.*, 2001; Mazzocco *et al.*, 2006; Temple & Carney, 1995) and executive function skill, including working memory, processing speed, and response inhibition (Bennetto *et al.*, 2001; Kirk *et al.*, 2005; Romans *et al.*, 1997; Temple *et al.*, 1996). In the next section, we explore the nature of poor math performance in fragile X and Turner syndromes and the implications of syndrome similarities and differences in understanding the underlying causes of MLD.

Syndrome models of variation in pathways to MLD

There are several approaches to exploring MLD in fragile X and Turner syndromes. One approach is to examine the factors that contribute to variability in math and related characteristics among individuals within a given syndrome. For example, such an approach may focus on whether the level of FMRP in fragile X or estrogen in Turner syndrome accounts for individual differences in math performance among females with the respective syndrome. Another complementary approach is to examine performance relative to other syndromes or in comparison to groups of children without a given syndrome, for example, comparing females with fragile X to those with Turner syndrome, or to typically developing children. Although examining variability both within and across diagnostic groups is helpful for addressing questions regarding the nature of MLD, the present chapter focuses on the latter approach.

Sources of variability across groups

In order to examine variability across groups, the present chapter discusses findings from three types of comparisons. The first type considers the performance of girls with fragile X or Turner syndrome relative to children from the general population. Evaluating fragile X and Turner syndrome relative to the general population provides a benchmark for evaluating whether performance in either syndrome varies beyond what is expected of children of a given age or grade without a known syndrome. The second type of comparison is between fragile X or Turner syndrome and a subset of children from the general population who meet criteria for MLD. These comparisons address whether areas of challenge reflect overall difficulty with math or a profile that is specific to the syndrome. The third type of comparison is between fragile X and Turner syndromes. Such comparisons are helpful for determining whether the areas of strength or challenge in math and related skills are specific to a given syndrome, or are common across the syndromes.

If the profile of skills were common across syndromes, syndrome-based research would represent MLD as a relatively homogeneous construct, meaning that a common underlying deficit or deficits may be associated with MLD, at least in these syndromes. Were this the case, we might also expect that the performance profiles observed in syndrome groups would be comparable to profiles observed among children with MLD who do not have any known genetic disorder. If, on the other hand, the nature of mathematics difficulties is syndrome specific, syndrome-based research provides models of different cognitive pathways to MLD. Whether these cognitive pathway models generalize to other children with MLD depends on the extent to which MLD subtypes themselves represent more homogeneous populations. As indicated earlier in this chapter, subtypes of MLD have been proposed, but the construct validity of these subtypes has not yet received replicated empirical support. Syndrome-based research is one possible source of such support, if – as we argue herein – group differences indicate syndrome-specific profiles of MLD.

Variability among subtypes of MLD

When making comparisons across groups, it is important to recognize that all groups are characterized by individual variability in performance. For example, not all children with MLD have difficulty with the same items or sets of items on a math test, and the source of the difficulty may vary for each child. Individual variability is particularly noteworthy in the field of MLD, because presently no commonly agreed upon core deficits have been established. Lack of readily identifiable core deficits has contributed to the difficulty among researchers in establishing a consensus definition to use when diagnosing MLD. Consequently, children in the general population with MLD represent a heterogeneous group whose etiology and characteristics may vary as a function of the criteria used to define MLD (Barbaresi *et al.*, 2005; Butterworth, 2005; Murphy *et al.*, 2007). Moreover, the current subtypes or classifications for defining MLD may not fully depict the range of possible math outcomes. For example, it is unclear whether late emerging math difficulties reflect MLD or difficulty with higher order skills, such as those related to mastery of algebra or geometry. Similarly, factors such as the comorbidity of reading disability or attention problems (e.g., ADHD), which are beyond the scope of the present chapter, may contribute to the manifestation of MLD.

Phenotypic variability despite genetic homogeneity

Fragile X and Turner syndromes are also associated with individual variability in the degree to which the corresponding behavioral phenotype is manifested; however, unlike children with MLD, individuals with these syndromes share a known common etiology. Thus, as a group, children with fragile X or Turner syndrome who also have MLD may represent a less heterogeneous group than children with MLD from the general population. As such, efforts to identify the distinct pathways that contribute to MLD among children with similar etiologies of MLD may inform our understanding of the different cognitive pathways leading to MLD in the general population. For example, exploring the contribution of visual–spatial deficits associated with Turner syndrome to math performance may inform which aspects of math are related to visual–spatial skills, and the extent to which visual–spatial deficits contribute to poor math performance in the general population.

In summary, the following sections present fragile X and Turner syndromes as potential models of the contribution that general cognitive functions, such as working memory and visual–spatial ability, can make to math performance. We begin by addressing the prevalence and persistence of MLD in fragile X and Turner syndromes, followed by a review of the profile of math and related skills in each syndrome, and a discussion of these syndromes as models of the pathways to MLD.

Next, we address the complexity associated with studying the contributions of cognitive dysfunction to mathematics learning and achievement.

MLD in fragile X and Turner syndromes

Prevalence and persistence

Fragile X and Turner syndromes may provide useful models of MLD, but only to the extent that MLD is both a prevalent and persistent characteristic of the syndrome. Documenting the prevalence and persistence of MLD in fragile X and Turner syndrome is an important initial step toward characterizing MLD in these syndromes, as it establishes that children with these syndromes are at risk for developing poor math performance. Indeed, math difficulty is present in fragile X and Turner syndrome as early as kindergarten (Mazzocco, 2001), suggesting that girls with fragile X or Turner syndrome have difficulty early in their formal schooling and with basic concepts, such as adding sets of numbers. Furthermore, the incidence of MLD during the school years is higher among girls with fragile X or Turner syndrome than the 6–10% reported in the general population (Mazzocco & McCloskey, 2005; Murphy *et al.*, 2006; Rovet, 1993). For example, using a standardized measure of early formal and informal math skills, the Test of Early Mathematics Ability-Second Edition (TEMA-2), we found that 87% of the girls with fragile X and 79% of the girls with Turner syndrome scored below the 25th percentile during at least one of their primary school years (kindergarten to third grade). Even when matched on IQ, girls with fragile X or Turner syndrome are 2.5 and 4.3 times more likely than their peers to meet criteria for MLD, respectively (Mazzocco, 2001).

To determine whether the observed difficulty in math was limited to early primary school or whether poor performance persisted over time, we also examined rates of persistence in our groups. In the general population, the persistence of MLD may be an important feature in defining MLD (Geary, 2004; Geary *et al.*, 2007), as not all children who meet criteria for MLD at one point in time continue to do so at subsequent evaluations (Shalev *et al.*, 1998; Silver *et al.*, 1999). Of the girls with fragile X or Turner syndrome in our study who met criteria for MLD, more than three-quarters (77% and 84%, respectively) met criteria a second time during the primary school years. Although the rate of MLD persistence was not statistically different from the normative group, 70% of whom met criteria for MLD more than once, girls with either syndrome who had persistent MLD were more likely than their peers to perform below the 10th percentile in formal and informal math skills (Murphy *et al.*, 2006). Taken together, these results suggest that the majority of girls with fragile X or Turner syndrome will meet criteria for MLD during their early school years and that difficulty with math is not simply a transitory delay (Murphy *et al.*, 2006).

Fragile X syndrome
Math skills

Poor math performance in fragile X is documented primarily through the use of mathematics achievement tests (e.g., Bennetto *et al.*, 2001; Brainard *et al.*, 1991; Grigsby *et al.*, 1990; Hagerman *et al.*, 1992; Mazzocco, 1998, 2001). Although critical as a first step in documenting poor math performance, achievement test scores depict overall performance across a range of skill sets and fail to reflect specific difficulty within a given domain. Mazzocco (2001), for example, found that kindergarten girls with fragile X demonstrated lower performance relative to an age-, grade-, and IQ-matched comparison group on the KeyMath-Revised Numeration and Geometry subtests, which include items ascertaining number sense (e.g., counting) and items measuring spatial relationships and qualities, respectively. However, differences were not found between the fragile X and comparison group on the KeyMath-Revised Measurement subtest, which assesses understanding of standard and nonstandard units of measurement. Consequently, poor math performance in fragile X may not encompass all mathematical domains and is not simply a function of global impairments in cognitive ability.

In order to further explore the nature of math difficulty in fragile X, we (Murphy *et al.*, 2006) compared primary school-age girls with fragile X or Turner syndrome to children from a normative group, and to children from a normative group who met criteria for MLD on individual items from several standardized measures (see Table 1). Consistent with our predictions, girls with fragile X syndrome were as accurate as their peers at reading and writing numbers. Also, they did not differ from their peers on items measuring rote counting, such as counting aloud from 1 to 41, counting backward by 1's, or counting by 10's.

Girls with fragile X were distinguished from their peers on the basis of statistically and clinically significant differences on items measuring aspects of number sense and basic addition. Although there are multiple aspects of number sense, we found three to be especially challenging for girls with fragile X syndrome relative to their peers: magnitude judgments, mental number line judgments, and understanding of counting principles. For instance, when asked to judge which of two presented quantities was more than the other, girls with fragile X had difficulty relative to children in the normative group. Although this implicates difficulty with understanding cardinal numbers, the difficulty occurred regardless of whether the quantities were presented visually (with item sets) or verbally (with number words). Accuracy in making verbal magnitude judgments also distinguished girls with fragile X from girls with Turner syndrome. Although the difference was not statistically significant (using an adjusted alpha of 0.01), the majority of girls with Turner syndrome (78%) made accurate magnitude judgments, compared to only about half (48%) of the girls with fragile X. For both verbal and visual magnitude

Table 1. Summary of implicated strengths and challenges in math and related skills in fragile X and Turner syndromes[a]

	Fragile X		Turner syndrome	
	Strength[b]	Challenge[b]	Strength[b]	Challenge[b]
Math[c]				
Number sense	Reading/writing numbers[††]	Visual/verbal magnitude judgments[*]	Reading/writing numbers	
	Rote Counting[††]:	Mental number line judgments	Visual/verbal magnitude judgments	
	Forward by 1s	Counting 8 pictured items[*]	Mental number line judgments	
	Backward by 1s	Applied Counting:	Rote counting	
	Forward by 10s	1-to-1 correspondence[†]	Applied counting:	
	Next number in series	Number constancy	1-to-1 correspondence	
		Identifying Nth in set	Number constancy	
			Identifying Nth in set	
Arithmetic operations		Adding sets less than 10	Fact retrieval (Accuracy)	Fact retrieval (Speed)
			Calculation (Untimed)	Calculation (Timed)
				Procedural errors on arithmetic problems

Related Skills[d]

Executive Function		Alignment errors on arithmetic problems
Working memory	Performance declines as working memory demands increase	Lower efficiency due to elevated response times & difficulty switching within and between tasks
Processing speed	Limited changes in brain activation in response to increasing task difficulty	Slower response times on verbal, visual–spatial, ocular motor tasks
Visual–Spatial Ability	Visual perceptual ability	Visual perceptual ability
	Difficulty recalling object location in array	Difficulty recalling objects in array
Language	Difficulty with linguistically complex word problems[*],[**]	Difficulty recalling objects location in array

[a] Table highlights areas of known strength and challenge as well as areas where evidence regarding math and related skills is lacking.

[b] Based on comparisons to children with no known syndrome: [*] Indicates area of challenge relative to Turner syndrome; [**] Finding is preliminary; [†] Indicates area of challenge relative to MLD; [††] Performance exceeds MLD.

[c] Information is based on Murphy et al. (2006); Rovet et al., (1994); Temple & Marriott (1998).

[d] Information is based on Kirk et al. (2005); Mazzocco et al. (2006); Rivera et al. (2002).

judgments, girls with fragile X did not differ from children in the normative group with MLD, suggesting that their performance is comparable to that of children from the general population who have difficulty in math.

Mental number line judgments, which require selecting which of two numbers was closer to a target number (e.g., Is 4 or 11 closer to 9?), were also challenging for girls with fragile X relative to their peers. Less than half of girls with fragile X demonstrated mastery of this skill relative to almost two-thirds of children in the normative sample. Of note, however, is that the accuracy of girls with fragile X on mental line judgments did not distinguish them from girls with Turner syndrome or children with MLD, suggesting that this difficulty may characterize poor math performance generally rather than being specific to fragile X.

The third aspect of number sense that distinguished girls with fragile X from their peers was knowledge of counting principles. This difficulty stands in contrast to the relative strength in rote counting skills (discussed previously). Specifically, girls with fragile X had more difficulty counting eight pictured items than their peers in the normative group or with Turner syndrome. Also, relative to peers, fewer girls with fragile X passed items requiring the application of counting principles, such as number constancy (e.g., recognizing that the total number of objects in a set does not change if the objects are rearranged), one-to-one correspondence (e.g., under-standing that each object in a set receives only one number name), and understanding ordinal numbers (e.g., identifying the fifth position in an array). Consequently, applied counting is an area of relative difficulty in fragile X that may contribute to poor performance on other tasks, such as addition, at least during the early primary school years. Indeed, we also found that girls with fragile X are distinguished from their peers on basic addition problems, such as adding sets of numbers less than 10.

When counting skills among girls with fragile X were evaluated relative to children with MLD, differences also emerged. For example, written representation and rote counting skills among girls with fragile X exceeded those of the MLD group. However, girls with fragile X performed more poorly than children with MLD on one-to-one correspondence when counting. This difference is particularly notewor-thy given that our study included first graders in the fragile X group, making this group, on average, older than the MLD group from our normative study. Despite differences in one-to-one correspondence, overall knowledge of applied counting principles, such as number constancy, cardinality, and identifying the Nth position in an array, did not distinguish girls with fragile X from children with MLD.

Considered together, our findings (Murphy *et al.*, 2006) suggest that the profile of relative strength in rote counting coupled with relative weakness in applied counting distinguished girls with fragile X from other children with MLD, who performed relatively poorly on both types of counting skills. It also distinguished girls with fragile X from girls with Turner syndrome, who did not differ from their peers from the normative group as markedly on rote or applied counting. Note, however, that the extent to which difficulty with applied counting persists through the school years in fragile X is unclear. Some evidence suggests that aspects of number sense, as measured by the ability to judge the accuracy of two operand equations (e.g., 2 + 3 = 5), is consistent with age-level expectations by adolescence (Rivera *et al.*, 2002). One implication of these findings is that early group differences in the profile of relative strengths and weaknesses may lead to distinct pathways of math skill acquisition, such that the same outcome (poor math achievement) may reflect different causes and require different approaches to intervention.

Relationship between math and related skills

Although counting-related difficulty appears to be a hallmark of math performance in young girls with fragile X, the source of this difficulty is unclear. Aspects of poor math performance in fragile X, including difficulty with applied counting, may arise as a function of deficits in specific areas of visual–spatial ability that are reported among girls with fragile X (Bennetto *et al.*, 2001; Cornish *et al.*, 1998; Jakala *et al.*, 1997; Kwon *et al.*, 2001). Alternatively, such difficulties may be attributable to deficits in aspects of executive function, such as working memory (Bennetto *et al.*, 2001; Kirk *et al.*, 2005). The subsequent sections address the possible contributions of visual–spatial ability and working memory to math performance in fragile X syndrome. Table 1 provides a summary of the most relevant strengths and challenges in math related skills that are implicated in fragile X.

Visual–spatial ability

In our own work (Mazzocco *et al.*, 2006), we find that aspects of visual–spatial ability, including the ability to distinguish individual shapes within a design and to recall the location of shapes within an array, are related to accuracy at detecting correct and incorrect counting among girls with fragile X. Furthermore, accuracy in recalling the location of shapes within an array is negatively correlated to formal and informal math skills, such as magnitude judgments and knowledge of counting rules; and accuracy of judging spatial orientation, distinguishing individual shapes embedded within a design, and determining what an incomplete figure looks like when completed are related to calculation skills. These relationships are not simply a function of IQ, and they distinguish girls with fragile X from girls with Turner syndrome.

On the one hand, the observed correlations between math and visual–spatial ability in fragile X support the notion that visual–spatial ability makes a contribution to math performance in fragile X. However, on our item analysis, girls with fragile X had difficulty relative to their peers on only 2 of the 19 spatial items. Moreover, these two spatial items were also the initial items in their domain set.

Consequently, poor performance on these items may reflect executive function difficulties, such as orienting to a new task, rather than visual–spatial deficits per se (Murphy *et al.*, 2006). Consistent with this notion, more girls with fragile X passed items assessing visual rather than verbal magnitude judgments (discussed previously), suggesting an actual *advantage* for visually presented over verbally presented information in fragile X (Murphy *et al.*, 2006). Thus, although visual–spatial and math skills are related in fragile X, visual–spatial deficits alone may be insufficient to account for the observed difficulty with mathematics. These findings also illustrate the complexity of the construct of visual–spatial ability, which we discuss further in the following section on Turner syndrome.

Executive function/working memory skills
Counting requires keeping track of the number tags used, tracking the items to be counted (ranging from counting with fingers to counting the number of people who are moving about a room), and may require inhibition of distracters (counting the apples in a bowl of mixed fruit). Success on these tasks would seem to require intact executive function skills. Findings across several studies are consistent with the notion of executive dysfunction associated with fragile X, including working memory deficits (Bennetto *et al.*, 2001; Kirk *et al.*, 2005; Kwon *et al.*, 2001; Tamm *et al.*, 2002). However, the precise contribution of executive function deficits to poor math performance in fragile X is unclear.

One way in which executive function deficits may influence performance is by limiting the ability to hold and manipulate information in working memory, an ability necessary for performing mathematics calculations or problem solving (Geary *et al.*, 2007). For example, Kwon and colleagues (2001) found that increasing the working memory load of a visual–spatial task resulted in decreased performance accuracy among girls with fragile X. In response to added task difficulty, females in the comparison group showed increases in brain activation; however, corresponding changes in brain activation were not observed among females with fragile X, suggesting that they do not or cannot regulate brain activation in response to increased working memory demands (Kwon *et al.*, 2001). Brain activation levels were correlated with performance accuracy in the comparison group, but not among females with fragile X. Indeed, there was an inverse correlation between brain activation and response time, but only when working memory load was increased, and only among females with fragile X. Thus, it is hardly the case that females with fragile X are simply "shutting down" or lacking in motivation to complete the more difficult task, despite behavioral indicators to the contrary. Consistent with this notion, Kirk and colleagues (2005) found that females with fragile X had relatively unchanged response times on a two-attribute naming task compared to a one-attribute naming task, a pattern that was opposite the response time increase observed in the comparison group.

How do these findings generalize to the challenges posed by mathematics? Rivera and colleagues (2002) report a similar pattern of findings among females with fragile X during a number-processing task. When asked to verify the accuracy of equations involving two or three operands (e.g., $2 + 3 = 5$, $2 + 3 - 4 = 1$), females with fragile X (ages 10 to 24 years) were as accurate as their peers when the equations involved two, but not three, operands. Poor performance on the three operand task in the group with fragile X coincided with a lack of increase in the level of brain activation between the two- and three-operand task, which the authors attributed to difficulty recruiting additional resources as task demands increase.

Identifying the effects of working memory demands is one step closer to uncovering potential cognitive correlates of poor math performance in females with fragile X. It would be an oversimplification to infer that females with fragile X cannot engage in working memory tasks, but these findings suggest that the threshold for working memory loads is lower in this group than in the general population.

Although the precise neural mechanisms are unclear, the behavioral results of both the Rivera and Kwon studies suggest a relationship between working memory demands and performance that may be specific to fragile X (see Table 1). Indeed both studies report a correlation between levels of FMRP protein and brain activation when working memory demands are high. Of note, however, is that in neither study were participants matched on IQ; and although IQ was used as a covariate, the range of IQ between the fragile X and comparison groups was widely disparate. Consequently, it is unclear whether the lack of activation in the group with fragile X is attributable to fragile X or to overall lower cognitive ability.

Moreover, the relationship between levels of brain activation and overall cognitive ability must be investigated if we are to address the specificity of fragile X in accounting for these difficulties. Indeed, we (Kirk et al., 2005) found that both a fragile X and an IQ-matched comparison group had considerable difficulty completing a task when the working memory demands were high compared to when they were low or moderate, consistent with the notion that FSIQ and working memory skills are correlated (as reviewed by Blair et al., 2005). However, there are limitations to this IQ/working memory correlation, suggesting that the two constructs represent distinct skills (Blair et al., 2005). This, too, is further exemplified by our findings that group differences in working memory, between the fragile X and comparison groups, persisted despite the relatively low IQs in both groups, particularly when working memory demands were moderate. On this moderately difficult task, the girls with fragile X made more errors than girls in their IQ-matched comparison group. Consequently, our findings suggest that working memory limitations in females with fragile X cannot be attributed solely to low FSIQ (Kirk *et al.*, 2005). We also conclude that working memory limitations are not linked to verbal memory span, based on recent evidence that 10-year-old girls with fragile X had digit spans comparable to those of IQ-matched peers, despite less efficient working memory performance among the former (Murphy & Mazzocco, in press).

Our recent longitudinal study examined math and working memory skills of girls with or without fragile X, from grades 1 to 7 (Murphy & Mazzocco, in press). We found that girls with fragile X and their grade- and IQ-matched peers both made gains in working memory efficiency over time. However, girls with fragile X demonstrated a slower growth rate and a lower threshold for the working memory load at which their performance efficiency was optimized. This difference in working memory threshold persisted at all grade levels examined. Working memory performance predicted both the level of math achievement attained and the rate of growth in math achievement. Thus, working memory limitations that are specific, in their severity, to fragile X may partly explain the pattern of mathematical abilities and disabilities in this group.

Turner syndrome
Math skills

Similar to girls with fragile X, girls with Turner syndrome, as a group, perform more poorly on measures of mathematics achievement than their peers (McCauley *et al.*, 1987; Molko *et al.*, 2003; Rovet, 1993; Rovet *et al.*, 1994). However, unlike fragile X, poor performance in Turner syndrome girls does not appear to be a function of a difficulty in number sense (Bruandet *et al.*, 2004; Murphy *et al.*, 2006; Rovet *et al.*, 1994; Temple & Marriott, 1998). Table 1 provides a summary of the relative strengths and challenges in specific aspects of mathematics performance implicated in Turner syndrome. Among adults and children with Turner syndrome, simple arithmetic, number comprehension and production, counting, and some aspects of understanding quantity (such as number comparison and estimation) represent areas of relative strength compared to other areas of mathematics (Bruandet *et al.*, 2004; Mazzocco, 2001; Murphy *et al.*, 2006; Temple & Marriott, 1998). We (Murphy *et al.*, 2006) found that girls with Turner syndrome in early primary school did not differ from their peers on individual items from the KeyMath-Revised Numeration subtest, or other items measuring basic number sense skills, such as rote and applied counting skills.

We also failed to find significant differences between girls with Turner syndrome and their peers on individual math items with strong visual–spatial components, such as items from KeyMath-Revised Geometry and Measurement subtests, and items measuring visual magnitude or mental number line judgments

(Murphy *et al.*, 2006). Of note, however, is that a lack of significant findings in areas of number sense and visual–spatial aspects of math may reflect the complexity of math, number sense, or visual–spatial ability rather than age or grade appropriate mastery of either area. Indeed, math, number sense, and visual–spatial ability do not represent unitary skills or sets of skills, rather each is a complex and multi-faceted construct (Berch, 2005; Geary, 1993, 2005; Temple & Carney, 1995).

Despite a consistent lack of differences between girls with Turner syndrome and their peers on aspects of number sense and math items with visual–spatial components, persons with Turner syndrome are distinguished from their peers in areas such as speed of arithmetic fact retrieval and response times on calculations (Bruandet *et al.*, 2004; Molko *et al.*, 2003; Rovet *et al.*, 1994). Response times among girls with Turner syndrome are especially long when the amount being added is large, for example adding 7 to a number vs. adding 2 (Molko *et al.*, 2003; Temple & Marriott, 1998). However, slower response times do not necessarily result in less accurate answers (Rovet *et al.*, 1994; Temple & Marriott, 1998). Slow fact retrieval may be accounted for in part by a general impairment in processing speed or by reliance on alternative strategies (e.g., finger counting) that require more time to execute than retrieval. These explanations are discussed in more detail later.

Another area that distinguishes math performance by girls with Turner syndrome vs. that of their peers is relatively weak multi-digit calculation skills. Such skills are characterized by frequent procedural errors, including neglecting to apply a procedure, such as carrying, use of an incorrect operation, or incomplete application of a procedure (e.g., Rovet *et al.*, 1994; Temple & Marriott, 1998). Rovet and colleagues (1994), for example, found that girls with Turner syndrome completed fewer items and had less adequate procedural knowledge of addition and division than age-, grade-, and verbal IQ-matched peers. In part, difficulty with calculation may be attributable to slow fact retrieval or working memory (discussed subsequently). Indeed, impairments in working memory are linked to poor math performance in children with MLD (Geary *et al.*, 2007; McLean & Hitch, 1999) and include increased reliance on counting strategies rather than retrieval, and high rates of procedural errors (Geary, 2004).

Relationship between math and related skills

Visual–spatial ability

Girls with Turner syndrome have overall poor math performance, as well as significantly lower performance on visual–perceptual and visual–motor tasks relative to their age- and grade-matched peers (Mazzocco, 2001; Rovet & Netley, 1982; Temple & Carney, 1995). See Table 1 for a summary of implicated strengths and challenges in math-related skills in Turner syndrome. As a result, visual–spatial deficits are suggested as a potential source of poor math performance in Turner syndrome (Mazzocco, 1998; Rovet, 1993). Indeed, girls with Turner syndrome are distinguished from their peers with fragile X or typical development on the basis of alignment errors made during written calculation (Mazzocco, 1998).

Despite preliminary and theoretical evidence to support a relationship between math and visual–spatial ability, lack of a consistent relationship between visual-spatial processing and procedural knowledge or math fact retrieval has led to the suggestion that poor math performance in Turner syndrome is independent of visual–spatial abilities per se (Rovet *et al.*, 1994; Temple & Marriott, 1998). Our failure to find significant differences between girls with Turner syndrome and their peers on math items with strong visual–spatial components is consistent with this notion (see Table 1). Moreover, even though performance is poor in both math and visual–spatial skills, we do not find consistent correlations between the two areas in Turner syndrome (Mazzocco *et al.*, 2006). For example, among girls with Turner syndrome, only one significant correlation emerged between math and visual-spatial ability: the ability to detect counting accuracy was correlated with accuracy at identifying shapes by spatial position and recognizing shapes embedded within a design. Although this correlation may indicate visual–spatial aspects of number, it may also reflect working memory skills associated with counting and not visual-spatial ability per se (Mazzocco *et al.*, 2006). As such, limited empirical evidence is available to support a direct relationship between poor math performance and visual–spatial ability in Turner syndrome, at least during the early school years. These findings are consistent with those for spina bifida (Barnes *et al.*, 2006; and Chapter 3), a disorder also associated with both MLD and visual–spatial deficits.

In interpreting the null findings, it is noteworthy that mathematics and visual-spatial abilities are both complex, multi-faceted constructs and that significant findings may emerge if specific aspects of math or spatial skills are assessed. Moreover, despite overlap in the proposed neuroanatomical pathways for math and visual–spatial skills, the precise pathways to be recruited during a task may vary, depending on the nature of the task. Many studies of the association between these constructs in Turner syndrome have focused on broadly defined visual-spatial or mathematics components, rather than specific aspects of spatial or mathematical ability. An exception is the work of Bruandet and colleagues (2004), which was based on Dehaene's triple code model of number processing (as reviewed by Dehaene *et al.*, 2005). This model posits the following three distinct neuroanatomical pathways: (1) a visual, Arabic number code that is involved in operations and calculations; (2) an auditory/verbal code that is involved in number or fact retrieval; and (3) a nonverbal quantity code relying on magnitude representation. The third of these pathways is thought to be most involved in both spatial skills and attention.

In the Bruandet *et al.* (2004) study, women with Turner syndrome had longer response times to identify quantities for large and small item sets, including sets of two, implicating deficiencies in the nonverbal quantity code. Although this code is believed to recruit visual–spatial related processes, there are other aspects of visual–spatial ability that are related to mathematics that are not deficient in persons with Turner syndrome. Of note is that the participants in Bruandet's study were adults, whereas the aforementioned studies involved children. Perhaps a more pronounced profile of spatially associated mathematics deficits emerges with age. On the one hand, the notion of a later-emerging spatial association with math is counter to the notion that early strategies (e.g., counting, comparing quantities when judging whether 9 or 7 is larger) are more heavily influenced by visual–spatial skills than are the more mature strategies that appear later (e.g., recall of math facts, comprehension of basic underlying principles). However, at present, information regarding the trajectory of math performance and strategy use among girls with Turner syndrome is limited. Furthermore, the nature of the math difficulty and its relationship to visual–spatial skills may change as new concepts, such as algebra and geometry, are introduced in later grades.

Executive function/working memory skills

Deficits in aspects of executive function, such as processing speed and working memory, have also been documented in Turner syndrome (see Table 1). However, similar to visual–spatial ability, executive function is a multifaceted construct rather than a unitary skill or set of skills. In the following section, we focus on processing speed and working memory, because these areas are implicated in poor math performance, especially fact retrieval and calculation deficits.

Processing deficits in Turner syndrome are documented for verbal processing tasks, such as rapid automatized naming (Mazzocco, 2001; Temple *et al.*, 1996); visuo-spatial processing tasks, such as mental rotation (Rovet & Netley, 1982); and in very basic behaviors such as involuntary eye movements (Lasker *et al.*, 2007), suggesting widespread impairments in processing speed. These deficits may contribute to poor math performance among girls with Turner syndrome relative to peers, especially in the area of fact retrieval. For example, slow processing speed may increase the amount of time needed to retrieve arithmetic facts from memory, which, in turn, may affect mastery of more complex mathematical concepts and problems, such as multidigit calculations. Of note, however, is that slow retrieval is associated with some, but not all arithmetic operations (Temple & Marriott, 1998), which is inconsistent with global processing deficits, at least with respect to arithmetic information.

Alternatively, rather than processing speed deficits per se, females with Turner syndrome may have a greater reliance on alternative strategies (e.g., finger counting) that require more time to execute than retrieval, and thereby lead to longer response times. Consistent with this notion, is the previously mentioned finding of Bruandet and colleagues (2004) that women with Turner syndrome take longer than their peers to identify quantities of two or more. Typically, small quantities from one to three can be rapidly identified without counting (a skill also referred to as subitizing). Thus, longer response times for identifying small quantities suggest that women with Turner syndrome may have a lower threshold than their peers for initiating counting, leading them to rely more heavily on alternative strategy use (such as direct counting of small item sets) than automatic retrieval (Bruandet *et al.*, 2004). In support of this possibility, patterns of brain activation observed among women with Turner syndrome relative to their peers suggest that women with Turner syndrome arrive at their responses on exact calculation problems by using a compensatory strategy rather than direct retrieval (Molko *et al.*, 2003). This strategy is fairly effective when the numbers being calculated are small, but is ineffective with large numbers, which may contribute to an apparent processing deficit on calculations (Molko *et al.*, 2003).

Although findings from behavioral and neuroimaging studies converge on slower response times among females with Turner syndrome, the extent to which slow processing, alternative strategy use, or some combination of the two best characterizes the performance deficits observed in Turner syndrome remains unclear. It is possible that the slower processing time leads to a reliance on external support, which in turn adds further to the response time. Longer latencies on relatively automatic tasks, such as rapid automatized naming (Mazzocco, 2001), oral fluency (Temple, 2002), and ocular motor behavior (Lasker *et al.*, 2007), do implicate a primary (but not necessarily exclusive) role of processing speed in poor math performance by females with Turner syndrome.

Several studies suggest that deficits in working memory and processing speed may contribute to the observed difficulties with calculation and to other areas of poor math performance in Turner syndrome (Buchanan *et al.*, 1998; Kirk *et al.*, 2005; Temple *et al.*, 1996). For example, in a study of 8- to 9-year-olds, we (Kirk *et al.*, 2005) found that girls with Turner syndrome were distinguished from IQ-matched peers by less efficient performance on both naming and working memory subtests of an executive function measure. On the naming subtest, girls with Turner syndrome took longer than their peers to complete the test, but were just as accurate. In contrast, when modest working memory demands were added, efficiency remained lower in the Turner syndrome group relative to peers, but both longer response time and lower accuracy contributed to the poor efficiency. Finally, when working memory demands were further increased, girls with Turner syndrome had lower efficiency relative to their peers, but this was attributable to more errors, not longer response times. Overall, the results across subtests suggest that both slow response time and difficulty changing responses within and between tasks contribute to the observed group differences on this measure. As such, in Turner syndrome, processing deficits, including accuracy of retrieval, may be altered when working memory demands are high (Kirk *et al.*, 2005).

Fragile X and Turner syndromes as models of the pathways to MLD

Comparisons between fragile X and Turner syndromes are also informative for understanding the nature of poor math performance, and the viability of these syndromes as models of existing MLD subtypes. Although few studies make direct comparisons between fragile X and Turner syndromes, the studies that do so suggest both similarities and differences in math and related skills (see Table 1).

Math skills

Our item analysis (Murphy *et al.*, 2006), indicated minimal syndrome differences in formal and informal math skills, except in the area of counting skills. More girls with Turner syndrome than with fragile X were correctly able to count eight pictured objects. Furthermore, girls with Turner syndrome demonstrated overall better mastery of counting rules, such as number constancy and cardinality, than girls with fragile X. No differences were found for rote counting, written representation, enumeration, or applied counting, such as identifying the fifth position in an array.

Lack of pronounced differences between fragile X and Turner syndrome may be due to our focus on children in early primary school. Indeed, the extent to which similarities and differences are maintained over the school years is unclear. For example, among girls 5–16 years of age, Mazzocco (1998) found that girls with Turner syndrome or fragile X were distinguished based on number and type of errors on calculation problems, number of unfamiliar problems attempted, and the cognitive skills that predicted performance. Also, among 7- to 12-year-old girls, girls with fragile X had more difficulty than girls with Turner syndrome at identifying correct and incorrect counting (Mazzocco *et al.*, 2006). Thus, there is some evidence to support a divergence in the profile of math skills between girls with fragile X or Turner syndrome over the school years.

Relationship between math and related skills

Along with documenting differences between fragile X and Turner syndrome in math, we have found that aspects of visual–spatial ability and executive function distinguish these two syndrome groups from each other and from their peers (see Table 1, Kirk *et al.*, 2005; Mazzocco *et al.*, 2006). For example, performance of girls with Turner syndrome is characterized by widespread deficits in visual perceptual ability, including difficulty recalling objects and their location in an array, and slower response times relative to peers; where as girls with fragile X have difficulty recalling the location of objects, but not the objects themselves relative to peers (Mazzocco *et al.*, 2006). As discussed previously, multiple correlations were observed between math performance and visual–spatial ability in fragile X, but only one such correlation between math and visual–spatial ability was observed among girls with Turner syndrome. These findings suggest important differences in the areas of visual–spatial ability that are challenging for girls with fragile X or Turner syndrome, and differences between syndromes in the relationship between visual–spatial ability and math.

Furthermore, behavioral data implicate different executive function difficulties in fragile X vs. Turner syndrome. We compared the eye movement behavior of girls with fragile X or Turner syndrome on a series of voluntary eye movement tasks, including memory-guided saccades that involve looking at a remembered location (Lasker *et al.*, 2007). These tasks are believed to reflect the function of the frontal eye field and dorsomedial prefrontal cortex, regions also linked to executive dysfunction. Females with either syndrome were slower and less accurate, relative to a comparison group, on voluntary eye movement tasks. However, effect sizes for the increase in response time (latency) relative to the comparison group were larger for the Turner syndrome group than for the fragile X group. Moreover, only the Turner syndrome group had significantly longer response times than females in either the fragile X or comparison groups on the involuntary eye movement task (which required looking at a target as soon as it appeared), implicating deficits in posterior parietal cortex function. Although these findings do not directly implicate poor math performance, they do point to differences in the neuropsychological pathways that may interfere with math performance.

Taken together, the profile of math-related skills associated with fragile X and Turner syndrome distinguishes these groups from each other and from their peers. As such, exploring these cognitive correlates and their relation to math performance in genetic syndromes can contribute to understanding MLD. One way in which syndromes can inform MLD is as models for examining possible subtypes of MLD and the corresponding mechanisms that contribute to poor math performance. For example, examining the relationship between specific visual–spatial deficits and math performance may inform the contribution of visual–spatial skills to math outcomes, thereby helping to determine the validity of the proposed visual–spatial subtype of MLD (Geary, 1993).

Alternatively, these syndrome models may exemplify how different domains of cognitive dysfunction influence mathematics learning and achievement regardless of whether difficulty in a specific area, such as visual–spatial ability, contributes to a "subtype" of MLD (Mazzocco & McCloskey, 2005). For example, poor performance on math calculation problems in Turner syndrome may be influenced by a number of factors, including the ability to manipulate information in working memory, difficulty with fact retrieval (which may be related to processing speed or reliance on alternative strategies), visual–spatial deficits that lead to improper problem alignment, or incomplete mastery of the procedures for calculating. In the following section, we explore the complexity of the associations between math and the cognitive correlates of MLD, such as visual–spatial ability, executive function, and language ability.

Exploring the complexity of cognitive correlates of MLD

One of the challenges associated with establishing pathways to MLD, and with assessing the potential role of cognitive correlates of MLD, is the complexity of mathematics and the cognitive correlates themselves (see Figure 1). For example, working memory, attention, inhibition, and processing speed, may act separately or together to influence math outcomes. Similarly, visual–spatial ability at a broad level encompasses multiple skills, such as visual processing, visual perception, visual construction, and spatial memory – each of which is composed of distinct or overlapping functions. These cognitive correlates may act directly to influence math performance; for example, poor visual perception is related to alignment errors on calculation problems in Turner syndrome (Mazzocco, 1998). These cognitive correlates may also act on math performance indirectly by influencing the acquisition and application of specific math skills, such as counting. For example, poor counting accuracy may reflect difficulty with counting or difficulty keeping track of the objects to be counted, which may reflect visual–spatial or working memory deficits. Although deficits in cognitive correlates, such as executive function and visual–spatial ability, are implicated in fragile X (Bennetto *et al.*, 2001; Cornish *et al.*, 1998; Kirk *et al.*, 2005; Kwon *et al.*, 2001) and Turner syndrome (Buchanan *et al.*, 1998; Romans *et al.*, 1997; Tamm *et al.*, 2003; Temple & Carney, 1995; Temple *et al.*, 1996), a necessary next step is to disentangle the relative contribution of each to math performance (Mazzocco & McCloskey, 2005).

The role of working memory ability in mathematics has received the most attention, both within fragile X and Turner syndrome (see Mazzocco & McCloskey, 2005, for a brief review), as well as in studies of MLD in the general population (e.g., Bull & Johnston, 1997; Geary *et al.*, 1991, 2004; Passolunghi & Siegel, 2004). However, deficits in working memory may be further compounded by deficits in other areas. For example, because of slow processing speed, the efforts to retrieve an answer may exhaust limited working memory resources available for problem solving, in essence taxing an already overloaded system (as reviewed by Geary *et al.*, 2007). As discussed previously, evidence of deficits in both processing

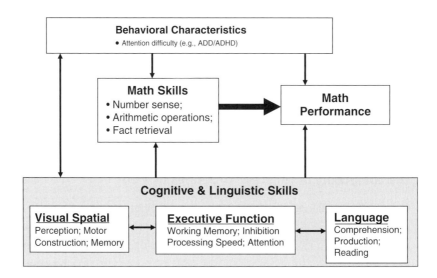

Figure 1.   Conceptual framework for evaluating the contribution of cognitive and behavioral correlates to mathematics learning disability (MLD) in fragile X and Turner syndromes. Note: given the complexity of each domain and the reciprocal relationships among domains, this figure is intended to broadly focus on the domains and relationships most relevant to the present discussion. This figure is not intended to be all-inclusive, as there are additional areas – such as attention or anxiety – that could influence and be influenced by these domains.

speed and working memory may contribute to the procedural errors observed among girls with Turner syndrome.

Along with studies of working memory, studies on spatial skills and language skills in fragile X, Turner syndrome, and MLD in the general population are ongoing. As discussed previously, a clear association has not been found between the visual–spatial and math deficits observed among girls with Turner syndrome, at least during the early school years. In part, lack of significant findings may be due to the complexity of the relationship between math and visual–spatial skills, or other factors, such as participant age and experimental design. Consequently, efforts to understand the relationship between visual–spatial ability and math in Turner syndrome and MLD in general may be augmented by focusing on neurodevelopmental disorders, such as Williams syndrome (discussed subsequently and see Chapter 8) and spina bifida (see Chapter 3), that are also associated with deficits in both math and visual–spatial ability.

Math and Williams syndrome

Among individuals with Williams syndrome, overall math performance is consistent with cognitive-level expectations (O'Hearn & Landau, 2007). Despite this overall consistency, a profile of strengths and challenges on specific math skills is evident relative to cognitive-level expectations. For example, O'Hearn & Landau (2007) found that adults with Williams syndrome were as good or better than a cognitive-level-matched comparison group on rote counting, visual and verbal magnitude judgments, number constancy, and reading and writing numbers. In contrast, individuals with Williams syndrome have difficulty with certain numerical tasks (e.g., understanding the cardinality principle; Ansari *et al.*, 2003; O'Hearn & Landau, 2007), a lower threshold for initiating counting when presented with small quantities (O'Hearn *et al.*, 2005), and impairments in visual estimation skills (Ansari *et al.*, 2007). Moreover, this difficulty with select aspects of math performance is concurrent with visual–spatial deficits.

One specific area that distinguishes individuals with Williams syndrome from cognitive-level-matched peers is accuracy at mental number line judgments, such as determining which of two numbers (e.g., 4 or 7) is closer to a target number (e.g., 6, O'Hearn & Landau, 2007). In part, difficulty with number line judgments may be related to visual–spatial deficits in Williams syndrome (O'Hearn & Landau, 2007), as the representation of numbers along a mental number line is thought to be influenced by spatial representation of quantity (see Fais & Fischer, 2005, for a review). However, a relationship between visual–spatial ability and math is not apparent in all areas. For example, Ansari and colleagues (2003) found that deficits in cardinality observed in children with Williams syndrome were correlated with language ability, whereas cardinality performance in the mental-age-matched comparison group was correlated with visual–spatial ability.

Consistent with the notion of a relationship between visual–spatial ability and math performance in Williams syndrome, O'Hearn *et al.* (2005) report that adults with Williams syndrome have a lower threshold than a cognitive-level-matched comparison group for initiating counting of small sets of numbers. This difficulty was related to the ability to visually track multiple objects, but not memory for fixed visual information. In contrast, Ansari and colleagues (2007) report that individuals with Williams syndrome did not differ from mental-age-matched peers on subitizing (i.e., rapidly identifying small quantities without counting), but do have more difficulty estimating quantities less than 12 when presented visually. Likewise, math performance among third graders with fragile X was significantly correlated with several (but not all) aspects of visual–spatial ability, including judgment of spatial orientation and the ability to determine what an incomplete figure would look like if completed, but not among girls with Turner syndrome (Mazzocco *et al.*, 2006). These findings are a mere hint of the complexities that underlie cognitive correlates of mathematics ability, yet they serve to illustrate the potential models of MLD to emerge from syndrome groups.

Math and Language

Just as spatial aspects of mathematics are not limited to problems in geometry, language aspects of mathematics may not be limited to word problems. A complete overview of the language–mathematics interplay is beyond the scope of this chapter (but see, Donlan, 2007). We briefly touch upon this topic to exemplify the potential importance of language in math.

To explore the relationship between language and math in fragile X and Turner syndromes, we examined the likelihood that girls with either syndrome were more likely to have difficulty with single-digit calculations when embedded within a complex word problem, a simple word problem, or a numeric equation. Overall, few differences emerged. However, girls with fragile X were more likely to have difficulty when the word problem was linguistically complex than when the same calculation was presented using simple language. In contrast, girls with Turner syndrome overall were not differentially influenced by word or numeric problems. Although preliminary, these results suggest a possible relationship between one aspect of language and math, at least in fragile X. It is noteworthy, however, that this relationship may be influenced by a variety of factors, including the ability to understand relative terms used in the problem (e.g., *greater than*, *some*, or *many*), the memory demands of the problem (e.g., whether the text of the problem is available while solving), the ability to track the multiple pieces of information presented in the problem, or the ability to focus on the critical elements of the problem. These factors may involve cognitive processes, such as working memory and processing speed, along with overall language ability.

Moreover, language, like executive function and visual–spatial ability, is a complex and multifaceted construct. Aspects of language include the knowledge of words and their meaning (semantic skills), an understanding of the rules for combining words to form phrases and sentences (syntactic skills), and the ability to use language to achieve goals (pragmatic skills). Efforts to understand the relative contribution of language to mathematics may benefit from focusing on fragile X, Turner, and other syndromes, such as Williams syndrome and Down syndrome, the latter of the two being a genetic syndrome associated with deficits in expressive language relative to cognitive ability (Chapman *et al.*, 1991). Both language ability and the nature of the visual–spatial deficits distinguish Williams and Down syndromes from each other (Bellugi *et al.*, 2000). Moreover, aspects of language also distinguish Down syndrome and fragile X from each other (Abbeduto & Murphy, 2004). Although the extent to which Williams and Down syndromes are associated with similar areas of math difficulty is unclear, cross-syndrome comparisons may be instrumental in clarifying the relationship between mathematical performance, language, cognitive ability, and specific cognitive processes, such as visual–spatial ability.

Conclusion

This chapter reviews the profile of math and math-related skills in fragile X and Turner syndrome, and suggests these syndromes as possible models for pathways leading to MLD. Although we have begun to explore the cognitive factors that contribute to math difficulty in these syndromes, empirically driven work is needed (Mazzocco & McCloskey, 2005; Dennis, Berch, & Mazzocco, 2009) and is under way. Continued efforts to examine the contributions of executive function, visual–spatial, and language ability to mathematics performance in these and other genetic syndromes will provide a means by which to evaluate current conceptualizations of MLD, thereby strengthening our understanding of the origins of poor math performance and subsequent routes for remediation.

REFERENCES

Abbeduto, L. & Murphy, M. M. (2004). Language, social cognition, maladaptive behavior, and communication in Down syndrome and fragile X syndrome. In M. Rice & S. Warren (Eds.), *Developmental Language Disorders: From Phenotypes to Etiologies* (pp. 77–97). Mahwah, NJ: Lawrence Erlbaum Associates.

Ansari, D., Donlan, C., & Karmiloff-Smith, A. (2007). Atypical and typical development of visual estimation abilities. *Cortex: Special Issue on Selective Developmental Disorders*, **6**, 758–68.

Ansari, D., Donlan, C., Thomas, M. S., Ewing, S. A., Peen, T., & Karmiloff-Smith, A. (2003). What makes counting count? Verbal and visuo-spatial contributions to typical and atypical number development. *Journal of Experimental Child Psychology*, **85**, 50–62.

Bailey, D. B., Jr., Hatton, D. D., & Skinner, M. (1998). Early developmental trajectories of males with fragile X syndrome. *American Journal of Mental Retardation*, **103**, 29–39.

Barbaresi, W. J., Katusic, S. K., Colligan, R. C., Weaver, A. L., & Jacobsen, S. J. (2005). Math learning disorder: Incidence in a population-based birth cohort, 1976–82, Rochester, Minn. *Ambulatory Pediatrics*, **5**, 281–9.

Barnes, M. A., Wilkinson, M., Khemani, E., Boudesquie, A., Dennis, M., & Fletcher, J. M. (2006). Arithmetic processing in children with spina bifida: Calculation accuracy, strategy use, and fact retrieval fluency. *Journal of Learning Disabilities*, **39**, 174–87.

Bellugi, U., Lichtenberger, L., Jones, W., Lai, Z., & St. George, M. (2000). The neurocognitive profile of Williams Syndrome: A complex pattern of strengths and weaknesses. *Journal of Cognitive Neuroscience*, **12**, 7–29.

Bennetto, L., Pennington, B. F., Porter, D., Taylor, A. K., & Hagerman, R. J. (2001). Profile of cognitive functioning in women with the fragile X mutation. *Neuropsychology*, **15**, 290–9.

Berch, D. B. (2005). Making sense of number sense: Implications for children with mathematical disabilities. *Journal of Learning Disabilities*, **38**, 289–384.

Blair, C., Zelazo, P. D., & Greenburg, M. T. (2005). The measurement of executive function in early childhood. *Developmental Neuropsychology*, **28**, 561–71.

Brainard, S. S., Schreiner, R. A., & Hagerman, R. J. (1991). Cognitive profiles of the carrier fragile X woman. *American Journal of Medical Genetics*, **38**, 505–8.

Bruandet, M., Molko, N., Cohen, L., & Dehaene, S. (2004). A cognitive characterization of dyscalculia in Turner syndrome. *Neuropsychologia*, **42**, 288–98.

Buchanan, L., Pavlovic, J., & Rovet, J. (1998). A reexamination of the visuospatial deficit in Turner syndrome: Contributions of working memory. *Developmental Neuropsychology*, **14**, 341–67.

Bull, R. & Johnston, R. S. (1997). Children's arithmetic difficulties: Contributions from processing speed, item identification, and short-term memory. *Journal of Experimental Child Psychology*, **65**, 1–24.

Butterworth, B. (2005). Developmental dyscalculia. In J. I. D. Campbell (Ed.), *Handbook of Mathematical Cognition* (pp. 455–467). New York: Psychology Press.

Chapman, R. S., Schwartz, S. E., & Kay-Raining Bird, E. (1991). Language skills of children and adolescents with Down syndrome: Comprehension. *Journal of Speech & Hearing Research*, **34**, 1106–20.

Cornish, L., Levitas, A., & Sudhalter, V. (2007). Fragile X syndrome: The journey from genes to behavior. In M. M. M. Mazzocco & J. L. Ross (Eds.), *Neurogenetic Developmental Disorders: Variation of Manifestation in Childhood* (pp. 73–103). Cambridge, MA: MIT Press.

Cornish, K., Munir, F., & Cross, G. (1998). The nature of the spatial deficit in young females with fragile X syndrome: A neuropsychological and molecular perspective. *Neuropsychologia*, **36**, 1239–46.

Cornish, K., Swainson, R., Cunnington, R., Wilding, J., Morris, P., & Jackson, G. (2004). Do women with fragile X syndrome have problems in switching attention? Preliminary findings from ERP and fMRI. *Brain and Cognition*, **54**, 235–9.

Crawford, D. C., Acuna, J. M., & Sherman, S. L. (2001). FMR1 and the fragile X syndrome: Human genome epidemiology review. *Genetics in Medicine*, **3**, 359–71.

Davenport, M. L., Hooper, S. R., & Zegar, M. (2007). Turner syndrome in childhood. In M. M. M. Mazzocco & J. L. Ross (Eds.), *Neurogenetic developmental disorders: Variation of Manifestation in Childhood* (pp. 3–45). Cambridge, MA: MIT Press.

Dehaene, S., Piazza, M., Pinel, P., & Cohen, L. (2005). Three parietal circuits for number processing. In J. I. D. Campbell (Ed.), *Handbook of Mathematical Cognition* (pp. 433–53). New York, NY: Psychology Press.

Dennis, M., Berch, D.B., Mazzocco, M.M.M. (2009). Mathematical learning disabilities in special populations: Phenotypic variation and cross-disorder comparisons. *Developmental Disabilities Research Reviews*, **15**, 80–9.

Donlan, C. (2007). Mathematical development in children with specific language impairments. In D. B. Berch & M. M. M. Mazzocco (Eds.), *Why Is Math So Hard for Some Children? The Nature and Origins of Mathematical Learning Difficulties and Disabilities* (pp. 151–72), Baltimore, MD: Brookes Publishing.

Ewart, A. K., Morris, C. A., Atkinson, D., *et al.* (1993). Hemizygosity at the elastin locus in a developmental disorder, Williams syndrome. *Nature Genetics*, **5**, 11–6.

Fais, W. & Fischer, M. H. (2005). Spatial representation of numbers. In J. I. D. Campbell (Ed.), *Handbook of Mathematical Cognition* (pp. 43–54). New York: Psychology Press.

Frangiskakis, J. M., Ewart, A. K., Morris, C. A., *et al.* (1996). LIM-kinase1 hemizygosity implicated in impaired visuospatial constructive cognition. *Cell*, **86**, 59–69.

Fuchs, L. S. & Fuchs, D. (2002). Mathematical problem-solving profiles of students with mathematics disabilities with and without comorbid reading disabilities. *Journal of Learning Disabilities*, **35**, 563–73.

Geary, D. C. (1993). Mathematical disabilities: Cognitive, neuropsychological, and genetic components. *Psychological Bulletin*, **114**, 345–62.

Geary, D. C. (1994). *Children's Mathematical Development: Research and Practical Applications.* Washington, DC: American Psychological Association.

Geary, D. C. (2004). Mathematics and learning disabilities. *Journal of Learning Disabilities*, **37**, 4–15.

Geary, D. C. (2005). Role of cognitive theory in the study of learning disability in mathematics. *Journal of Learning Disabilities*, **38**, 305–7.

Geary, D. C., Brown, S. C., & Samaranayake, V. A. (1991). Cogntive addition: A short longitudinal study of strategy choice and speed-of-processing differences in normal and mathematically disabled children. *Developmental Psychology*, **27**, 787–97.

Geary, D. C., Hoard, M. K., Byrd-Craven, J., & DeSoto, M. C. (2004). Strategy choices in simple and complex addition: Contributions of working memory and counting knowledge for children with mathematical disability. *Journal of Experimental Child Psychology*, **88**, 121–51.

Geary, D. C., Hoard, M. K., Nugent, L., & Byrd-Craven, J. (2007). Strategy use and working memory capacity. In D. B. Berch & M. M. M. Mazzocco (Eds.), *Why Is Math So Hard for Some Children? The Nature and Origin of Mathematical Learning Difficulties and Disabilities* (pp. 83–105), Baltimore, MD: Brookes Publishing.

Greenough, W. T., Klintsova, A. Y., Irwin, S. A., Galvez, R., Bates, K. E., & Weiler, I. J. (2001). Synaptic regulation of protein synthesis and the fragile X protein. *Proceedings from the National Academy of Sciences of the United States of America*, **98**, 7101–06.

Grigsby, J. P., Kemper, M. B., Hagerman, R. J., & Myers, C. S. (1990). Neuropsychological dysfunction among affected heterozygous fragile X females. *American Journal of Medical Genetics*, **35**, 28–35.

Hagerman, R. (1999). *Neurodevelopmental Disorders: Diagnosis and Treatment.* Oxford, UK: Oxford University Press.

Hagerman, R. J. (2002). The physical and behavioral phenotype. In R. J. Hagerman & P. J. Hagerman (Eds.), *Fragile X Syndrome: Diagnosis, Treatment, and Research* (pp. 3–109). Baltimore, MD: The Johns Hopkins University Press.

Hagerman, R. J., Jackson, C., Amiri, K., Silverman, A. C., O'Connor, R., & Sobesky, W. (1992). Girls with fragile X syndrome: Physical and neurocognitive status and outcome. *Pediatrics*, **89**, 395–400.

Jakala, P., Hanninen, T., Ryynanen, M., *et al.* (1997). Fragile X: Neuropsychological test performance, CGG triplet repeat lengths, and hippocampal volumes. *Journal of Clinical Investigation*, **100**, 331–8.

Kirk, J. W., Mazzocco, M. M. M., & Kover, S. T. (2005). Assessing executive dysfunction in girls with fragile X or Turner syndrome using the Contingency Naming Test (CNT). *Developmental Neuropsychology*, **28**, 755–77.

Kwon, H., Menon, V., Eliez, S., *et al.* (2001). Functional neuroanatomy of visuospatial working memory in fragile X syndrome: Relation to behavioral and molecular measures. *American Journal of Psychiatry*, **158**, 1040–51.

Lasker, A., Mazzocco, M. M. M., & Zee, D. (2007). Ocular motor indicators of executive dysfunction in females with fragile X or Turner syndrome. *Brain and Cognition*, **63**, 203–20.

Lyon, M. F. (1972). X-chromosome inactivation and developmental patterns in mammals. *Biological Reviews of the Cambridge Philosophical Society*, **47**, 1–35.

Martin, N. D., Snodgrass, G. J., & Cohen, R. D. (1984). Idiopathic infantile hypercalcaemia– a continuing enigma. *Archives of Disease in Childhood*, **59**, 605–13.

Mazzocco, M. M. M. (1998). A process approach to describing mathematics difficulties in girls with Turner syndrome. *Pediatrics*, **102**, 492–6.

Mazzocco, M. M. M. (2001). Math learning disability and math LD subtypes: Evidence from studies of Turner syndrome, fragile X syndrome, and neurofibromatosis Type 1. *Journal of Learning Disabilities*, **34**, 520–33.

Mazzocco, M. M. M., Bhatia, N., & Lesniak-Karpiak, K. (2006). Visuospatial skills and their association with math performance in girls with fragile X or Turner Syndrome. *Child Neuropsychology*, **12**, 87–110.

Mazzocco, M. M. M. & McCloskey, M. (2005). Math performance in girls with Turner or fragile X syndrome. In J. I. D. Campbell (Ed.), *Handbook of Mathematical Cognition* (pp. 269–97). New York, NY: Psychology Press.

Mazzocco, M. M. M., Pennington, B. F., & Hagerman, R. J. (1993). The neurocognitive phenotype of female carriers of fragile X: Additional evidence for specificity. *Journal of Developmental and Behavioral Pediatrics*, **14**, 328–35.

McCauley, E., Kay, T., Ito, J., & Treder, R. (1987). The Turner syndrome: Cognitive deficits, affective discrimination, and behavior problems. *Child Development*, **58**, 464–73.

McLean, J. F. & Hitch, G. J. (1999). Working memory impairments in children with specific arithmetic learning difficulties. *Journal of Experimental Child Psychology*, **74**, 240–60.

Mervis, C. B., & Morris, C. A. (2007). Williams syndrome. In M.M.M. Mazzocco and J.L. Ross (Eds.), *Neurogenetic Developmental Disorders: Variation of Manifestation in Childhood* (pp. 199–262). Cambridge, MA: MIT Press.

Molko, N., Cachia, A., Riviere, D., *et al.* (2003). Functional and structural alterations of the intraparietal sulcus in a developmental dyscalculia of genetic origin. *Neuron*, **40**, 847–58.

Murphy, M.M, & Mozzocco, M.M.M. (in press). The trajectory of mathematics skills and working memory thresholds in girls with fragile X syndrome. Cognitive Development. In press.

Murphy, M. M., Mazzocco, M. M. M., Gerner, G., & Henry, A. E. (2006). Mathematics learning disability in girls with Turner syndrome or fragile X syndrome. *Brain and Cognition*, **61**, 195–210.

Murphy, M. M., Mazzocco, M. M. M., Hanich, L., & Early, M. (2007). Cognitive characteristics of children with Mathematics Learning Disability (MLD) varies as a function of criterion used to define MLD. *Journal of Learning Disabilities*, **40**, 458–78.

O'Hearn, K. & Landau, B. (2007). Mathematical skill in individuals with Williams Syndrome: Evidence from a standardized mathematics battery. *Brain and Cognition*, **64**, 238–46.

O'Hearn, K., Landau, B., & Hoffman, J. E. (2005, April). *Subitizing in People with Williams Syndrome and Normally Developing Children*. Paper presented at the Society for Research in Child Development, Atlanta, GA.

Oostra, B. A. (1996). Fragile X syndrome in humans and mice. *Acta Geneticae Medicae Et Gemellologiae*, **45**, 93–108.

Passolunghi, M. C. & Siegel, L. S. (2004). Working memory and access to numerical information in children with disability in mathematics. *Journal of Experimental Child Psychology*, **88**, 348–67.

Rivera, S. M., Menon, V., White, C. D., Glaser, B., & Reiss, A. L. (2002). Functional brain activation during arithmetic processing in females with fragile X syndrome is related to FMR1 protein expression. *Human Brain Mapping*, **16**, 206–18.

Romans, S. M., Roeltgen, D. P., Kushner, H., & Ross, J. L. (1997). Executive function in girls with Turner's syndrome. *Developmental Neuropsychology*, **13**, 23–40.

Rousseau, F., Heitz, D., Tarleton, J., *et al.* (1994). A multicenter study on genotype-phenotype correlations in the fragile X syndrome, using direct diagnosis with probe StB12.3: The first 2,253 cases. *American Journal of Human Genetics*, **55**, 225–37.

Rovet, J. F. (1993). The psychoeducational characteristics of children with Turner syndrome. *Journal of Learning Disabilities*, **26**, 333–41.

Rovet, J. F. (2004). Turner syndrome: A review of genetic and hormonal influences on neuro-psychological functioning. *Child Neuropsychology*, **10**, 262–79.

Rovet, J. & Netley, C. (1982). Processing deficits in Turner's syndrome. *Developmental Psychology*, **18**, 77–94.

Rovet, J. F., Szekely, C., & Hockenberry, M. N. (1994). Specific arithmetic calculation deficits in children with Turner syndrome. *Journal of Clinical and Experimental Neuropsychology*, **16**, 820–39.

Scholock, Luckasson, Shogren, *et al.* (2007).

Semel, E. & Rosner, S. R. (2003). *Understanding Williams syndrome: Behavioral patterns and interventions*. Mahwah, NJ: Lawrence Erlbaum Associates.

Shalev, R. S., Manor, O., Auerbach, J., & Gross-Tsur, V. (1998). Persistence of developmental dyscalculia: What counts? *Journal of Pediatrics*, **133**, 358–62.

Silver, C. H., Pennett, D.-L., Black, J. L., Fair, G. W., & Balise, R. R. (1999). Stability of arithmetic disability subtypes. *Journal of Learning Disabilities*, **32**, 108–19.

Strømme, P., Bjørnstad, PG, & Ramstad, K. (2002). Prevalence estimation of Williams syndrome. *Journal of Child Neurology*, **17**, 269–71.

Tamm, L., Menon, V., Johnston, C. K., Hessl, D. R., & Reiss, A. L. (2002). fMRI study of cognitive interference processing in females with fragile X syndrome. *Journal of Cognitive Neuroscience*, **14**, 160–71.

Tamm, L., Menon, V., & Reiss, A. L. (2003). Abnormal prefrontal cortex function during response inhibition in Turner syndrome: Functional magnetic resonance imaging evidence. *Biological Psychiatry*, **53**, 107–11.

Tassabehji, M., Metcalfe, K., Fergusson, W. D., *et al.* (1996). LIM-kinase deleted in Williams syndrome. *Nature Genetics*, **13**, 272–3.

Temple, C. M. (2002). Oral fluency and narrative production in children with Turner's syndrome. *Neuropsychologia*, **40**, 1419–27.

Temple, C. M. & Carney, R. A. (1993). Intellectual functioning of children with Turner syndrome: A comparison of behavioural phenotypes. *Developmental Medicine and Child Neurology*, **35**, 691–8.

Temple, C. M. & Carney, R. A. (1995). Patterns of spatial functioning in Turner's syndrome. *Cortex*, **31**, 109–18.

Temple, C. M., Carney, R. A., & Mullarkey, S. (1996). Frontal lobe function and executive skills in children with Turner's syndrome. *Developmental Neuropsychology*, **12**, 343–63.

Temple, C. M. & Marriott, A. J. (1998). Arithmetical ability and disability in Turner's Syndrome: A cognitive neuropsychological analysis. *Developmental Neuropsychology*, **14**, 47–67.

Waber, D. P. (1979). Neuropsychological aspects of Turner's syndrome. *Developmental Medicine and Child Neurology*, **21**, 58–70.

8

A developmental approach to genetic disorders

Sarah J. Paterson

Introduction

In recent years, several researchers have attempted to apply the adult neuropsychological model to neurodevelopmental disorders. In the adult model, localized brain damage gives rise to a juxtaposed pattern of impaired and intact abilities. When applied to neurodevelopmental disorders, this approach fails to capture the role of development itself in the formation of the final phenotype. An alternative to this common strategy is a neuroconstructivist approach that considers the contribution of the infant start state, the entire developmental trajectory, and underlying cognitive processes to the phenotypic outcome. Results from studies of language and number in infants and toddlers with Williams syndrome and Down syndrome, along with a briefer discussion of face processing, will be presented in support of this position. The application of this approach to other developmental disorders such as autism will also be discussed.

The traditional adult neuropsychological approach to disorder is a static one, in contrast to a neuroconstructivist perspective, which emphasizes the importance of development and of studying early development and not just the endstate in older children and adults. A theoretically driven investigation of the cognitive processes underlying behavior as well as the use of converging measures to describe these processes are crucial aspects of understanding neurodevelopmental disorders from a neoconstructivist approach.

Three developmental disorders, i.e., Williams syndrome, Down syndrome, and autism, will be used to illustrate the developmental neoconstructive approach. The

The empirical work by Paterson and colleagues, presented in this chapter, was conducted while the author was a graduate student at the Neurocognitive Development Unit, Institute of Child Health, University College London. It was a supported PhD Studentship to the author from the Down Syndrome Association and by grants to A. Karmiloff-Smith from The Williams Syndrome Foundation, UK, Medical Research Council, and the Healthcare Foundation. I wish to thank Annette Karmiloff-Smith and everyone who was at the NDU for many stimulating discussions that have contributed greatly to my thinking about development, and J. P. Nawyn for his helpful comments on an earlier draft of this chapter.

majority of studies to be discussed concern the first two groups. These groups have proven very valuable to the study of atypical development because they exhibit uneven and different cognitive profiles in the adult endstate, despite similar overall cognitive ability. Given that the groups differ in their strengths and weaknesses, one can conduct cross-syndrome, cross-domain research to investigate whether certain aspects of atypical development are syndrome-specific or occur as a result of general cognitive impairment. One can also compare the adult endstate with the infant state to demonstrate that the infant start state is very different from the mature phenotype and that one cannot make assumptions about the endstate of a disorder from infant performance or vice versa.

The domains of language, number, and face processing are of particular interest here because several studies have collected data from both adults and infants and toddlers, allowing both the beginning of the developmental trajectory and the endstate to be characterized within each domain. The results from these studies will demonstrate that the pattern of abilities seen in early development can change drastically as a consequence of even small perturbations in the process of development and will therefore highlight the importance of examining the entire developmental trajectory in attempting to understand the cognitive phenotypes of neurodevelopmental disorders.

Different approaches to developmental disorder

There is a long and successful tradition of investigating brain–behavior relations by studying adults with acquired brain injuries. Lesions in particular areas of the brain have helped scientists understand the functional contributions of local brain areas. For example, a stroke patient may have a lesion in the fusiform face area and will not be able to recognize faces but may function normally on other cognitive tasks, such as reading or drawing. Christine Temple (1997) characterizes the objective of case studies in clinical cognitive neuropsychology as follows: "to propose selective deficits of a common modular architecture of a developmental system." This implies that the cognitive system is made up of a number of specialized systems or modules, and that an impairment in behavior points to impairment in the underlying specialized system. Such an approach has, of course, led to many useful findings and provides a solid starting point for the investigation of the developmental process. However, this method is inappropriate for the study of developmental disorders, because it does not consider the process of change over development. Nor does it fully accept that the infant brain is not just a miniature version of the adult.

In contrast, the neuroconstructivist approach emphasizes the role of development in shaping the mature phenotype (Elman *et al.*, 1996; Karmiloff-Smith, 1998).

The very process of development is thought to create the cognitive outcomes seen in adulthood, as in the case when low-level biases toward particular types of stimuli develop into specialized circuitry over the course of development. So, for example, from birth infants appear to be biased to seek out face-like stimuli and thereby provide the developing cortical circuits with ample face stimuli. In turn, this exposure will lead to the specialized circuitry for face processing seen later in development (Morton and Johnson, 1991). By this view, functional specialization is an outcome of development and is not present from the outset. In order to study development this way, it is necessary to investigate cognitive ability from as early as possible in development so that its developmental trajectory can be charted. In addition, it is important to consider the processes underlying a particular behavior. A score on a standardized measure may be achieved in a variety of ways, and some strategies may lead to success in some domain but weakness in another. As an example, a focus on detail might be useful when discriminating between two faces but might slow down one's response when trying to reconstruct a group of blocks into a pattern. Because it appears that cognitive functioning is widely distributed in the brain, particularly as skills are developing, it is highly likely that several domains are affected by a particular disorder. However, overt behavioral impairment may be more obvious in some domains than in others. A seemingly generalized problem with neural circuitry, such as a difference in the pathways that encode rapidly presented stimuli, might have a noticeable behavioral effect on a skill such as speech processing, which relies heavily on this process, but would have much less obvious behavioral impact on a skill such as face processing, which does not draw upon those resources (Karmiloff-Smith, 1998).

The state of the infant brain, both in terms of structure and function, cannot and should not be derived from the adult brain (Elman *et al.*, 1996; Karmiloff-Smith, 1998; Paterson *et al.*, 1999). This is true for both the intact adult brain and the lesioned brain. Although a lesion in adulthood may have an effect on a particular function at that time, it cannot be inferred that this area necessarily subserves such a function during development. Johnson (2000) suggests an interactive specialization approach, in which the different pathways in the brain develop over time, with changes both within and between pathways that lead to increasing specialization. This approach differs from a maturational perspective in which functional competence is dependent on the maturation of particular brain areas that subserve that function. In the more developmental view, the contribution of different brain areas and circuits to cognitive function will vary over time. For example, as infants acquire more vocabulary, their electrophysiological responses to known words become much more localized to the left hemisphere (Neville *et al.*, 1991). Earlier in development it is likely that several brain circuits are attempting to process words and so responses are more widespread.

Several investigators have shown that areas involved in the development of a function are not the same as those required for its maintenance. For example, Bates (1997) has shown that early in language development, damage to the right hemisphere has a bigger impact on comprehension than damage to the left hemisphere, contradicting what we would expect based on the adult model. The localization of various cognitive functions changes as they develop. Areas associated with attention, for example, move from the posterior areas to more anterior areas throughout development (Posner & Petersen, 1990).

Despite many examples of change across development, there are some areas of cognition that appear to be rather well-developed even in infancy, such as object perception (e.g., Kellman & Spelke, 1983) and there are skills, for example part–whole processing, that exhibit similar types of impairment after brain injury in both adults and children (Stiles, 1998). However, this does not rule out the possibility that these areas underwent a developmental process. Changes may occur very early in development, or could occur very rapidly. It is also important not to forget that a portion of development is harder to characterize because it occurs even before birth. In both the visual and auditory systems, neural networks are already forming during gestation, aided by spontaneous neural activity (Katz & Shatz, 1996). Given these findings, taking a developmental approach and avoiding assumptions that the functional structure of the brain is pre-existing in the infant is likely to help us elucidate structure function relations more thoroughly.

Populations studied

Williams syndrome (WS) is a rare neurodevelopmental disorder caused by a hemizygous submicroscopic deletion of some 28 genes on chromosome 7q11,23 (Donnai and Karmiloff-Smith, 2000). It occurs in approximately 1 in 20,000 live births, although see Strømme *et al.* (2002) for a much higher prevalence estimate of 1 in 7500. Clinical features of WS include several physical abnormalities accompanied by mild to moderate mental retardation and a specific personality profile. IQs are generally in the 50s and 60s. The cognitive profile of the mature WS phenotype is very distinctive and is characterized by marked strengths and weaknesses. Several studies have suggested that, despite general cognitive impairment, face processing and vocabulary skills are *relatively* good, whereas number and visuo-spatial constructive ability is poor (e.g., Järvinen-Pasley *et al.*, 2008; Mervis *et al.*, 1999).

Down syndrome (DS) is more common, occurring 1 in 800 births. It results from defects on the 21st chromosome, the most common of which is trisomy 21 (47 XX or 47 XY) in which an extra chromosome 21 is present. Trisomy 21 is found in approximately 95% of people with DS. DS gives rise to clear physical characteristics and learning disabilities, with IQs in a similar range to those found in WS. Previous work suggests that the pattern of strengths and weaknesses in the DS cognitive profile is nearly opposite that found in WS. Individuals with DS have particular difficulties with language and with number, but are less impaired on tasks that rely on spatial abilities (e.g., Klein & Mervis, 1999; see Chapter 6).

Autism is a complex developmental disorder that gives rise to a distinctive cognitive profile. Individuals with autism exhibit particular difficulty in the social domain, have difficulties with communication, and exhibit restricted or repetitive behaviors (American Psychiatric Association, DSM-IV, 2000). In addition to these impairments, some aspects of visual processing are atypical. Gaze and face processing are particularly impaired (Klin *et al.*, 2002, 1999). Some researchers have argued that individuals with autism may demonstrate an over-reliance on featural processing (Frith, 1989). There is increasing evidence to suggest neurological and genetic bases for autism (see O'Roak & State, 2008, for a review, and Chapter 2). However, unlike for DS and WS, it is not yet possible to diagnose autism with genetic testing. This has meant that it is challenging to diagnose children younger than 3 years old, the time at which many of the socio-communicative symptoms become more apparent. Despite this difficulty, more recent work with preschoolers has revealed that, early in development, in addition to the core symptoms of autism, more general nonverbal and motor delays are also present (Volkmar *et al.*, 2005; Zwaigenbaum *et al.*, 2005). In the general population, the prevalence rates of autism have been estimated conservatively as 1:150, with about four times as many males as females affected (CDC, 2007).

There are, of course, numerous neurodevelopmental disorders that would benefit from investigation using a more developmental approach, and such work is already being conducted in fragile X syndrome (Scerif *et al.*, 2005). However, for the purpose of this chapter, the three disorders described above will be the focus. DS and WS are of particular interest here because, as is discussed in the following sections, their cognitive profiles differ in adulthood. One group is much poorer at number than the other and the opposite is true for language. It is important to bear in mind that, despite this difference in the endstate, it is the developmental processes themselves that are crucial to understanding how these differences arise.

Before turning to cognition however, it is necessary to briefly consider the importance of genetics for development. In considering these three disorders and the role of genes in their cognitive outcomes, it is important not to over simplify. The pathway from genes to brains to behavior is extremely complex. Genes code for proteins, not behavior. By taking a developmental approach, we attempt to consider what effects changes in the genotype might have on developmental processes and how small changes in the genes can lead to marked changes at the level of behavior. The complexity of this process is well illustrated by fragile X syndrome. Despite being a single gene disorder, in which the FMR1 gene is silenced, leading to reduction in the amount of the protein FMRP (O'Donnell & Warren, 2002), the cognitive profile of this disorder of this disorder is not straightforward (see Chapter 1). There are certainly no single gene to behavior mappings. Indeed, fragile X syndrome also provides a good example of the role of developmental processes and timing in shaping the behavioral phenotype. Gene and protein expression is not static and changes over the course of development (Tamanini *et al.*, 1997; see Scerif & Karmiloff-Smith, 2005, for a more thorough discussion of this and the developmental approach to genes and cognition). Such changes in gene expression over development underscore the importance of charting the whole developmental trajectory and considering the impact of timing of both environmental and biological events on development.

The relationship between genetic and behavioral variability is also important to consider. Why do individuals who share very similar genetic deletions exhibit very different cognitive abilities? Despite the majority of individuals having a similar sized deletion, the degree of cognitive impairment is relatively heterogeneous in WS. This may be due in part to familial genetic influences which work together with the genetics of the disorder. Just as in typical development, an individual might be likely to be at the higher end of a distribution such as intelligence because genetic factors in the family predispose individuals to high intelligence. A genetic disorder may not allow them to reach their full potential but might still cause them to be in the upper range of performance for that disorder. In addition, environmental influences both within and outside the individual should be considered. Genes interact with other genes to control biological processes, so genetic variability outside the area associated with a particular disorder can also contribute to development (Gray *et al.*, 2006; Scerif and Karmiloff-Smith, 2005). It is important to keep the role of genes in mind as development in three cognitive domains is considered.

Examples from early language development

Several investigators have used WS as an example of the modularity of language, perhaps most notably, Steven Pinker (1994). He states that "although IQ is measured at around 50, older children and adolescents with WS are described as hyperlinguistic with selective sparing of syntax, and grammatical abilities that are close to normal in controlled testing." Pinker suggests that language is spared in the face of general cognitive impairment. However, many recent studies from a number of laboratories have demonstrated that the pattern of strengths and weaknesses is much more complex and that language is not completely "spared" in this population. For example, impairments have been found in the formulation of the past tense (Thomas *et al.*, 2001), in processing ungrammatical sentences (Karmiloff-Smith *et al.*, 1998), and in the use of grammatical gender in Italian (Volterra *et al.*, 1996). While there may be a relative strength in language, compared to the profile seen in DS for example, the process by which language is acquired may be very different, and there are clear deficits within the language domain even in the adult endstate (see Brock, 2007, for a review).

It is true that adults with WS generally outperform adults with DS, matched on overall cognitive ability, on receptive vocabulary tests. For example, in a study using the British picture vocabulary test, the adult WS group exhibited a significantly smaller discrepancy between test age and vocabulary age than an adult DS group, matched on CA and MA (Paterson, 2000). However, both WS and DS groups are language delayed in early childhood (Klein & Mervis, 1999; Paterson *et al.*, 1999; Singer Harris *et al.*, 1997). Paterson and colleagues (1999) investigated receptive vocabulary using a preferential looking paradigm. They tested 15 infants and toddlers with WS (mean CA, 30.4 months; mean MA, 16.5 months), 22 with DS (mean CA, 29.7 months; mean MA, 15.6 months), and 17 MA- and 17 CA-matched controls. They found that the degree of language delay in both disorders was similar, with the pattern seen in WS and DS groups like that seen in MA-matched controls. Data from a parent questionnaire, the MacArthur Communicative Development Inventory (CDI-Words and Gestures), demonstrate language delay in the WS and DS groups, but also suggest that the profile of language abilities in infants and toddlers is atypical (Paterson *et al.*, 2000). While the WS and DS groups are both delayed in expressive and receptive vocabulary, the advantage of comprehension over expressive language comprehension advantage seen in typically developing toddlers is much reduced in the WS group. For a given level of comprehension, production in the WS groups was surprisingly high, suggesting that early in development a firm foundation of understanding on which to build a productive vocabulary may be lacking. Indeed, parents of children with WS have sometimes asked for an extra column on the CDI: "says but does not understand" (see also Singer Harris *et al.*, 1997). The DS group was behaving very much like MA-matched controls, whereas the profile of language comprehension and expression in the WS group looked like neither CA- nor MA-matched controls. In sum, individuals with WS outperform individuals with DS in language by adolescence and adulthood. In early childhood, in contrast, the groups are equally delayed in language, yet their language profiles differ; toddlers with DS show a delayed but typical developmental profile with an advantage of comprehension over expression, whereas toddlers with WS show a delayed but atypical developmental profile with no comprehension advantage (see Chapter 5 for a discussion of syntactic performance in WS).

Given this discontinuity across development, it is important to ask how these skills develop. Several studies have now been conducted which suggest that individuals with WS acquire language in an atypical manner. This difference begins even before the infant can produce language, in speech processing. Nazzi *et al.* (2003) investigated speech segmentation in toddlers with WS and DS using a headturn preference procedure (Jusczyk & Aslin, 1995). In this task, infants are familiarized with bisyllabic words such as CANdle and then tested with four passages, two containing the target words and two containing unfamiliar words that the child was not exposed to during the familiarization phase) with the same stress pattern, e.g., KINGdom. If the infant is able to segment the word from fluent speech, it is expected that he or she will listen significantly longer to the passages containing the familiar words. Using this technique, it has been demonstrated that at 7.5 months, typically developing infants can segment words with a strong–weak structure (the dominant stress pattern in English), from fluent speech, and that at 10.5 months they can segment words with the less common weak–strong pattern, such as "guiTAR" (Jusczyk *et al.*, 1999). However, despite having mental and chronological ages of 19 months and 33 months, respectively, well beyond the level at which typically developing infants can segment even the less common stress pattern, the toddlers with WS were unable to reliably segment the weak–strong words from fluent speech. In order to segment the more common strong–weak words successfully, the infant can use cues from prosody or stress, placing a word boundary before the strong syllable. For example, segmenting before a boundary works in this case: "the |CANdle| was on the |TABle|," but not in this one: "the gui| TAR IS on the table." In the latter example with a weak–strong word, segmenting using a strong syllable as a word boundary yields "taris," which is nonsense in English. The segmentation of these weak strong words requires a more sophisticated strategy that relies on distributional or statistical information to group syllables together. The ability to segment these words requires knowledge that is acquired by implicit learning of statistical properties in the language, for example, which syllables are likely to follow other syllables and which syllable pairings are not acceptable in the infant's particular language (Jusczyk *et al.*, 1999; Saffran *et al.*, 1996;). As the results demonstrate, the performance of toddlers with WS is seriously delayed. This is particularly striking if one considers that relatively few exposures to connected speech are thought to be necessary for typically developing infants to derive word boundaries (Saffran *et al.*, 1996). It is likely that children with WS are using a different strategy with which to acquire weak–strong words, particularly given the finding that such words were already in their vocabularies (Nazzi *et al.*, 2003). The toddlers with WS might acquire weak–strong words by repeated exposure to words in isolation or perhaps these individuals can segment weak–strong words, but require much more time to segment the speech stream than was provided in laboratory conditions. In either case, this delay in segmentation is likely to have an impact on the efficiency with which new words are acquired.

Differences across syndromes have also been reported in the social cognitive precursors to language. Joint attention is a core social cognitive skill that plays a very important role in early language acquisition (Bates *et al.*, 1979). Joint attention is "the ability to coordinate attention with a social partner" (Mundy *et al.*, 2000, p. 325) and is triadic involving the infant, adult, and an object. It can be either initiated by the infant, calling an adult's attention to an object the infant is looking at, or the infant can follow the attention of an adult. From the results discussed below, it is apparent that this skill develops atypically in WS.

In an observational study, Mervis *et al.* (1999) found that, in typical development, referential pointing emerges before the use of referential language or labels, but that the opposite is true in WS. These children have several words before they begin to point. This is noteworthy because pointing is a useful strategy to elicit labels from caregivers. These results are expanded upon in a study of 13 toddlers with WS (mean age 31 months) using the Early Social Communication Scales (Mundy and Hogan, 1996). Laing and her colleagues (Laing *et al.*, 2002) found that children with WS were impaired both at responding to and initiating joint attention when compared with MA-matched controls. While they were able to interact successfully in a dyad, enjoying the attention of an adult, they had difficulty with triadic interaction involving an object and another person. In particular, they had problems with shifting attention between the object and the person. This skill is important for acquiring new labels, for example, either by following the point of a caregiver or pointing out an object to a caregiver. Interestingly, studies of visual attention also suggest that infants with WS may have difficulty in shifting attention, exhibiting "sticky fixation" (Brown *et al.*, 2003). This impairment may well contribute to difficulties with triadic joint attention. Laing *et al.* (2002) also demonstrated that the infants with WS point less than controls and also follow points less often. It is important to note that this is not merely a function of their cognitive delay, because children with DS produce points like their typically developing counterparts (Franco & Wishart, 1995).

In addition to exhibiting differences in the precursors to language, people with WS appear to learn new words differently from their typically developing counterparts. The relationship between cognitive milestones and those in language acquisition is atypical in WS. For example, in typical development, the ability to sort objects into categories precedes the vocabulary spurt, whereas in WS, the vocabulary spurt often considerably precedes the ability to categorize. A discrepancy of 6–12 months was found from the onset of the vocabulary spurt to the emergence of exhaustive sorting. Indeed, some children with WS had a vocabulary of more than

500 words before they began spontaneous sorting of objects into categories (Mervis & Bertrand, 1997). These results suggest that individuals with WS might be focusing less on semantics in their word learning than their typically developing and DS counterparts. It appears that they are acquiring labels before acquiring the notion of object kinds or categories on which to map them. This finding is supported by results from a study of name-based categorization in 2- to 6-year-olds with WS (Nazzi & Karmiloff-Smith, 2002). In contrast to typically developing 20-month-olds (Nazzi & Gopnik, 2001), the young children with WS could not categorize unfamiliar objects on the basis of nonsense labels, which they had been taught prior to testing. This was despite the fact that their vocabularies were much larger than those of the younger typically developing infants. It is possible that the children with WS are learning the phonological sequences of labels for objects but have only a shallow referential understanding of them (Karmiloff-Smith *et al.*, 2003).

Individuals with WS do not use the same constraints for word learning as typically developing infants or infants with DS. In a study of older WS children and adults, differences were found in the use of lexical constraints such as the *whole object constraint* and the *taxonomic constraint* when learning a new word. Unlike normal 3-year-olds, people with WS are equally likely to assume that a label refers to part of a novel object as to the whole. In contrast, typically developing children are more likely to use the whole label for an object with which they aren't familiar and to assume a label corresponds to a part if they are familiar with the whole object label (Stevens & Karmiloff-Smith, 1997). In other words, the WS group tends not to obey the *whole object constraint* in language acquisition. WS individuals also made little use of the *taxonomic constraint*. When they were presented with a novel object that was given a novel name and were then asked to give another object with the same label, WS subjects did not show a bias toward objects from the same taxonomic category, such as shape. Again this constraint is used by typically developing 3-year-olds (Golinkoff *et al.*, 1994). These particular constraints seem to be relatively late appearing in development and, given the delay in language acquisition in WS, it may be that these individuals never acquire such constraints.

Taken together, these results from studies of early language and language acquisition highlight the importance of both a developmental approach and a fine-grained analysis of the processes underlying test results (Karmiloff-Smith, 1998; Karmiloff-Smith *et al.*, 2003). They demonstrate that one cannot assume that the relative strength of WS language in adulthood indicates the presence of an intact language system in the face of general cognitive impairment. As we have seen, several studies have reported language delay early in development and a close examination of the process of language acquisition suggests that its developmental trajectory is somewhat atypical. Even before they produce language, infants with

WS appear to have difficulty segmenting words out of the speech stream. As they develop, they do not exhibit the normal relationship between cognitive and language milestones, which is seen in typical development and in other atypically developing groups, such as DS. The developmental trajectory of children with WS, is such that they begin to acquire language before they have the cognitive insights that are important for bootstrapping language in normal development. For example, understanding that objects can be put into distinct categories, provides a useful semantic building block for acquiring words as labels for these categories. In addition to these cognitive differences, anomalies in their social interaction likely play a role in atypical language acquisition. The less efficient joint attention skills of infants with WS mean that many typical opportunities for object labeling are not available to them. They must therefore find other opportunities for word learning. Later in life, a fine-grained analysis of language reveals that, despite seemingly good vocabulary, adults with WS still learn new words in a different way and continue to exhibit subtle language deficits (see Thomas & Karmiloff-Smith, 2005, for a review). If one were to rely solely on good test performance in adulthood, information about differences in these cognitive processes across development would be missed.

Number studies

In the following section, Paterson presents data from the number domain to again highlight the importance of carefully studying skill development when building models of and making inferences about cognition from neurodevelopmental disorders. In the neuropsychological literature, there are many adult lesion studies that show how impairment of specialized cognitive systems can lead to deficits in specific aspects of numeracy or number understanding. For example, some patients cannot perform number tasks such as calculation and subitizing, but have no difficulty with spoken number language (Cipolotti *et al.*, 1991). While these findings are interesting, it is important to note that they do not tell us anything about how the number system developed; they merely describe the result of insult to an otherwise normal, mature brain. In contrast, in neurodevelopmental disorders, the brain develops differently both pre- and postnatally, so it is likely that the cognitive processes underlying skills such as number processing are also very different from those seen in adult patients with lesions (Karmiloff-Smith, 1998; Karmiloff-Smith *et al.*, 2002, 2003).

In order to chart the development of number ability in atypical developmental populations, Paterson *et al.* (1999) assessed individuals with WS and DS. In adulthood, these groups both have difficulty with number, but when asked about their children's difficulties, parents of individuals with WS have expressed particular concerns about number. There is a slightly larger literature on numeracy in adults with DS, and their difficulties appear to be related to overall cognitive ability. For example, studies of counting have suggested that developmental level, not DS per se, is a good indicator of success (Caycho *et al.*, 1991; Nye *et al.*, 1995).

Most studies to date have found number skills in WS to be poor. Udwin *et al.* (1996) measured numerical ability using the arithmetic subscale of the WISC-R and WISC-III at 12 years and again at 21 years of age. They found that performance remains at a plateau in WS, at around the level of an 8-year-old, i.e., well below chronological age. Number performance is worse than would be expected when compared to the extent of their overall cognitive impairment.

Given these general difficulties with number seen in adults with WS and DS, it appears important to investigate more specific number abilities both in adulthood and at the outset of development, in infancy. In order to chart development, it is necessary to attempt to choose tasks that tap into similar processes in both the adult and infant. This is not always possible, of course, either because such tests cannot be constructed or because the way in which stimuli are processed changes dramatically over the course of development. However, such tasks are a very useful tool in both charting developmental trajectories and in trying to investigate how the relationship between behavior and the possible brain areas on which the behavior relies change over development.

Paterson and colleagues (Paterson *et al.*, 1999, 2006) conducted studies of number in adults and infants with WS and DS. Sensitivity to changes in numerosity was measured in 13 infants with WS (mean CA, 31 months; mean MA, 16.9 months), 22 with DS (mean CA, 31 months; mean MA, 15.6 months), and in 16 MA- and 14 CA-matched controls. Participants were familiarized with three pairs of displays, with each display containing two objects. The displays were made up of changing sets of objects, so it could be established that infants were not responding merely to new objects in the test phase but were extracting numerosity. Care was also taken to vary the spatial extent and layout of the displays, so that infants could not rely solely on the area of the display covered to make their discrimination (Clearfield & Mix, 1999). After familiarization with sets of two, infants were presented with one card displaying new objects but the old numerosity (two) and another displaying new objects and a novel numerosity (three). If infants were sensitive to the difference in numerosity, then one would expect the mean looking time to the novel numerosity to be longer than that to the familiar numerosity, even though the objects were novel in both cases. Some have argued that this sensitivity to small numerosities is based on non numerical object tracking skills. To do this task, infants could keep track of individual objects and compare their representations of the objects in one array with the objects in the other to detect a mismatch (Huttenlocher *et al.*, 1994; Uller *et al.*, 1999). That said, the ability to parse arrays of several objects into separate entities, which can then be given numerical tags, is a useful building block for number and may bootstrap typical development in this domain (Carey, 1998).

Given the number difficulties of both groups in adulthood, it was predicted that, if initial states can be directly inferred from endstates, then both the WS and DS groups would show impairment on this small number discrimination task. The results did not support this oft-held assumption. Rather, they indicated that the CA-matched, MA-matched, and WS groups looked significantly longer at the novel numerosity and were therefore likely to be extracting numerosity information from the displays. By contrast, the infants with DS looked equally long at both the novel and familiar displays and did not appear to extract numerosity. This difference was not an artifact of familiarization time, because looking time in both the WS and DS groups decreased by a similar amount across the six familiarization trials and infants with DS showed a novelty preference in other tasks. It seems, therefore, that one of the precursors of number (sensitivity to changes in numerosity) is present in infants with WS but not in those with DS. This is striking given the adult data presented below. As we shall see, the pattern of number ability found in infancy does not reflect that seen in adulthood.

Numerosity discrimination in the mature phenotype was assessed using a task that was as similar as possible to the infant task, so that comparisons could be made across development (Paterson *et al.*, 2006). Participants with WS (mean CA, 20;9 years; and mean MA, 6;9 years), with DS (mean CA 24;3 years; and mean MA, 5;9 years) and MA- and CA-matched controls were tested using a computerized numerosity comparison task (Dehaene, 1989). Participants were asked to press a key that corresponded to the larger of two displays, which were presented simultaneously on a screen. The pairs of displays were made up of randomly arranged dots. The numerical distance between the two stimuli in each pair varied, so in some pairs the numerosities were close, for example, 2 and 3, and in others the numerosities were far apart, for example, 2 and 7. This was done so that the presence of the symbolic distance effect (SDE) in responses could be examined. This is a very robust effect and arises because individuals take longer to respond to close pairs than to far pairs (Moyer & Landauer, 1967). It is likely that the SDE results from variability in the magnitude representation. If the representation of the mental number line in the brain is relatively fuzzy (Dehaene & Cohen, 1994), then it will be easier to distinguish the larger of two numbers if they are far apart because overlapping activation is reduced.

Results from this task indicated that MA-matched, CA-matched, and DS groups exhibited the symbolic distance effect, whereas the WS group did not. In addition, the WS group was the least accurate in their responses. These data suggest that individuals with WS might represent number atypically and be less affected by the semantics of numerosity, as represented by the mental number line. Although the DS group appeared to lack one of the basic prerequisites for number in infancy, they have acquired a basic conception of numerosity by adulthood. On the other hand, the infants with WS were able to discriminate small set sizes in infancy, but they followed a different trajectory in subsequent learning, because they fail to display the competency with number seen in the adults with DS.

A battery of number tasks typically used with neuropsychological patients was given to the participants to examine a wider variety of number skills. The tasks included seriation, matching dots to Arabic numerals, saying what number comes before or after another, and basic arithmetic. The DS group performed significantly better overall than the WS group, despite poorer language skills. Although individuals with WS were able to count by rote, at least to 20, they had difficulty when they had to manipulate numbers and not merely reproduce a verbal string by rote. Impairments were seen even when participants were asked to put numbers in the correct order. These problems with ordering numbers suggest that the links between representations of magnitude and their lexical and numerical symbols are weak. The individuals with WS also had difficulty with reading multidigit numbers. This difficulty seems to result from poor transcoding, i.e., the switch from written Arabic codes to spoken numbers and may arise from either a poorly specified representation of numerosity, or from the fact that these individuals may not rely on an understanding of the semantics of number to guide their responses.

Atypical development has also been demonstrated by data from an estimation task with children and adults. Ansari *et al.* (2007) studied individuals' abilities to estimate or say how many dots were on rapidly presented arrays. They found that children and adults with WS were particularly poor at estimating numerosity when the number of dots presented was 7 or above. More interestingly, however, they found that the development trajectory of this ability was different between groups. The improvement in accuracy seen between childhood (mean age 9 years) and adulthood in WS (mean age 28) was much smaller than that seen in only 1 year (between age 4/5 and 6/7) in the typically developing group. Not only was development slower in the WS group, it was also qualitatively different. The variability of responses to this task decreased with age in both groups. However, in the WS group, the variability was less likely centered around the correct response than in the typically developing groups. Ansari and colleagues suggest that the poor performance of the WS group at estimating the number of dots in rapidly presented arrays might arise from difficulty in mapping cognitive representations of amount to a verbal "five" or symbolic "5" outputs. This could be due to a lack of clear cognitive representations of numerosity on which to base these other outputs. A similar difficulty may also give rise to problems demonstrated with tasks from the number battery in the Paterson *et al.* study. Ansari's data highlight the importance of investigating the developmental trajectory and not just the end state. Atypically developing individuals might not only exhibit slowed development but also a qualitatively different path.

These data also highlight the importance of characterizing the infant phenotype. If the adult profile had been used to derive the infant profile, the presence of different starting states and divergent developmental trajectories would not have been discovered. In summary, while infants with WS appear to be able to extract numerosity information from a visual display, adults with WS are impaired on a numerosity comparison task. The opposite is true for DS. In the DS group, it appears numerosity understanding is delayed in infancy, but by adulthood, people with DS are using similar numerical processes to normal controls. By contrast, it is likely that individuals with WS are using a different strategy to deal with numerosity throughout development, which they continue to rely on unsuccessfully for tasks involving more complex numerical processing, such as the conversion of an analog magnitude representation of number into its corresponding symbolic representation, such as an Arabic numeral.

Further research into developmental trajectories of numerical cognition might lead to better understanding of how it is that infants with WS can discriminate numerosities, and what causes their difficulties in later life. An impairment in their magnitude representation or their access to it is a recurring candidate (Ansari *et al.*, 2003; Paterson *et al.*, 2006). Alternatively, or perhaps in addition, adults with WS may be relying on a feature-based strategy to encode and compare numerosities. By this approach, known as the object files model, infants individuate objects in each array, putting each object into a new internal memory file. Then they compare their representations of the objects in one array with the objects in the other and detect a mismatch (Carey, 1998; Huttenlocher *et al.*, 1994; Simon, 1997; Uller *et al.*, 1999). This strategy would work for small numerosities but would break down for numerosities larger than 4, after which there are too many records to maintain in memory. This strategy could lead to success in the infant task but would lead to difficulties with more complex tasks faced in later childhood and adulthood that require the manipulation of larger quantities.

Face processing

In addition to the importance of studying the process of development, it is also important to consider very carefully the nature of the behavior being measured. Studies of atypically developing populations have revealed that similar levels of performance can arise from very different underlying cognitive processes and/or different neural pathways. This final section will discuss some studies of face processing conducted with individuals with WS and autism. The comparison between these groups provides an excellent illustration of the importance of going beyond standardized test scores in order to characterize underlying cognitive processing skills and developmental trajectories.

Several studies have reported that individuals with WS exhibit relatively good face processing skills despite generally poor visuo-spatial skills. Studies have shown WS subjects scoring within the normal range on standardized tests of face processing such as the Benton Facial Recognition Test (Deruelle *et al.*, 1999; Karmiloff-Smith, 1997; Udwin and Yule, 1991). As happened in the language domain, this had led to claims that face processing is a spared ability (Bellugi *et al.*, 1990). However, it is important to investigate the cognitive processes underlying these scores, because they may reveal that face processing is not as typical as it seems. It has been suggested that individuals with Williams syndrome rely more on individual features than the configural relationship between features when processing faces and other objects, such as cars or houses (Deruelle *et al.*, 1999; Karmiloff-Smith *et al.*, 1997). However, other studies have challenged this view (Deruelle *et al.*, 2003; Tager-Flusberg *et al.*, 1993; see Karmiloff-Smith *et al.*, 2004, for a discussion). Whatever strategy is used, it appears that the developmental trajectory for face processing in WS is atypical (Karmiloff-Smith *et al.*, 2004). As discussed in the section on language, in order to characterize the process of development fully, it is necessary to examine changes in a domain right from the outset through to adulthood, and to compare the developmental progression of the atypically developing group with that of controls at many stages of development. Karmiloff-Smith *et al.* (2004) did just that, enabling them to compare older children and adults with WS, from 12 to 54 years old, against the typical trajectory of face recognition built from data from typically developing children ranging from 2 to 11 years old. One main difference found between the trajectories for typically developing children and individuals with WS concerned the emergence of the inversion effect, which reflects the fact that faces are more difficult to process when they are upside down and therefore cannot be processed on the basis of configural information. Karmiloff-Smith *et al.* (2004) found that typically developing children become more sensitive to inversion as they get older. However, this was not the case for individuals with WS.

This difference in face processing between groups is also present at the neural level. In two different studies, electrophysiological responses of individuals with WS to faces were atypical. They did not show the typical increase in amplitude of the N170 component to inverted faces (Grice *et al.*, 2001), and the early part of their ERP waves (100–200 ms after onset of the stimulus) to faces was abnormal (Mills *et al.*, 2000). Even more interestingly, their responses also differed from those of individuals with autism. Individuals with autism are thought to rely heavily on featural processing, perhaps like their counterparts with WS (Deruelle *et al.*, 1999;

Frith, 1989). However, in contrast to the WS group, people with autism perform poorly on face processing tasks (e.g., Deruelle *et al.*, 2004; Grelotti *et al.*, 2002; Klin *et al.*, 1999). Despite the possibility that both may have similar underlying visual processing styles, their behavioral outcomes are rather different. At the electrophysiological level, although both groups exhibit a reduced inversion effect in the amplitude of the N170 (Grice *et al.*, 2001), they show differences in gamma band neural oscillations. These are low frequency oscillations in EEG, which are thought to be related to visual binding processes (Singer and Gray, 1995). Grice *et al.* (2001) hypothesized that given the atypical visual processing seen in WS and autism, gamma band oscillations to visual stimuli might also be atypical. This was the case. However, the nature of the responses of the two atypically developing groups differed. The group with autism exhibited gamma bursts to faces, like normal controls, but there was no difference in their gamma response to upright vs. inverted faces. The WS group, on the other hand, had no clear gamma bursts in either condition.

Individuals with WS appear to perform normally in standardized face tasks, whereas people with autism perform poorly. Despite this, both groups exhibit similar responses in one aspect of their electrophysiological response to faces. The possible decrease in second-order configural processing in both groups clearly does relate to their behavioral competency, pointing to the fact that individuals can shape their own development by seeking out certain environments. Individuals with WS are social and show great interest in faces beginning in infancy (Bertrand *et al.*, 1993; Laing *et al.*, 2002). This interest and thus great exposure might drive their competence. On the other hand, individuals with autism show little interest in faces and, therefore, do not build up this "expertise." Instead, they have to rely solely on general visual perception mechanisms to process faces, leading to less optimal recognition (Klin *et al.*, 2003).

In sum, these data demonstrate that, despite seemingly normal performance of individuals with WS on behavioral tests of face processing, both the cognitive processes and their underlying neural bases are different from those seen in controls and in people with autism. The results emphasize the great importance of taking a multi-modal approach to developmental disorders and examining development at many levels.

Conclusions

As this brief survey of studies on the developmental trajectory of language, number, and face processing has shown, atypical cognitive development is extremely complex and, although it seems obvious, the process of development must be taken into account when developing theories of development (Karmiloff-Smith, 1998). The adult neuropsychological model, with its static notion of impaired and intact cognitive domains, does not fit the developmental data. Atypical development must be traced right from its origins in infancy through to the adult endstate.

In the language domain, we have seen that, although language is relatively good in adults with WS, early language acquisition is seriously delayed as in individuals with DS. In addition, it appears that right from the outset the process by which individuals with WS acquire language is different from both typically developing infants and other atypically developing groups. In many cases they do not appear to follow the normal sequence of language milestones, nor do they appear to place the same emphasis on certain aspects of language, such as word meaning when learning new words.

For number, we see a complete dissociation in performance from infancy to adulthood in WS. While these individuals appear to be successful at discriminating small numerosities in infancy, they have significant impairments in adulthood. In contrast, individuals with DS have difficulties in infancy but appear to follow the expected trajectory, albeit at a slower pace. In this domain too we see that a possible reliance on a strategy of concentrating on local elements, which yields success in another domain, may be detrimental for number. It appears that an individual with WS may be very focused on individual dots in arrays and are slow to process the overall numerosity of the array.

The work on face processing further emphasizes the importance of going beyond test scores when interpreting developmental data. These studies show that very different cognitive processes can underlie similar test performance. While face processing in WS might seem "intact," the process by which these individuals achieve their normal test performance may not be typical. In fact, inspection of electro-physiological data reveals that, at this level, there are marked differences not only between the WS and typically developing groups but also between autism and WS.

It is important to remember that the brains of children with genetic disorders *develop differently* right from the outset at embryogenesis. Small changes in gene dosage can have cascading effects both on the expression of other genes and the production of proteins. The complexity of genetic effects should not be taken for granted, and it is important to remember that genes code for proteins and not for neurons or specific cognitive abilities. Even tiny changes in the genome may mean that these children have differences in brain anatomy, neurochemistry, and even in the timing of periods of brain growth. Small differences in neuronal wiring, for instance, may cause them to have different biases toward certain stimuli and this may lead to the use of different processing strategies (Elman *et al.*, 1996; Karmiloff-Smith, 1998). As we have seen with the example of featural processing, a strategy that is helpful in one domain may cause problems if employed atypically in another domain. Small, seemingly general biases or strategies can lead to a distinct pattern of cognitive strengths and weaknesses.

In future work, we must gather converging data from a variety of sources, because, as these studies have shown, findings at one level of description, for example from electrophysiology, can paint an extremely different picture from those at another level such as performance on a standardized test. It is also important to try and develop measures that are as sensitive as possible in order to try examine areas in which, despite seemingly normal performance on more coarse behavioral measures, the participant has compensated for weakness over the course of development. For example, while accuracy on a particular task may be within the normal range, a measure of reaction time might reveal slower performance and thereby point to a deficit that has been compensated (Karmiloff-Smith, 1998).

These findings stress the importance of tracing cognitive abilities from the infant start state and studying the process of development rather than making assumptions using data from the endstate, which has so often been the case. The studies suggest that, despite similar starting states in many disorders, complex interactions between subtle in-built biases and the environment can lead to remarkable differences in the endstate. If one takes a rigidly static view of WS and DS, the following scenario would arise. Adults with WS do well on standardized test of vocabulary, which suggests that vocabulary is a spared ability, whereas adults with DS perform poorly. If one were to characterize infants in these groups by this view, one would expect those with DS to be delayed and those with WS to be like typically developing infants. Infants with WS would, therefore, be likely to receive very little early intervention because in this group, even if there is a little delay, language will end up being intact. In contrast, by taking a more dynamic approach, we can see that development is different right from the outset in several different areas of language and in related cognitive skills that normally play a role in language development. Furthermore, careful dissection of cognitive processes in adulthood, even in an area of relative skill, reveals subtle impairments. By this dynamic view, early intervention could be aimed at helping these children use the strategies that work for them to bolster development. With careful design of tasks and a multi-modal approach, we should be able to build upon these findings to take a truly developmental approach to developmental disorder.

REFERENCES

American Psychiatric Association. (2000). *Diagnostic and Statistical Manual of Mental Disorders*, 4th edn. Text Revision. Washington, DC: American Psychiatric Association.

Ansari, D., Donlan, C., & Karmiloff-Smith, A. (2007). Typical and atypical development of visual estimation abilities. *Cortex*, **6**, 758–68.

Ansari, D., Donlan, C., Thomas, M. S., Ewing, S. A., Peen, T., & Karmiloff-Smith, A. (2003). What makes counting count? Verbal and visuo-spatial contributions to typical and atypical number development. *Journal of Experimental Child Psychology*, **85**, 50–62.

Bates, E. (1997). Plasticity, localization and language development. In S. H. Broman & J. M. Fletcher (Eds.), *The Changing Nervous System: Neurobehavioral Consequences of Early Brain Disorders* (pp. 214–53). New York: Oxford University Press.

Bates, E., Benigni, L., Bretherton, I., Camaioni, I., & Volterra, V. (1979). *The Emergence of Symbols, Cognition, and Communication in Infancy*. New York: Academic Press.

Bellugi, U., Bihrle, A., Jernigan, T., Trauner, D., & Doherty, S. (1990). Neuropsychological, neurological, and neuroanatomical profile of Williams syndrome. *American Journal of Medical Genetics*, **6**, 115–25.

Bertrand, J., Mervis, C. B., Rice, C. E., & Adamson, L. (1993). Development of joint attention by a toddler with Williams syndrome. Paper presented at the Gatlinburg Conference on Research and Theory in Mental Retardation and Developmental Disabilities, Gatlinburg, TN.

Brock, J. (2007). Language abilities in Williams syndrome: A critical review. *Development and Psychopathology*, **19**, 97–127.

Brown, J. H., Johnson, M. H., Paterson, S. J., Gilmore, R., Longhi. E., & Karmiloff-Smith, A. (2003). Spatial representation and attention in toddlers with Williams syndrome and Down syndrome. *Neuropsychologia*, **41**, 1037–46.

Carey, S. (1998). Knowledge of number: Its evolution and ontogeny. *Science*, **282**, 641–2.

Caycho, L., Gunn, P., & Siegal, M. (1991). Counting by children with Down's syndrome. *American Journal on Mental Retardation*, **95**, 575–83.

CDC. (2007). Prevalence of autism spectrum disorders-autism and developmental disabilities monitoring network, 14 Sites, United States, 2002. *MMWR Surveillance Summaries*, **56**, 12–28.

Cipolotti, L., Butterworth, B., & Denes, G. (1991). A specific deficit for numbers in a case of dense acalculia. *Brain*, **114**, 2619–37.

Clearfield, M. W. & Mix, K. S. (1999). Number versus contour length in infants' discrimination of small visual sets. *Psychological Science*, **10**, 408–11.

Dehaene, S. (1989). The psychophysics of numerical comparison: A reexamination of apparently incompatible data. *Perception and Psychophysics*, **45**(6), 557–66.

Dehaene, S. & Cohen, L. (1994). Dissociable mechanisms of subitizing and counting: Neuropsychological evidence from simultanagnosis patients. *Journal of Experimental Psychology: Human Perception and Performance*, **20**, 958–75.

Deruelle, C., Mancini, J., Livet, J. O., Casse-Perrot, C. & de Schonen, S. (1999). Configural and local processing of faces in children with Williams syndrome. *Brain and Cognition*, **41**, 276–98.

Deruelle, C., Rondan, C., Gepner, B., & Tardif, C. (2004). Spatial frequency and face processing in children with autism and Asperger syndrome. *Journal of Autism and Developmental Disorders*, **34**, 199–210.

Deruelle, C., Rondan, C., Mancini, J., & Livet, M. (2003). Exploring face processing in Williams syndrome. *Cognitie, Creier, Comportanent*, **7**, 157–71.

Donnai, D. & Karmiloff-Smith, A. (2000). Williams syndrome: From genotype through to the cognitive phenotype. *American Journal of Medical Genetics: Seminars in Medical Genetics*, **97**(2), 164–71.

Elman, J., Bates, E., Johnson, M. H., Karmiloff-Smith, A., Parisi, D., & Plunkett, K. (1996). *Rethinking Innateness: A Connectionist Perspective on Development*. Cambridge, MA: MIT Press.

Franco, F. & Wishart, J. G. (1995). Use of pointing and other gestures by young children with Down syndrome. *American Journal on Mental Retardation*, **100**(2), 160–82.

Frith, U. Autism: Explaining the Enigma. Oxford: Blackwell; 1989.

Golinkoff, R. M., Mervis, C. B., & Hirsh-Pasek, K. (1994). Early object labels: The case for a developmental lexical principles framework. *Journal of Child Language*, **21**(1), 125–55.

Gray, V., Karmiloff-Smith, A., Funnell, E., & Tassabehji, M. (2006). In-depth analysis of spatial cognition in Williams syndrome: A critical assessment of the role of the LIMK1 gene. *Neuropyschologia*, **44**(5), 679–85.

Grelotti, D. J., Gauthier, I., & Schultz, R. T. (2002). Social interest and the development of cortical face specialization: What autism teaches us about face processing. *Developmental Psychobiology*, **40**, 213–25.

Grice, S. J., Spratling, M. W., Karmiloff-Smith, A., *et al.* (2001). Disordered visual processing and oscillatory brain activity in autism and Williams syndrome. *Neuroreport*. **12**(12), 2697–700.

Huttenlocher, J., Jordan, N. C., & Levine, S. C. (1994). A mental model for early arithmetic. *Journal of Experimental Psychology: General*, **123**(3), 284–96.

Järvinen-Pasley, A., Bellugi, U., Reilly, J., *et al.* (2008). Defining the social phenotype in Williams syndrome: A model for linking gene, brain, and cognition. *Development and Psychopathology*, **20**, 1–35.

Johnson, M. H. (1997). *Developmental Cognitive Neuroscience: An Introduction*. Oxford: Blackwell.

Johnson, S. C. (2000). The recognition of mentalistic agents in infancy. *Trends in Cognitive Sciences*, **4**, 22–8.

Jusczyk, P. W., & Aslin, R. N. (1995). Infants' detection of the sound patterns of words in fluent speech. *Cognitive Psychology*, **29**, 1–23.

Jusczyk, P. W., Houston, D. M., & Newsome, M. (1999). The beginnings of word segmentation in English- learning infants. *Cognitive Psychology*, **39**, 159–207.

Karmiloff-Smith, A. (1997). Crucial differences between developmental cognitive neuroscience and adult neuropsychology. *Developmental Neuropsychology*, **13**, 513–24.

Karmiloff-Smith, A. (1998). Development itself is the key to understanding developmental disorders. *Trends in Cognitive Sciences*, **2**, 389–98.

Karmiloff-Smith, A., Brown, J. H., Grice, S., & Paterson, S. J. (2002). Dethroning the myth: Cognitive dissociations and innate modularity in Williams syndrome. *Developmental Neuropsychology*, **23**, 227–43.

Karmiloff-Smith, A., Grant, J., Berthoud, I., Davies, M., Howlin, P., & Udwin, O. (1997). Language and Williams Syndrome: How intact is "intact"? *Child Development*, **68**, 246–62.

Karmiloff-Smith, A., Scerif G., & Ansari, D. (2003). Double dissociations in developmental disorders? Theoretically misconceived, empirically dubious. *Cortex*, **39**, 161–3.

Karmiloff-Smith, A., Scerif, G., & Thomas, M. (2002). Different approaches to relating genotype to phenotype in developmental disorders. *Developmental Psychobiology*, **40**, 311–22.

Karmiloff-Smith, A., Thomas, M., Annaz, D., *et al*. (2004). Exploring the Williams syndrome face processing debate: The importance of building developmental trajectories. *Journal of Child Psychology and Psychiatry*, **45**(7), 1258–74.

Karmiloff-Smith, A., Tyler, L. K., Voice, K., *et al.* (1998). Linguistic dissociations in Williams syndrome: Evaluating receptive syntax in on-line and off-line tasks. *Neuropsychologia*, **36**(4), 342–51.

Katz, L. C., & Shatz, C. J. (1996). Synaptic activity and the construction of cortical circuits. *Science*, **274**, 1133–8.

Kellman, P. J., & Spelke, E. S. (1983). Perception of partly occluded objects in infancy. *Cognitive Psychology*, **15**, 483–524.

Klein, B. P., & Mervis, C. B. (1999). Contrasting patterns of cognitive abilities of 9- and 10-year olds with Williams syndrome or Down syndrome. *Developmental Neuropsychology*, **16**, 177–96.

Klin, A., Jones, W., Schultz, R. T., & Volkmar, F. (2003). The enactive mind, or from actions to cognition: Lessons from autism. *Philosophical Transactions of the Royal Society of London. B. Biological Science*, **358**(1430), 345–60.

Klin, A., Jones, W., Schultz, R. T., Volkmar, F., & Cohen, D. J. (2002). Visual fixation patterns during viewing of naturalistic social situations as predictors of social competence in individuals with autism. *Archives of General Psychiatry*, **59**, 809–16.

Klin, A., Sparrow, S. S., de Bildt, A., Cicchetti, D. V., Cohen, D. J., & Volkmar, F. R. (1999). A normed study of face recognition in autism and related disorders. *Journal of Autism & Developmental Disorders*, **29**, 499–508.

Laing, E., Butterworth, G., Ansari, D., *et al.* (2002). Atypical linguistic and socio-communicative development in toddlers with Williams syndrome. *Developmental Science*, **5**(2), 233–46.

Mervis, C. B., & Bertrand, J. (1997). Developmental relations between cognition and language: Evidence from Williams syndrome. In: L. B. Adamson & M. A. Romski (Eds.), *Research on Communication and Language Disorders: Contributions to Theories of Language Development* (pp. 75–106). New York: Brookes.

Mervis, C. B., Morris, J., Bertrand, J., & Robinson, B. F. (1999). Williams syndrome: Findings from an integrated program of research. In H. Tager-Flusberg (Ed.), *Neurodevelopmental Disorders* (pp. 65–110). Cambridge, MA: MIT Press.

Mills, D. L., Alvarez, T. D., St. George, M., Appelbaum, L. G., Bellugi, U., & Neville, H. (2000). Electrophysiological studies of face processing in Williams syndrome. *Journal of Cognitive Neuroscience*, **12**(Suppl.), 47–64.

Morton, J., & Johnson, M. H. (1991). CONSPEC and CONLERN: A two-process theory of infant face recognition. *Psychological Review*, **98**, 164–81.

Moyer, R. S. & Landauer, T. K. (1967). Time required for judgments of numerical inequality. *Nature*, **215**, 1519–20.

Mundy, P., Card, J., & Fox, N. (2000). EEG correlates of the development of infant joint attention skills. *Developmental Psychobiology*, **36**, 325–38.

Mundy, P. & Hogan, A. (1996). *A Preliminary Manual for the Abridged Early Social Communication Scales (ESCS)*. Available through the University of Miami, Department of Psychology, Coral Gables, Florida: www.psy.miami.edu/

Nazzi, T. & Gopnik, A. (2001). Linguistic and cognitive abilities in infancy: When does language become a tool for categorization? *Cognition*, **80**, B11–B20.

Nazzi, T. & Karmiloff-Smith, A. (2002). Visual- and name-based object categorization by children with Williams syndrome. *Neuroreport*, **13**, 1259–62.

Nazzi, T., Paterson, S., & Karmiloff-Smith, A. (2003). Early word segmentation by infants and toddlers with Williams syndrome. *Infancy*, **4**(2), 251–72.

Neville, H., et al. (1991). Syntactically based sentence processing classes: Evidence from event-related brain potentials. *Journal of Cognitive Neuroscience*, **3**, 151–65.

Nye, J., Clibbens, J., & Bird, G. (1995). Numerical ability, general ability and language in children with Down's Syndrome. *Down's Syndrome: Research and Practice*, **3**(3), 92–103.

O'Donnell, W. T., & Warren, S. T. (2002). A decade of molecular studies of fragile X syndrome. *Annual Review of Neuroscience*, **25**, 315–38.

O'Roak, B. & State, M. (2008). Autism genetics: Strategies, challenges, and opportunities. *Autism Research*, **1**, 4–17.

Paterson, S. (2000). *The Development of Language and Number Understanding in Williams Syndrome and Down Syndrome: Evidence from the Infant and Mature Phenotypes*. Unpublished doctoral thesis, University College London.

Paterson, S. J., Brown, J. H., Gsodl, M. K., Johnson, M. H., & Karmiloff-Smith, A. D. (1999). Cognitive modularity and genetic disorders. *Science*, **286**(5448), 2355–8.

Paterson, S., Girelli, L., Butterworth, B., & Karmiloff-Smith, A. (2006). Are numerical difficulties syndrome specific? Evidence from Williams syndrome and Down Syndrome. *Journal of Child Psychology and Psychiatry*. **47**(2), 190–204.

Pinker, S. (1994). *The Language Instinct*. New York, NY: Harper Collins Publishers, Inc.

Posner, M. I. & Petersen, S. E. (1990). The attention system of the human brain. *Annual Review of Neuroscience*, **13**, 25–42.

Saffran, J. R., Newport, E. L., & Aslin, R. N. (1996). Word segmentation: The role of distributional cues. *Journal of Memory and Language*, **35**, 606–21.

Scerif, G. & Karmiloff-Smith, A. (2005). The dawn of cognitive genetics? Crucial developmental caveats. *Trends in Cognitive Sciences*, **3**, 126–35.

Scerif, G., Karmiloff-Smith, A., Campos, R., Elsabbagh, M., Driver, J., & Cornish, K. (2005). To look or not to look? Typical and atypical development of oculomotor control. *Journal of Cognitive Neuroscience*, **4**, 591–604.

Simon, T. J. (1997). Reconceptualizing the origins of number knowledge: A non-numerical account. *Cognitive Development*, **3**, 349–72.

Singer, W. & Gray, C. M. (1995). Visual feature integration and the temporal correlation hypothesis. *Annual Review of Neuroscience* **18**, 555–86.

Singer Harris, N. G., Bellugi, U., Bates, E., Jones, W., & Rossen M. (1997). Contrasting profiles of language development in children with Williams and Down syndrome. *Developmental Neuropsychology*, **13**(3), 345–70.

Stevens, T. & Karmiloff-Smith, A. (1997). Word learning in a special population: Do individuals with Williams syndrome obey lexical constraints? *Journal of Child Language*, **24**, 737–65.

Stiles, J. (1998). The effects of early focal brain injury on lateralization of cognitive function. *Current Directions in Psychological Science*, **7**(1), 21–6.

Strømme, P., Bjørnstad, P. G., & Ramstad, K. (2002). Prevalence estimation of Williams syndrome. *Journal of Child Neurology*, **17**, 269–71.

Tager-Flusberg, H. (1993). What language reveals about the understanding of mind in children with autism. In Baron-Cohen, S., Tager-Flusberg, H., & Cohen, D. (Eds.). *Understanding Other Minds: Perspectives From Autism* (pp. 138–57). Oxford, England: Oxford University Press.

Tamanini, F., Willemsen, R., van Unen, L., *et al*. (1997). Differential expression of FMR1, FXR1 and FXR2 proteins in human and brain testis. *Human Molecular Genetics*, **6**, 1315–22.

Temple, C. M. (1997). Cognitive neuropsychology and its applications to children. *Journal of Child Psychology and Psychiatry*, **38**, 27–52.

Thomas, M. S. C., Grant, J., Barham, Z., *et al*. (2001). Past tense formation in Williams syndrome. *Language and Cognitive Processes*, **2**(16), 143–76.

Thomas, M. S. C., & Karmiloff-Smith, A. (2005). Can developmental disorders reveal the component parts of the human language faculty? *Language Learning and Development*, **1**(1), 65–92.

Udwin, O., Davies, M., & Howlin, P. (1996). A longitudinal study of cognitive abilities and educational attainment in Williams syndrome. *Developmental Medicine and Child Neurology*, **38**, 1020–9.

Udwin, O. & Yule, W. (1991). A cognitive and behavioural phenotype in Williams syndrome. *Journal of Clinical and Experimental Neuropsychology*, **13**, 232–44.

Uller, C., Carey, S., Huntley-Fenner, G., & Klatt, L. (1999). What representations might underlie infant numerical knowledge? *Cognitive Development*, **14**(1), 1–36.

Volkmar, F., Chawarska, K., & Klin, A. (2005). Autism in infancy and early childhood. *Annual Review of Psychology*, **56**, 12.1–12.22.

Volterra, V., Capirci, O., Pezzini, G., Sabbadini, L., & Vicari, S. (1996). Linguistic abilities in Italian children with Williams syndrome. *Cortex*, **32**, 663–77.

Zwaigenbaum, L., Bryson, S., & Rogers, T. (2005). Behavioral manifestations of autism in the first year of life. *International Journal of Developmental Neuroscience*, **23**(2–3), 143–52.

9

The use of strategies in embedded figures: Tasks by boys with and without organic mild mental retardation: A review and some experimental evidence

Anastasia Alevriadou and Helen Tsakiridou

The field dependent–independent cognitive style and role of simultaneous and successive processes

Educators and researchers have long recognized the unique differences among individuals and the effects these differences can have on learning. Concern for these differences led to research on the cognitive variables or cognitive styles that individuals possess (Tamaoka, 1985). Green (1985) defines cognitive style as consistencies in the ways in which people perceive, think, respond to others, and react to their environment. He contends that cognitive styles are bipolar, value neutral, consistent across domains, and stable over time. With nearly 5,000 references in the literature, field dependence/independence has received the most attention by researchers of all the cognitive styles (Chinien & Boutin, 1993; Harold, 1996; Kent-Davis & Cochran, 1989).

The Field Dependent–Independent cognitive style was hypothesized by Herman Witkin (e.g., Witkin, 1950; Witkin & Goodenough, 1981) and refers to the extent to which a person is dependent vs. independent in organization of the surrounding perceptual field. Measures of cognitive style provide a more extensive and more functional characterization of the child than could be derived from IQ tests alone (Messick, 1984).

A principal measure of field dependence–independence is the Embedded Figures Test (e.g., Children's Embedded Figures Test by Karp & Konstadt, 1971; The Diagnostic Embedded Figures Test by Aalders & Pennings, 1981), in which children locate a previously seen simple figure within a larger, complex figure (pattern). Bowd (1976) stated that embedded figures tests are the most widely used measures designed to assess field dependence–independence in children.

Witkin (1950) noted that field-dependent individuals tend to operate in a global manner and be distracted by background elements, while field-independent individuals tend to abstract an item from the surrounding field, following a more analytical approach, which means greater aptitude for restructuring (i.e., imposing organization on received information). Children with mental retardation show a field-dependent mode of perceiving (Shah & Frith, 1993; Witkin & Goodenough, 1981). Nesbit and Chambers (1976), using the Children's Embedded Figures Test, found that children with cultural–familial mental retardation performed significantly worse than their MA-matched peers without mental retardation. Similarly, Bice *et al.* (1986) showed that boys without mental retardation were more field-independent than those with mental retardation. The difference is that boys with mental retardation remain field-dependent, while boys without mental retardation start as field-dependent and become more field-independent, as they get older (Alevriadou *et al.*, 2004).

The results from many studies (Pascual-Leone & Goodman, 1979; Span, 1973) are equivocal with respect to the role of information-processing strategies in the Embedded Figures Test. For example, Span (1973) examined the written reports of 35 participants on problem solving strategies employed while trying to solve the Embedded Figures Test. The participants were divided into three groups based on their written reports: participants that used globalizing strategies; those that used analyzing strategies; and those who were unable to explain their approach. It seems that the bipolar dimension of the global vs. analytical way of perceiving (Witkin *et al.*, 1962) is too limited, particularly for interpreting the results of children and special populations (Alevriadou *et al.*, 2004; Hardy *et al.*, 1987).

A growing body of research (Palmer, 1977; Pennings, 1988) converges on a theory in which executive strategies for a successful solution can be located on a bipolar dimension, with simultaneous (holistic, synthetic, figurative strategies at one extreme and successive (analytic, serialistic) strategies at the other extreme. From a theoretical point of view, both modes of processing are in accordance with the definitions of simultaneous and successive processing in the model of cognitive abilities proposed by Das and colleagues (Das, 2002; Das *et al.*, 1979; Naglieri *et al.*, 1990).

Simultaneous processes allow the individual to integrate stimuli into groups in which each component of the stimulus array must be interrelated with every other element. Simultaneous processing has the element of surveyability, because the components of the task are interrelated and accessible to inspection either through examination of the actual stimuli during the activity or through memory of the stimuli. Successive processes provide the integration of stimuli into a serial order in which the elements form a chainlike progression. The distinguishing quality of successive processing is that the elements are related only linearly (Das *et al.*, 1979; Naglieri *et al.*, 1990).

Das *et al.* (1979) anticipated that simultaneous processing would be manifested in tests of field-dependence, although Naglieri (1989) suggested that the possibility of applying simultaneous or successive strategies could be minimized or maximized by the form of the presented task or the instruction given. Span (1980) suggested, by analogy to Zaporozhets' studies on training of visualization strategies (Zaporozhets, 1965), that the development of actions in embedded figures tasks might be conceptualized as a process of internalization in which different stages are distinguished. Actions executed in the earliest stage on a sensory–motor level are followed by external models. In a later stage, they are carried out on a mental level with an internal representation. Initially, the actions on a mental level are executed slowly and successively in an extensive manner. Later on, these actions are shortened and executed simultaneously. To enable research on typically developing children's use of restructuring strategies in solving embedded figures tasks, Pennings (1988) introduced a new administration procedure. He used (1) the simultaneous strategy, (2) the successive strategy, (3) the externalized-successive strategy, and (4) the global-manipulatory strategy.

In the externalized-successive strategy, the children carry out the successive strategy in a sensory–motor way. First, the children have to place iron bars, which have a bright color on one end, on the simple figure in a counter-clockwise fashion. Then, they have to identify and copy the same figure in the complex pattern using an identical set of bars. In the global-manipulatory strategy, the child moves a transparent, cutout of the simple figure over the different configurations, with which a complex pattern has been constructed, until he or she thinks that the cutout covers the hidden figure.

In the administration procedure, the four strategies that a child can apply are induced by means of prescriptions (i.e., sets of directions about what he or she has to do to solve an embedded figures task). The four sets of problem-solving instructions are presented in a fixed sequence from (1) to (4). Pennings (1988) proposed that a person with a high level of knowledge and operations would be able to solve a task using the simultaneous strategy instructions, whereas a person with a relatively low level can, after a failure, make use of the instructions for strategies (2), (3), or (4). His hypotheses were justified, as relatively high frequencies of global-manipulatory strategy use were found in 5-year-old typically developing children, which decreased in favor of the externalized-successive and successive strategies in the 7-year-old typically developing children. In the second investigation, Pennings (1990) predicted that the four strategies could be scaled on one restructuring-in-perception variable. Development follows a path from the global-manipulatory to the simultaneous strategy, going through the externalized-successive and the successive strategy in that order.

Strategy competencies and deficits in individuals with mental retardation

Previous research has shown that individuals with mental retardation are less likely to develop, use, monitor, regulate, evaluate, and transfer cognitive strategies than typically developing individuals (Belmont & Mitchell, 1987; Pressley & Hilden, 2006). Their difficulties in planning strategies are reflected in their low scores on measures of simultaneous and successive processes (Bardos, 1987; Das *et al.*, 1979), suggesting that individuals with mental retardation are strategically deficient (Bray, 1987). In contrast to a substantial literature showing deficiencies in the use of verbally based strategies, more recent studies (Bray *et al.*, 1994; Fletcher & Bray, 1995; Fletcher *et al.*, 2003) suggest that children with mental retardation show competence on tasks allowing external representation as a memory cue. Bray *et al.* (1994) showed that 11-year-old children with mental retardation and 7-year-old children without mental retardation used more object-oriented external strategies (pointing, holding, and moving the objects) than did 11-year-old children without mental retardation. But as they grow older, children without mental retardation start to rely on both internal (verbal) and external strategies, particularly children older than age 7. This pattern of results indicated that individuals with mental retardation have strategy capabilities that are underestimated by the use of verbally based tasks. In tasks that allow external representation, children and adolescents with mental retardation demonstrate considerably more strategy competency than they do on verbally based tasks.

Bray *et al.* (1997) noted that relatively few studies of memory strategies have included children with mental retardation in more than one age group. Bray *et al.* (1985) found that the proportion of subjects with mental retardation using rehearsal increased from 19% to 31% between 11-, 15-, and 18-years of age, indicating that there are developmental changes in strategy competency in adolescents with mental retardation. In a similar study of individuals without mental retardation in the same age range, the proportion of individuals using a selective rehearsal strategy increased from 25% to 75%, indicating that the rate of change in strategy use is greater in adolescents without mental retardation (Bray *et al.*, 1985). Virtually all of these studies have shown that children with mental retardation display a developmental increase in strategy capabilities (Bray *et al.*, 1985; Brown & Barclay, 1976). In addition to these cross-sectional studies of strategy development, there has been one longitudinal study of children with mental retardation. Turner *et al.* (1996) tested a group of 10-year-old students with and without mental retardation each year for 3 years on several memory tasks. Developmental changes were consistent across the two groups. Although the number of cross-sectional studies is very small and there is only one longitudinal study, the results of these studies provide consistent evidence for developmental changes in the strategy competency of children and adolescents with mental retardation. These children show a developmental progression from little strategy use to more widespread use of strategies. The rate of progress for individuals without mental retardation was faster than for those with mental retardation, although individuals with mental retardation demonstrated a consistent rate of development (Bray *et al.*, 1997). As Bray *et al.* (1997) have contended, to understand strategy capabilities, investigators must more fully explore developmental changes in both the strengths and the weaknesses of individuals with mental retardation rather than focusing nearly exclusively on their deficits.

The present study was designed to assess the development of strategies used for solving embedded figures tasks in boys with and without mental retardation of lower and higher mental age. In this study, the etiology of the subjects' mental retardation was restricted to organic mental retardation of nongenetic origin and the participants were all males due to well-documented gender differences in cognitive style (e.g., Diamond *et al.*, 1983; Johnson & Mead, 1987; Kerns & Berenbaum, 1991).

Method

Participants

The sample of the study consisted of 60 young individuals. To test the strategies used, the 60 participants were further subdivided into four groups (n = 15) matched on mean mental age, using the Raven's Colored Progressive Matrices (Raven, 1965): two groups of boys with mental retardation (Group A and Group B) and two groups of typically developing boys (Group C and Group D). Group A and Group C were matched on mental age at 5.7 years. Group B and Group D were matched on mental age at 8.1 years. Each pair of groups differed significantly in mean chronological age.

Group A was composed of 15 boys with organic mild mental retardation ranging in chronological age from 9 to 11 years *(M = 9.8 years, SD = 0.65)*, with a mean mental age of 5.7 years *(SD = 0.83)*. Six of the participants were premature and had anoxia at birth, three had postnatal head trauma, two had encephalitis, one was infected with rubella in utero, and three had epilepsy. All of the boys were receiving special education, and none were living in institutional settings.

Group C consisted of 15 boys without mental retardation with chronological ages ranging from 5 to 5.4 years (M = 5.2 years, SD = 0.35) and a mean mental age of 5.7 years (SD = 0.85). All participants were recruited from preschool/kindergarten classes.

Group B was composed of 15 boys with organic mild mental retardation ranging in chronological age from 11 to 14 years *(M = 13.0 years, SD = 1.47)*. The mean mental age was 8.1 years (*SD* = 0.52). Seven of the participants were premature and had anoxia at birth, three had postnatal head trauma, two had encephalitis, and the remaining three had epilepsy. All boys were attending special classes and none were living in institutional settings.

Group D consisted of 15 boys without mental retardation with chronological ages ranging from 7.0 to 7.7 years (*M* = 7.4 years, *SD* = 0.23). All of the boys were recruited from primary schools. The mean mental age for this group was 8.1 years (*SD* = 0.43).

Groups A and C were the lower mental age groups (*M* = 5.7 years) and groups B and D were the higher mental age groups (*M* = 8.1 years).

Instrumentation

A modified version of The Diagnostic Embedded Figures Test by Aalders and Pennings (1981) (see Pennings, 1990) was used for the measurement of field dependence–independence. It consisted of six geometric patterns with six different accompanying simple figures. There were two training items which served to acquaint participants with the task and with the four sets of instructions. The purpose of the six test items was to determine which set of instructions participants used to successfully solve the problems.

The lines of the simple figure and the hidden figure within the complex pattern had lengths of 2, 4, and 6 cm, and all of the lines (of the simple as well as the complex figure) were 4 mm in width. All drawings had been printed with black ink on white paper (30 × 21 cm). Each pair of simple figure and complex pattern were drawn on one page, with the simple figure in the upper left quadrant, above the complex pattern in the lower right quadrant of the page. Each item was placed in a plastic cover and kept in a ring binder.

Internal consistency reliability coefficients for the modified version by Aalders and Pennings were .88 and .90 for Groups A and C, and .92 and .86 for Groups B and D, respectively. A coefficient alpha reliability estimate of .88 was found overall for the participants of this study.

Instruction

The instructions were exactly the same as those used by Pennings (1988). The test was individually administered to the participants in a quiet room. The administration was divided into two phases: an introduction phase and a diagnosis phase. In the first phase, the child was introduced to the task with a demonstration item, and to each of the strategies with four sets of instructions and four different practice items. In the second phase, the participants were administered six items with four sets of standardized instructions to induce strategies (1) to (4). The instructions given were as follows:

(1) The experimenter removed the cover sheet from the simple figure and said: "Now you may first have a look at the small figure. Try to remember the entire figure as well as possible." After 10 seconds, the experimenter removed the cover sheet from the complex pattern by shifting it upward over the simple figure and said "Look if you can see the hidden figure lying somewhere and trace it."

(2) "You may see both the small and the large figure. Try to find line after line of the small figure. When you have found the hidden figure completely, you may point it out."

(3) The experimenter removed the cover sheet from the simple figure and said: "You may first place the bars on the lines of the small figure." The experimenter then gave the child an identical set of bars, removed the cover sheet from the complex pattern and said: "You may take these bars and use them to find the hidden figure."

(4) The experimenter removed the cover sheet and said: "This cutout fits exactly in the small figure. You may move it over the large figure until you see the lines of the hidden figure along all sides of the cutout."

For each item, it was investigated with which instruction it was possible to find the solution. The instruction inducing the simultaneous strategy was given first (working time: 5 seconds). If the participant was not able to solve the item under these conditions, then he was presented with the same task again, but with the instruction to induce the successive strategy (working time: 55 seconds). If the participant failed again, the instruction belonging to the externalized-successive strategy was given (working time: 75 seconds). Finally, if he made an error, the same task was given but using the instructions for the global-manipulatory strategy (working time: 45 seconds).

Scoring

The strategy that the child used to successfully solve each of the six tasks was recorded for every participant. The experimenter recorded (1), (2), (3), or (4) for each task.

Results

For the independent variables, boys were categorized according to group (1: with mental retardation, 2: without mental retardation) and mental age (1: lower, 2: higher). The dependent variable was the strategy the boys used to solve the six embedded figures tasks: (1) the simultaneous strategy, (2) the successive strategy, (3) the externalized-successive strategy, and (4) the global-manipulatory strategy.

A hierarchical log linear model with backward elimination was used for each of the six tasks to test for interaction effects among the variables. The hierarchical log linear model after backward elimination of nonsignificant effects provided the best model, which, was then considered and applied in a custom logit model. In the logit model, strategy was the dependent variable, and group and mental age were the independent variables. For the analysis of the data, the statistical package SPSS 12 was used.

The log linear analysis revealed significant main effects of group and mental age for four out of six tasks, significant interaction between group and mental age for two tasks, and both significant main effects and interactions between group and mental age for one task. Detailed presentation of the results is described below.

Effect of group

For tasks 1, 2, 4, and 5, there was a significant main effect of group (Table 1). As it can be seen in Table 2 , boys without mental retardation used the first strategy more frequently than boys with mental retardation to solve task 1 (26:16), task 2 (26:18), task 4 (24:9), and task 5 (20:5). Only boys with mental retardation used the fourth strategy in tasks 1, 2, and 4; and 10 boys with mental retardation compared to 2 boys without mental retardation used the fourth strategy in task 5.

Effect of mental age

There was a main effect of mental age for tasks 1, 2, 4, and 5 (Table 1). Namely, boys of higher mental age used the first strategy more often than boys of lower mental age to solve task 1 (26:16), task 2 (27:17), task 4 (22:11), and task 5 (17:8). The fourth

Table 1. Significant log linear models of the data in six embedded figures tasks

Model	Task 1			Task 2			Task 3		
	L	df	p	L	df	p	L	df	p
Null	25.78	10	0.004	22.05	10	0.020	25.82	10	0.004
Due to Group	15.84	3	0.001	11.28	3	0.010			
Due to Mental Age	9.75	3	0.021	9.20	3	0.030			
Due to Group x Mental age							12.74	4	0.010
	Task 4			Task 5			Task 6		
	L	df	p	L	df	p	L	df	p
Null	46.40	10	0.000	39.67	10	0.000	36.79	10	0.000
Due to Group	29.35	3	0.000	22.56	3	0.000			
Due to Mental Age	12.63	3	0.006	13.18	3	0.004			
Due to Group x Mental Age				11.68	4	0.02	010.9	4	0.028

Table 2. Observed frequencies in strategies used by group and mental age in six embedded figures tasks

Task	Mental age	Group	Strategy			
			1	2	3	4
1	Lower	MR	5	2	2	6
		No MR	11	3	1	0
	Higher	MR	11	1	1	2
		No MR	15	0	0	0
2	Lower	MR	5	4	0	6
		No MR	12	3	0	0
	Higher	MR	13	1	0	1
		No MR	14	1	0	0
3	Lower	MR	4	6	1	4
		No MR	7	4	1	3
	Higher	MR	6	3	2	4
		No MR	15	0	0	0
4	Lower	MR	2	3	5	5
		No MR	9	6	0	0
	Higher	MR	7	2	1	4
		No MR	15	0	0	0
5	Lower	MR	3	4	3	5
		No MR	5	5	3	2
	Higher	MR	2	2	6	5
		No MR	15	0	0	0
6	Lower	MR	0	6	1	8
		No MR	8	6	1	0
	Higher	MR	7	1	0	7
		No MR	10	2	0	3

strategy was used more times by boys of lower mental age than by boys of higher mental age to solve task 1 (6:2), task 2 (6:1), task 4 (5:4), and task 5 (7:5) (Table 2).

Interactions

There was a significant interaction between group and mental age for tasks 3, 5, and 6 (Table 1). More specifically, in task 3, although more higher mental age boys without mental retardation (15 boys) used the first strategy than did lower mental age boys without mental retardation (7 boys), there was no difference between the lower and higher mental age groups with mental retardation (4:6). In task 5, although the first strategy was used by all the higher mental age boys without mental retardation and only by five lower mental age boys without mental retardation, it was used by approximately the same number of lower and higher mental age boys with mental retardation (2:3). Finally, for task 6, fewer boys with mental retardation of lower mental age used the first strategy than boys with mental retardation of higher mental age (0:7), whereas the number of boys without mental retardation using the first strategy did not significantly differ as a function of lower or higher mental age (8:10).

Discussion

The theoretical frame of reference in which four solution strategies are distinguished is very different from the theory on the embedded figures tasks of Witkin *et al.* (1962). The logit-model analysis of the data for the six embedded figures tasks showed very interesting results. For four of the six tasks, we found a significant difference in strategy profiles related to group. Boys without mental retardation showed relatively high frequencies of the simultaneous strategy, and to a lesser degree the successive strategy. Only a very small number of boys without mental retardation used the global-manipulatory strategy. In contrast, boys with mental retardation had high frequencies of the externalized-successive and the global manipulatory strategy. Although individuals with mental retardation have often been described as nonstrategic (Ellis, 1970), it appears from this investigation that boys with mental retardation are able to use, at least, the external strategies (the externalized successive strategy and the global-manipulatory strategy).

This finding is consistent with other studies (Bray *et al.*, 1994; Fletcher & Bray, 1995) that support the use of external strategies by individuals with mental retardation. Previous studies (Bebko & Luhaorg, 1998; Bray *et al.*, 1997) suggest that, although in nonlinguistic effortful tasks persons with mental retardation are often quite strategic, differences in organizational and elaborational strategies between samples with and without mental retardation are often not entirely eliminated. Even preschoolers without mental retardation use external representation and a variety of other types of strategies (successive and simultaneous). From the other side, the cognitive potential of children with mental retardation requires more external support, like holding and manipulating objects (third and fourth strategy). The pattern of strategy competency is also consistent with the idea that individuals with mental retardation may be restricted in the use of some strategies (the simultaneous strategy and to a lesser degree the successive strategy) due to working memory capacity needed for using these strategies (Spitz, 1979). For the simultaneous strategy, the boys have to keep in mind the shape, size, and position of the simple figure as a whole, whereas for the successive strategy, only a line of the simple figure must be held in mind.

The hypothesized differences in restructuring strategies in relation to mental age were confirmed. For four of the six tasks, we found a significant difference in strategy profiles that was related to mental age. Greater increases in strategy use were found in the higher mental age group than the lower mental age group. This finding is consistent with the study of Henry (2008), who suggested that the development of coding strategies in children with mental retardation is linked to increases in mental age.

According to the type of strategies used, 13–87% of the boys with mental retardation of higher mental age used the simultaneous strategy across the six tasks (instead of 0–33% in the lower mental age), whereas 67–100% of the boys without mental retardation of the same mental age used the strategy across the six tasks (instead of 33–80% in the lower mental age). It is very interesting that, although boys with mental retardation of higher mental age use mainly the simultaneous strategy, a large number of them (7–47%) still use the global-manipulatory strategy, probably showing some kind of cognitive inertia (Dulaney & Ellis, 1997; Ellis & Dulaney, 1991). Some boys with mental retard-ation of higher mental age may continue to be perseverative in their thinking. It is also possible that the group by mental age interaction, found in some tasks, occurs primarily when the simultaneous strategy is emerging in boys without mental retardation in higher mental age but has not yet developed in those with mental retardation.

Our results are consistent with previous findings (Bray *et al.*, 1997; Fletcher & Bray, 1995), showing a developmental progression in external strategy use by children with mental retardation. Those of higher mental age (8.1 years) used the simultaneous strategy more times (except task for 5) than those of lower mental age (5.7 years). The rate of progress for individuals without mental retardation was faster than for those with mental retardation, but there was consistent evidence of development for the individuals with mental retardation. Bray *et al.* (1985) found that the proportion of individuals with mental retardation using rehearsal strategies increased from 19% to 31%, whereas the proportion of individuals without mental retardation using such strategies increased from 25% to 75%. In our sample, the proportion of boys with mental retardation using the simultaneous strategy increased from 16.5% to 50%, whereas the proportion for boys without mental retardation using the strategy increased from 56.5% to 83.5%. The use of the simultaneous strategy found in both groups of higher mental age imparts a devel-opmental character to the differences, suggesting an improvement with increased cognitive maturity. That is not to say that individuals with mental retardation do not also have areas of weakness.

The role of visual selective attention seems to be of great importance, espe-cially if we take into consideration that persons with mental retardation are more distracted by the presence of irrelevant information in the stimulus (the simple figure on the embedded figures tasks is "hidden" within the complex figure) than are individuals without mental retardation (Cha & Merrill, 1994; Merrill & Taube, 1996). The selection of one stimulus over another is likely to involve not only facilitation or excitatory processes directed toward the selected target but also inhibition or suppression processes that operate to minimize responding to nontarget stimuli (Tipper, 1985). The individuals with mental retardation are less efficient in suppressing non-target information than those without mental retardation. Hence, this may result in performance decrements across a variety of tasks (Cha & Merrill, 1994). The ability of visual selective attention has not been fully developed in young children. But as they get older, individuals with mental retardation exhibit poorer selection skills and smaller suppression effects than do children without mental retardation (Hagen & Huntsman, 1971). In our study, as the figures became more complex (especially in tasks 5 and 6), needing greater amounts of suppression and selective skills, most of the boys with mental retardation used externalized-successive and the global manipulatory strategy, even in the higher mental age group.

Motivational factors can also partially explain the differences found in strategy use between boys with and without mental retardation (Merighi, Edison, & Zigler, 1990; Saldaňa, 2004). Strategy use is viewed as a complex cognitive phenomenon that is influenced by strategy knowledge and by motivational factors necessary to energize these strategies. One key factor hypothesized to affect strategy use is the history of failure in independent problem solving (Weisz, 1979). The greater the history of failure that children with mental retardation experience in applying their own solutions to problems, the greater the amount of outer-directedness (or reliance mainly on external cues rather than on their internal cognitive abilities to solve a task or problem) they show compared to children without mental retardation (Bybee & Zigler, 1998). Researchers generally report declines in outer-directedness among children without mental retardation at higher mental ages (MacMillan & Wright, 1974; Yando & Zigler, 1971). As children without mental retardation get older, they become more inner-directed and field independent, trusting their own solutions to problems. On the contrary, declines in outer-directedness are found much less consistently in children with mental retardation of higher mental age (Bybee & Zigler, 1998).

Feuerstein (1980) noted that persons with mental retardation don't use strategies spontaneously. His intervention program aims at transforming the passive cognitive style of individuals with mental retardation into one that is more characteristic of autonomous and independent thinkers, using mediated learning experiences. For example, spatial dimensions, which are critical in field dependence–independence tests, are among the cognitive functions whose development is strongly dependent upon mediated learning experiences, because they are based mainly upon relational thinking.

Analytically, the mediating agent (i.e., the teacher, the parent) selects and organizes environmental stimuli so as to facilitate successful cognitive processes. The mediator selects stimuli that are most appropriate and then frames, filters, and schedules them. Through this process of mediation, the cognitive structure of the child with mental retardation is affected. The child acquires behavior patterns, learning sets and operational structures (i.e., approaches to mentally organizing, manipulating, and acting upon information gained from external and internal sources). Thus, the effects of mediated learning experiences may be conceptualized as inducing in the child with mental retardation a great variety of orientations and strategies that become crystallized in the form of sets and habits and constitute the prerequisites for the modification of their cognitive style (Feuerstein, 1980). This theorization lends credibility to several reports on the effectiveness of mediated learning on individuals with mental retardation (e.g., Feuerstein *et al.*, 1979; Lifshitz & Rand, 1999).

The use of strategies has valuable implications for special education (Bray *et al.*, 1997). It appears that the knowledge of individual and group differences in strategy use, based on embedded figures tests, has not been exploited in the field of special education. External representation and other types of strategies that develop in young children (holding, searching) may be rich areas for future investigation of strategy competency in individuals with mental retardation, including those with neurogenetic disorders. The investigation and theoretical discussion of competencies along with deficits may result in the discovery and appropriate attention to a continuum of strategic behaviors and a clearer understanding of the factors that influence the discovery and use of strategies. As Bray *et al.* (1997) have contended, to understand strategy capabilities, investigators must more fully explore developmental changes in both the strengths and the weaknesses of individuals with mental retardation rather than focusing almost exclusively on their deficits. Furthermore, many researchers (Dermitzaki *et al.*, 2008; Saldaňa, 2004) are interested in investigating self-regulatory strategic behavior and metacognitive skills. Older and more recent studies have shown that, when instruction of individuals with mental retardation emphasizes self-regulated use of strategies, enhanced strategy use, improved performance, and motivation enhancement may occur (Agran *et al.*, 2005; Fletcher & Bray, 1995). Such an approach will make important contributions to a general theory of the cognitive nature of mental retardation. Furthermore, it might contribute to the development of appropriate educational interventions for children with intellectual disabilities of both acquired and genetic origins (Dermitzaki *et al.*, 2008).

REFERENCES

Aalders, A. P. R. & Pennings, A. H. (1981). Het verborgen-figuren diagnosticum. [The diagnostic embedded figures test]. *Pedagogische Studien*, **58**, 265–75.

Agran, M., Sinclair, T., Alper, S., Cavin, M., Wehmeyer, M., & Hughes, C. (2005). Using self-monitoring to increase following-direction skills of students with moderate to severe disabilities in general education. *Education and Training in Developmental Disabilities*, **40**, 3–13.

Alevriadou, A., Hatzinikolaou, K., Tsakiridou, H., & Grouios, G. (2004). Field dependence-independence of normally developing and mentally retarded boys of low and upper/middle socioeconomic status. *Perceptual and Motor Skills*, **99**, 913–23.

Bardos, A. N. (1987). *Differentiation of normal, reading disabled, and developmentally handicapped students using the Das-Naglieri cognitive processing tasks.* Unpublished doctoral dissertation, Ohio State University, Columbus, Ohio.

Bebko, J. M. & Luhaorg, H. (1998). The development of strategy use and metacognitive processing in mental retardation: Some sources of difficulty. In J. Burack, R. Hodapp, & E. Zigler (Eds.), *Handbook of Mental Retardation and Development* (pp. 382–407). Cambridge, UK: Cambridge University Press.

Belmont, J. M. & Mitchell, D. W. (1987). The general strategies hypothesis as applied to cognitive theory in mental retardation. *Intelligence*, **11**, 91–105.

Bice, T., Halpin, G., & Halpin, G. (1986). A comparison of the cognitive styles of typical and mildly retarded boys with educational recommendations. *Education and Training of the Mentally Retarded*, **33**, 93–7.

Bowd, A. (1976). Item difficulty on the Children's Embedded Figures Test. *Perceptual and Motor Skills*, **43**, 134.

Bray, N. W. (1987). Why are the retarded strategically deficient? *Intelligence*, **11**, 45–8.

Bray, N. W., Fletcher, K. L., & Turner, L. A. (1997). Cognitive competencies and strategy use in individuals with mild mental retardation. In W. E. MacLean, Jr. (Ed.), *Handbook of Mental Deficiency, Psychological Theory and Research*, 3rd edn. (pp. 197–217). Hillsdale, NJ: Erlbaum.

Bray, N. W., Hersh, R. E., & Turner, L. A. (1985). Selective remembering during adolescence. *Developmental Psychology*, **21**, 290–4.

Bray, N. W., Saarnio, D. A, Borges, L. M., & Hawk, L. W. (1994). Intellectual and developmental differences in external memory strategies. *American Journal on Mental Retardation*, **99**, 19–31.

Bray, N. W., Turner, L. A., & Hersh, R. E. (1985). Developmental progressions and regressions in the selective remembering strategies of EMR individuals. *American Journal of Mental Deficiency*, **90**, 198–205.

Brown, A. L. & Barclay, C. R. (1976). The effect of training specific mnemonics on the meta-mnemonic efficiency of retarded children. *Child Development*, **47**, 71–80.

Bybee, J. & Zigler, E. (1998). Outer-directedness in individuals with and without mental retardation: A review. In J. Burack, R. Hodapp, & E. Zigler (Eds.), *Handbook of Mental Retardation and Development* (pp. 461). Cambridge, UK: Cambridge University Press.

Cha, K. H. & Merrill, E. (1994). Facilitation and inhibition effects in visual selective attention processes of individuals with and without mental retardation. *American Journal on Mental Retardation*, **98**, 594–600.

Chinien, C. A. & Boutin, F. (1993). Cognitive style FOil: An important learner characteristic for educational technologists. *Journal of Educational Technology Systems*, **21**, 303–11.

Das, J. P. (2002). A better look at intelligence. *Current Directions in Psychological Science*, **11**(1), 28–33.

Das, J. P., Kirby, J. R., & Jarman, R. F. (1979). *Simultaneous and Successive Cognitive Processes*. New York: Academic Press.

Dermitzaki, I., Stavroussi, P., Bandi, M., & Nisiotou, I. (2008). Investigating ongoing strategic behaviour of students with mild mental retardation: Implementation and relations to performance in a problem solving situation. *Evaluation and Research in Education*, **21**, 96–110.

Diamond, R., Carey, S., & Back, K. J. (1983). Genetic influences on the development of spatial skills during early adolescence. *Cognition*, **13**, 167–85.

Dulaney, C. & Ellis, N. R. (1997). Rigidity in the behavior of mentally retarded persons. In W. E. Maclean (Ed.), *Ellis' Handbook of Mental Deficiency, Psychological Theory and Research* (pp. 175–195). Mahwah, NJ: Erlbaum.

Ellis, N. R. (1970). Memory processes in retardates and normals. In N. R. Ellis, (Ed.), *International Review of Research in Mental Retardation* (Vol. 4, pp. 132). New York: Academic Press.

Ellis, N. R. & Dulaney, C. (1991). Further evidence for cognitive inertia of persons with mental retardation. *American Journal on Mental Retardation*, **95**, 613–21.

Feuerstein, R. (1980). *The Instrumental Enrichment Method: An Intervention Program for Cognitive Modifiability*. Baltimore: University Park Press.

Feuerstein, R., Rand, Y., Hoffman, M., & Miller, R. (1979). Cognitive modifiability in retarded adolescents: Effects of instrumental enrichment. *American Journal of Mental Deficiency*, **83**, 539–50.

Fletcher, K. L. & Bray, N. W. (1995). External and verbal strategies in children with and without mild mental retardation. *American Journal on Mental Retardation*, **99**(4), 363–75.

Fletcher, K. L., Huffman, L. F., & Bray, N. W. (2003). Effects of verbal and physical prompts on external strategy use in children with and without mild mental retardation. *American Journal on Mental Retardation*, **108**(4), 245–56.

Green, K. (1985). *Cognitive, Style: A Review of the Literature*. Chicago: Johnson O'Connor Research Foundation.

Hagen, J. & Huntsman, N. (1971). Selective attention in mental retardation. *Developmental Psychology*, **5**, 151–60.

Hardy, R. C., Eliot, J., & Burlingame, K. (1987). Stability over age and sex of children's responses to embedded figures test. *Perceptual and Motor Skills*, **64**, 399–406.

Harold, L. D. (1996). *Interaction of cognitive style and learner control of presentation mode in a hypermedia environment*. Unpublished doctorate dissertation, Virginia Polytechnic Institute and State University, Blacksburg, VA.

Henry, L. (2008). Short-term memory coding in children with intellectual disabilities. *American Journal on Mental Retardation*, **113**, 187–200.

Johnson, E. S. & Mead, A. C. (1987) Developmental patterns of spatial ability: An early sex difference. *Child Development*, **58**, 725–40.

Karp, S. A. & Konstadt, N. (1971). The Children's Embedded Figures Test (CEFT). In H. A. Witkin, P. K. Oltman, E. Raskin, & S. A. Karp (Eds.), *Manual for the Embedded Figures Test* (pp. 21–26). Palo Alto, CA: Consulting Psychologists Press.

Kent-Davis, J. & Cochran, K. F. (1989). An information processing view of field dependence-independence. *Early Child Development and Care*, **51**, 31–47.

Kerns, K. & Berenbaum, S. (1991). Sex differences in spatial ability in boys. *Behavior Genetics*, **21**, 383–96.

Lifshitz, H. & Rand, Y. (1999). Cognitive modifiability in adult and older people with mental retardation. *Mental Retardation*, **37**, 125–38.

MacMillan, D. & Wright, D. (1974). Outer-directedness in boys of three ages as a function of experimentally induced success and failure. *Journal of Experimental Psychology*, **66**, 919–25.

Merighi, J., Edison, M., & Zigler, E. (1990). The role of motivational factors in the functioning of mentally retarded individuals. IN R. M. Hodapp, J. A. Burack, & E. Zigler (Eds.), *Isues in the Developmental Approach to Mental Retardation* (pp. 114–34). Cambridge, UK: Cambridge University Press.

Merrill, E. & Taube, M. (1996). Negative priming and mental retardation: The processing of distractor information. *American Journal on Mental Retardation*, **101**, 63–71.

Messick, S. (1984) The nature of cognitive styles: Problems and promise in educational practice. *Educational Psychologist*, **19**, 59–74.

Naglieri, J. A (1989). A cognitive processing theory for the measurement of intelligence. *Educational Psychologist*, **24**, 185–206.

Naglieri, J. A, Das, J. P., & Jarman, R. F. (1990). Planning, attention, simultaneous, and successive processes as a model of assessment. *School Psychology Review*, **19**(4), 423–42.

Nesbit, W. C. & Chambers, J. (1976). Performance of MA-matched nonretarded and retarded children on measures of field dependence. *American Journal of Mental Deficiency*, **80**(4), 469–72.

Palmer, S. E. (1977). Hierarchical structure in perceptual representation. *Cognitive Psychology*, **9**, 441–74.

Pascual-Leone, J. & Goodman, D. (1979). Intelligence and experience: A neo- Piagetian approach. *Instructional Science*, **8**, 301–67.

Pennings, A. H. (1988). The development of strategies in embedded figures tasks. *International Journal of Psychology*, **23**, 65–78.

Pennings, A. H. (1990). An item response model for describing the use of strategies in embedded figures tasks. In H. Mandl, N. Bennett, E. De Corte, & H. F. Friedrich (Eds.), *Learning and Instruction: European Research in an International Context* (Vol. 2, pp. 231–45). Oxford, UK: Pergamon.

Pressley, M. & Hilden, K. (2006). Cognitive strategies. In W. Damon & R. M. Lerner, (Eds. in Chief), and D. Kuhn & R. S. Siegler (Vol. Eds.), *Handbook of Child Psychology: Vol 2. Cognition, Perception and Language*. 6th edn. (pp. 511–56). Hoboken, NJ: John Wiley and Sons.

Raven, J. C. (1965) *Guide to Using the Colored Progressive Matrices*. London: Lewis.

Saldaňa, D. (2004). Interactive assessment of metacognition: Exploratory study of a procedure for persons with severe mental retardation. *European Journal of Psychology of Education*, **19**(4), 349–64.

Shah, A. & Frith, U. (1993). Why do autistic individuals show superior performance on the block design task? *Journal of Child Psychology and Psychiatry*, **34**, 1351–64.

Span, P. (1973). *Structuring Tendency as an Aspect of Cognitive Style*. Unpublished doctoral dissertation. State University of Utrecht, Utrecht.

Span, R. (1980). *Restructuring as a Cognitive Task*. Paper presented at the Annual Meeting of the AERA, Boston, MA.

Spitz, H. H. (1979). Beyond field theory in the study of mental deficiency. In N. R Ellis (Ed.), *International review of research in mental retardation*, 2nd edn. (pp. 121–41). Hillsdale, NJ: Erlbaum.

Tamaoka, K. (1985). *Historical Development of Learning Style Inventories from Dichotomous Cognitive Concepts of Field Dependence and Field Independence to Multi-dimensional Assessment*. (ERIC *Document* Reproduction Service No. ED 339 729).

Tipper, S. (1985) The negative priming effect: Inhibitory effects of ignored primes. *Quarterly Journal of Experimental Psychology*, **37A**, 571–90.

Turner, L. A, Hale, C., & Borkowski, J. G. (1996). Influence of intelligence on memory development. *American Journal on Mental Retardation*, **100**, 468–80.

Weisz, J. (1979). Perceived *control* and learned helplessness among mentally retarded and nonretarded boys: A developmental analysis. *Developmental Psychology*, **15**, 311–9.

Witkin, H. A. (1950) Individual differences in ease of perception of embedded figures. *Journal of Personality*, **19**, 1–15.

Witkin, H. A, Dijk, R B., Faterson, H. F., Goodenough, D. R., & Karp, S. A. (1962). *Psychological Differentiation*. New York, NY: Wiley.

Witkin, H. A. & Goodenough, D. R. (1981) *Cognitive Styles: Essence and Origins*. New York: International Universities Press.

Yando, R. & Zigler, E. (1971). Outer-directedness in the problem-solving of institutionalized and nonistitutionalized typically developing and retarded boys. *Developmental Psychology*, **4**, 277–88.

Zaporozhets, A. V. (1965). The development of perception in the preschool child. *Monographs of the Society for Research in Child Development*, **30**, 82–101.

Index

A-bar movements 111–113, 117
A-chain deficit hypothesis 117
A-movements 111–113, 117
academic skills, spina bifida 57
adaptive function 57
aging
   cognitive, spina bifida 73–74
   language, Down syndrome 135–137
Angelman's syndrome 21–22
applied behavior analysis (ABA) 35–37
arithmetic
   errors 69–70, 152, 159
   speed of fact retrieval 152, 159, 161–163
articulatory problems, Down syndrome 125
ASD *see* autistic spectrum disorders
Asperger's syndrome 20
   developmental trajectory 33
   early language development 87–88
Assessment of Basic Language and Learning (ABBLS) 36–37
ataxia 9
attention
   joint *see* joint attention
   orienting, spina bifida 58–59
   shifting, Williams syndrome 183
   visual selective 209–210
attention deficit hyperactivity disorder (ADHD), *FMR1*
     premutation carriers 6
autism 19–42, 179
   adult outcomes 32
   broader phenotype (BAP) 23, 98
   early language development 87–88
   face processing 189–191, 192
   FMR1 premutation carriers 6
   fragile X syndrome 5, 21–22
   genetics 21–24, 97–99
   initial outcome studies 28–29
   interventions 34–39
   mechanisms of improvement 39–42
   neuroanatomical findings 24–28, 96–97
   optimal outcome 33–34
   phenomenology 19–21
   recovery hypothesis 39–40
   stability of early diagnosis 31–32
   subgroups 32–33
   underconnectivity theory 92, 93
   weak central coherence theory 92, 93
autistic disorder, diagnostic criteria 20

autistic spectrum disorders (ASD) 19–42
   adult outcomes 32
   changes in symptoms over time 29–30
   diagnostic criteria 19–20
   early language development 86–90
   epidemiology 21
   FMR1 premutation carriers 6
   genetics 21–24, 97–99
   initial outcome studies 28–29
   interventions 34–39
   language and communication 85–100
   language processing 91–94
   mechanisms of improvement 39–42
   neuroanatomical findings 24–28
   optimal outcome 33–34
   overlap with language disorders 90–99
   phenomenology 19–21
   predictors of language outcomes 88–90
   stability of early diagnosis 31–32
   subgroups 32–33

babbling, infant 124–125
   Down syndrome 124–125
   interactive 125
   reduplicated 125
behavioral interventions, autism 35–37
behavioral phenotypes, comparisons xv
brain injuries, acquired 176, 177
bridging inferences 64
broader autism phenotype (BAP) 23, 98

calculations
   difficulties with 69–70, 152, 159, 163
   slow response times 159
case conflicts 112
case errors 116
case marking 112–113
Chiari II hindbrain malformation 53–54
Children's Embedded Figures Test 199
chronological age (CA) controls
   embedded figures task study 203–204
   Williams syndrome 106, 107, 109, 111
cognitive aging, spina bifida 73–74
cognitive function
   genetic influences on development 179–180,
     192–193
   localization during development 178

cognitive style
   defined 199
   field dependent/independent 199–201
   interventions in mental retardation 210–211
communication impairment, autistic spectrum disorders
      19–20, 85–100
counting skills 69, 154–155, 163
critical period (CP), language development 132–134

Dehaene's triple code model of number processing 160
Denver model 37
developmental disorders 175–193
   approaches to studying 176–178
   genetic influences 179–180, 192–193
   mathematics learning disability 143–144
   see also specific disorders
developmental interventions, autism 37
developmental language disorder *see* specific language
      impairment
developmental perspectives xv, 175–193
   early language development 180–185
   embedded figures task strategies 202–203, 209
   face processing 189–191
   genetics and 179–180
   number ability 185–189
   populations studied 178–180
   rationale 176–178
diabetes 54–55
Diagnostic Embedded Figures Test 199, 204
discourse, Down syndrome 131–132
Down syndrome (DS) 122–137, 178–179, 193
   critical period for language development 132–134
   genetics 122
   interindividual variability 134–135
   language aging 135–137
   mathematics learning disability 168–169
   mental growth 123
   mosaicism 122–123
   number ability 185–189, 192
   prelinguistic development 123–125
   speech and language development 123–135, 181–182, 192

educational interventions, mental retardation 211
embedded figures tasks 199–211
   information-processing strategies 200–201
   strategies used in mental retardation 202–203, 205–211
   study methodology 203–205
   study results 205–208
environmental factors
   autism 22
   development in spina bifida 67–69
epicanthal folds 134–135
ethnic variations, spina bifida 54
executive function, and math performance 152
   fragile X syndrome 156–158
   Turner syndrome 161–163, 164
eye movement behavior 164

faces
   processing 177, 189–191, 192
   visual attention to 41

fenobam 12
field dependent/independent cognitive style
      199–201
Floor Time 37
FMR1 gene 3–13
   full mutation 4, 144
   mRNA toxicity 5–7, 9, 10–11
   premutation 4, 5–8
      female carriers 7–8
      male carriers 8
      screening 12
   product *see* fragile X mental retardation protein
folic acid supplementation 54
fragile X-associated tremor/ataxia syndrome (FXTAS) 3–4,
      9–11
   diagnostic criteria 9
   female premutation carriers 8, 10
   pathological features 10–11
   radiological features 10
   screening 12
   treatment 11–12
fragile X mental retardation 1 gene *see FMR1* gene
fragile X mental retardation protein (FMRP) 4,
      5–8, 144
fragile X syndrome (FXS) 3, 144–145, 179
   autism 5, 21–22
   cascade testing and screening 12
   executive function/working memory 156–158, 164
   female cognitive phenotypes 144–145
   mathematics learning disability 143–144, 147–148,
      151–158
      compared to Turner syndrome 163–165
      language skills and 168–169
      phenotypic variability 149
      prevalence and persistence 150
      profile of math skills 151–155
      role of math related skills 155–158
   molecular biology 4, 180
   phenotypes 4–5
   treatment 11–12
   visual spatial ability 155–156, 163–164

genetic influences, development 179–180, 192–193
gesture production 86
glucose metabolism, genes 54–55
grammatical abilities
   assessment 109
   development in Down syndrome 129–130
   Williams syndrome 107, 108–109, 118
gross motor skills, interventions in spina bifida 72

heterogeneity, genes, brain and behavior xiv

idiom comprehension, spina bifida 62, 66
imitation skills, language outcomes in ASD and 89–90
intellectual disabilities (ID) *see* mental retardation
intelligence (IQ)
   autistic spectrum disorders 21, 31
   Down syndrome 122–123
   spina bifida 56
interactive specialization approach 177

joint attention
    autistic spectrum disorders 20, 89–90
    Williams syndrome 183

lamin A/C 11
Landau–Kleffner syndrome 21
language
    aging, Down syndrome 135–137
    math performance and 168–169
    predictors of outcomes in ASD 88–90
    processing, ASD and language disorders 91–94
language development
    autism spectrum 86–90
    changes in localization 178
    critical period 132–134
    developmental approach 180–185
    Down syndrome 123–135, 181–182, 192
    Williams syndrome 105–118, 180–185, 192
    within-syndrome variability 134–135
language disorders
    autism spectrum 19–20, 34, 85–100
    behavioral phenotypes 94–96
    language processing 91–94
    overlap with ASD 90–99
    see also specific language impairment
learning disabilities
    FMR1 premutation carriers 6
    spina bifida 57, 61–62, 69
lexical development
    constraints on 127
    Down syndrome 126–128
    long-term memory and 128
    segmenting 127
    short-term memory and 128
life span perspectives xv
    language in Down syndrome 122–137
    mathematical cognition in spina bifida 69–71
lithium 12
locomotion interventions, spina bifida 72
long-term memory (LTM), Down syndrome 128

macrocephaly 24–25
mathematics learning disability (MLD) 143–169
    complexity of cognitive correlates 165–168
    fragile X syndrome *see under* fragile X syndrome
    framework for studying 146–147
    individual variability 149
    models of pathways to 163–165
    neurodevelopmental disorders 143–144
    spina bifida 69–71, 160
    subtypes 147, 149
    syndrome-based approaches to studying 147–150
    Turner syndrome *see under* Turner syndrome
    Williams syndrome 144, 166–167, 168–169
mean length of utterances (MLU) 129, 132–134
mediated learning 210–211
memory strategies, embedded figures tasks 202–203
mental age (MA)
    assessment, Williams syndrome 110
    controls 107–108, 109, 110, 111, 203–204
    decline, Down syndrome 135–136

Down syndrome 123
    embedded figure task strategies and 206–207, 209
    lexical development and 126
mental retardation (MR) (intellectual disability; ID)
    autistic spectrum disorders 21
    critical period for language development 132–134
    development of educational interventions 211
    Down syndrome 122–123
    embedded figures tasks
        strategies used 202–203, 205–211
        study methodology 203–205
        study results 205–208
    field-dependent perception 200
    mediated learning 210–211
    speech and language development 126–128,
        130–131
    spina bifida 56
    X-linked 3
methylenetetrahydrofolate reductase (MTHFR) gene 54
mirror neuron system 27–28
morphosyntactic development, Down syndrome 129–130,
    132–134
motivational factors, embedded figures task 210
myelomeningocele *see* spina bifida myelomeningocele

neuroconstructivist approach 175, 176–178
neurofibromatosis 21–22
neuropsychological model, adult 175, 176
number processing, Dehaene's triple code model 160
number skills
    developmental approach 185–189
    Down syndrome 185–189, 192
    fragile X syndrome 151–155
    spina bifida 69
    Turner syndrome 152, 158–159
    Williams syndrome 167, 185–189, 192

obesity 54–55
object categorization 183–184
object-cleft sentences 111–118
on-line processing 63
ovarian insufficiency, primary (POF) 4, 7–8, 12

parenting style and quality
    interventions 72
    spina bifida 68–69
passive voice understanding
    Down syndrome 130
    Greek language test sentences 111–113
    Williams syndrome 113–118
peer training 38–39
perseverative behaviors, autism 19–20, 31–32
pervasive developmental disorder (PDD) 20
pervasive developmental disorder – not otherwise specified
    (PDD-NOS) 20, 31, 36
    early language development 87–88
    overlap with language disorders 94–96
phonological development, Down syndrome 126, 132–134
pointing, referential 20, 183
pragmatic language impairment (PLI) 94
    overlap with autism spectrum 94–96

pragmatics, Down syndrome 130–131
prelinguistic development, Down syndrome 123–125
primary ovarian insufficiency (POF) 4, 7–8, 12
processing speed deficits 152, 161–163
processing strategies
    embedded figures tasks 200–201
    mental retardation 202–203, 205–211
prosody, Down syndrome 126

reading comprehension impairments, spina bifida
        61–67, 73
rehearsal strategies, embedded figures task
        202–203, 209
relationship development intervention (RDI) 37
repetitive behaviors, autism 19–20, 31–32
response times, Turner syndrome 159, 161–163
Rett's disorder 20, 21–22

SCERTS model 37
segmentation, lexical input 127, 182–183
seizures 21
semantic structural development, Down
        syndrome 129
sentence comprehension
    assessment methodology 111–113
    Williams syndrome 110–118
short-term memory (STM), Down syndrome 128
simultaneous processes, embedded figures tasks
        200–201
situation models 64–66
social isolation 19–20
social motivation impairment, autism 39–41
social stories 38
socio-economic status (SES), spina bifida outcome and 57,
        67–68
specific language impairment (SLI) (developmental
        language impairment) 94
    autism spectrum and 23, 94, 95–99
    genetics 97–99
    language processing 92–94
    neuroanatomical findings 96–97
    semantic-pragmatic subtype see pragmatic language
        impairment
speech
    development, Down syndrome 125–126
    intelligibility, Down syndrome 133
spina bifida myelomeningocele (SBM) 53–74
    associative vs. assembled processing 59–67
    behavioral phenotype 56–67
    clinical care and intervention 72–74
    core cognitive deficits 57–59
    environmental factors 67–69
    features 53–54
    genotype 54–55
    genotype–phenotype relations 55–56
    in utero repair 54
    longitudinal and life span studies 67–71
    mathematical cognition 69–71, 160
    neuroimaging 55–56
story processing, Down syndrome 131–132
subject-cleft sentences 111–118

subject–verb–object (SVO) word order sentences
        111–113
successive processes, embedded figures tasks
        200–201
suppression of irrelevant word meaning 63–64
surface-level representations 62–63
syntactic abilities, Williams syndrome 106–109

taxonomic constraint 184
TEACCH 36, 38
Test for Reception of Grammar (TROG) 107, 109
text-based representations 63–64
theta-role
    assessment 112–113
    conflicts 112
    errors 116, 117
timing deficits, spina bifida 58
treatment and education of autistic and related
        communication handicapped children (TEACCH)
        36, 38
tremor 9
trisomy 21 see Down syndrome
tuberous sclerosis 21–22
Turner syndrome 145–146
    executive function/working memory 161–163, 164
    mathematics learning disability 143–144, 147–148, 152,
        158–167
        compared to fragile X syndrome 163–165
        language skills and 168–169
        phenotypic variability 149
        prevalence and persistence 150
        profile of math skills 158–159
        role of related skills 159–163
    visual spatial ability 158–161, 163–164

underconnectivity theory, autism 92, 93

visual perception, spina bifida 60
visual spatial ability, and math performance 152,
        164–165, 166
    fragile X syndrome 155–156, 163–164
    spina bifida 69
    Turner syndrome 158–161, 163–164
    Williams syndrome 167–168
vocabulary
    expressive 181
    learning new words 183–184
    receptive 181

weak central coherence theory, autism 92, 93
wh-questions 111–113
    comprehension in Williams syndrome 113–118
    production in Williams syndrome 108
whole object constraint 184
Williams syndrome (WS) 146, 178, 193
    face processing 189–191, 192
    language development 105–118, 180–185, 192
    mathematics learning disability 144, 166–167,
        168–169
    number skills 167, 185–189, 192
    phenotypic variability 180

Williams syndrome (WS) (cont.)
  sentence comprehension 110–118
  story telling ability 131
  study methodologies 109
  syntactic abilities 106–109
words, learning new 183–184

working memory, and math performance 152, 165–166
  fragile X syndrome 156–158
  spina bifida 71
  Turner syndrome 161–163

X-linked mental retardation (MR) 3